THE HEALERS

A history of medicine in Scotland

DAVID HAMILTON

Edinburgh
CANONGATE

First published in 1981
by Canongate Publishing Ltd.
17 Jeffrey Street, Edinburgh

Paperback edition 1987

ISBN 0 86241 152 1

The publisher acknowledges subsidy of the Scottish Arts Council towards the publication of this volume.

Designed by Ruari McLean
Typeset in 10 on 13 Bembo and
I.T.C. Zapf Chancery Bold
Printed and bound in Great Britain
by Billing & Sons Ltd., Worcester

British Library Cataloguing in Publication Data

Hamilton, David, *1939* –
The healers: a history of medicine in
Scotland.—2nd ed.
1. Medicine—Scotland—History
I. Title
610′.9411 R495

ISBN 0-86241-152-1

For
Haldane Tait
and
Edward Walker

ACKNOWLEDGEMENTS AND THANKS

It is a pleasure to record the help of those who advised on all or part of the text. Dr Haldane Tait, Peter Chiene, Sir John Brotherston, Rev. J.H. Hamilton, Dr Joseph Wright and Mr Douglas Clark gave detailed help with the text. I am also grateful to colleagues in the University of Glasgow for their expert advice in areas of their special interest, namely Dr Ian Cowan, Dr Olive Checkland, Dr Helen Brock and Dr Christina Larner. Dr E.A. Underwood's published work has been most useful and he also answered many additional questions. In addition the recent increase in interest in Scottish social history and science has produced works of relevance to medicine. I have drawn heavily on the publications of the Department of Economic History in the University of Edinburgh, notably those of Professor M.W. Flinn and Professor T.C. Smout, and have extensively used the series of papers by Dr J.B. Morrell of the School of Studies in Social Sciences of University of Bradford.

The help of the librarians and staff of the following institutions is also gratefully acknowledged: the Mitchell Library Glasgow; University of Glasgow library; University of Edinburgh library; Baillies Library Glasgow; the Scottish Record Office, and the libraries of the Royal College of Physicians and Surgeons of Glasgow, the Royal College of Surgeons of Edinburgh and the Royal College of Physicians of Edinburgh. My final thanks go to my secretary Ms Irene White.

Contents

Introduction

Scotland offers almost unique opportunities for medical historians. For a conventional history, there is a rich stock of famous doctors and their discoveries. There are also the contributions of four ancient universities and three equally old colleges of physicians and surgeons. For historians of public health there is the famous struggle against the problems of the industrial revolution and the lives and works of the great sanitary reformers in Glasgow and Edinburgh. For the social historian there are equal opportunities in the diversity of the health care in the Highlands and Lowlands, the rich traditions of Scottish folk medicine and the interactions of Scottish and English medical practice. Much else can be learnt in relating Scotland's great innovative periods to her cultural and political state at the time. It is perhaps surprising therefore that there are no up-to-date accounts of any of these aspects of health and health care in Scotland. The earlier classic work by J.D. Comrie *History of Scottish Medicine* covers the area of interest only up to the start of the present century and there are now many new sources available and new questions to be asked.

In writing this short account of Scottish medicine I have given a broad account of Scottish health and her healers and have put together the main medical, social and legislative events. Throughout, I have distinguished the three levels of health care – care for the rich, the working class and the poor – and I hope this approach sheds light on even familiar events. In addition, there are neglected areas of Scottish medical history. There has been no complete analysis of why Scottish medicine and medical education led the way in 18th century Britain and Europe or why Scottish doctors were the pace-setters in the medical services of England, the Empire and the armed forces. Nor is there a convincing account of the reasons for the decline in Scottish medical education in the early 19th century. The medical services under the Poor Law in Scotland have not been described, and the Scottish voluntary hospitals await a detailed history of their separate traditions. Lastly, the absence of any recent texts on Scottish medicine has led to an unfortunate notion that there is nothing interesting or unusual about health and health care in Scotland in the 20th century. These areas of neglect are explored in this book.

The primary sources relevant to health care in Scotland are reasonably good throughout the period and are particularly good in the 18th century. But there are some gaps elsewhere. The medieval records are poor in Scotland as a result of much early destruction by fire, flood, shipwreck and war. In early Scotland painters and engravers were few and the forces of Calvinism after the Reformation continued to discourage these vanities: we have few illustrations of early Scottish medicine. Health care in the gaelic-speaking areas and the Highlands remains mysterious, since their historians preferred oral to written records. Much of Scottish Victorian medical journalism and biography is pious and superficial, a tradition which spilled over into the 20th century. Lastly, most recent writing on health care in Britain refers, on closer inspection, to England only.

To help the general reader, I have tried to avoid technical language or extensive biography and in doing so I may have done less than justice to individual contributions to research and development. However, this aspect of Scottish medicine is well described elsewhere particularly by Comrie, whose book will always be an unrivalled source of reference.

It was tempting to end this book at the start of the 20th century at a time when commentators consider that the centralisation of government obliterated most regional differences. However, recent events have suggested that a separate Scottish approach to medicine may still exist. Hence an attempt has been made to look at 20th century British medicine from a Scottish viewpoint, an approach which has been rewarded by the discovery of a large amount of neglected material, notably the Highlands and Islands Medical Scheme, the Cathcart Report and the Scottish Emergency Medical Service during the Second World War.

Thus the aim of this short work is to give the reader a straightforward historical account of the health problems and attempts at their solutions in Scotland. Though Scotland made unique contributions to progress in these areas, these were changes which eventually affected all countries. This book, therefore, also tells part of the whole history of medicine.

David Hamilton
Glasgow 1981

1
The dark ages

Of the earlier inhabitants of Scotland we know little and can reconstruct little of the life of the people from the scraps of archeological evidence available.[1] The earliest known inhabitants of Scotland are those who occupied a site at Morton in Fife about 6000 BC, and the evidence there suggests they were a nomadic people, skilled at hunting and fishing even for large fish. In Neolithic times a more settled people appeared and about 2200 BC a well constructed stone habitation existed at Skara Brae in Orkney. The numerous later Bronze Age settlements however give little clue regarding the life of the people, but suggest the increasing importance of agriculture. We can only guess about the health and health care of these primitive people – probably the main threats to health and life were famine and war. The results of warfare could be not only death in battle but also slavery and famine since the victors would remove or destroy the crops. Even in peace time, crop failure would be an ever present threat. Another terrifying event in early times may have been human sacrifices carried out to placate or to win favours from the gods.

Direct evidence on health and health care is, however, absent. Evidence from excavated bones is scanty since they are poorly preserved in the Scottish soils, though healing fractures and other bony injuries suggestive of war wounds have been found.[2] Teeth are better preserved and good dental health existed in prehistoric Scotland.[3] Of great interest is the find near Rothesay, Bute, of a skull dating from the early Bronze Age which shows that during life a trepan hole – an earlier form of trephining – had been made through the skull, probably in an attempt to cure insanity, epilepsy or headaches.[4] This form of therapy is seen in many primitive societies and was practised in Scotland up to the 16th century.[5,6] This surgical operation would be carried out in the belief that disease resulted from the possession of the sufferer by evil spirits and that an easy route of exit from the body helped an early departure of the spirit. The operation of trepanning is not easy and the early tribes almost certainly had medicine men who had these skills. In other medical problems this animistic explanation of disease was clearly not applicable. War wounds, burns or accidental injuries, together with the accidents of childbirth, were clearly mechanical problems and their management could be reasonably left to folk healers or be dealt with by traditional methods.

While life at this time in Scotland would be short and brutish for the people, it is possible that they were spared some of the health problems found later. Firstly, the impenetrable nature of the marsh and forest made regular travel impossible and this may have prevented the spread of epidemic disease. The second blessing possessed by the early peoples was their abundant supply of fresh spring water which, if sensibly used, would not be polluted with bacteria from human excretion. Moreover, the small, slowly growing population may have been self-sufficient in food by hunting in the forest and fishing in the rivers open to all. Thirdly, the simple housing and dress of the inhabitants of Scotland in the Dark Ages may have left her free of some of the other threats to health posed by urban life in Scotland of a later date – typhus from body lice and the plague spread by the black rat and its fleas.

Of the early medicine men in Scotland we know little and there is even controversy over the presence in Scotland of the Druids at the time when this cult was strong elsewhere in Europe.[7] The serpent-like tracery in Celtic carvings and the Roman historian's description of human sacrifices carried out by the defending army of Calgacus prior to the battle of Mons Graupius AD 84 are suggestive of druidical beliefs and rituals.[8] If the Druids were active in Scotland, they would have provided divination, astrology and herbs and charms for disease in man and animals. Certainly, centuries later Columba encountered healers called the Magi at the court of King Brudei, who may have been the last remnants of the Druids ruthlessly put down in England by Emperor Claudius.[9]

The first descriptions of the inhabitants of Scotland also come from the Romans. When they withdrew from Scotland about the year AD 211, having occupied it from AD 81, they left behind them a wild and barbaric land. Baffled and demoralised by the successful guerrilla warfare against them, the Romans under Severus had latterly caught only glimpses of their opponents, and the Roman historians give us a brief description of the land and inhabitants of Scotland.[10] The tribes were barbaric, usually going naked and they used the most primitive of tools. The land of Scotland was apparently an inhospitable place, mostly forest, peat bog and marsh, a terrain unsuited to the Roman army.

In fighting off the Romans, the dwellers of Scotland had however denied themselves exposure to the advanced civilisation of the invaders, not least their considerable knowledge of disease, health care and sanitation. Roman surgery was sophisticated and their surgical methods and instruments were not improved upon in Europe until 1000 years later. Roman views on internal medicine were relatively less progressive, since they had set aside the earlier Greek natural explanations of disease and the sensible Hippocratic approach to therapy and modified it to include a role for the Roman gods of healing. The Roman army in Scotland had advanced medical arrangements and their camps had well developed sanitary systems. Three surgeons were attached to each legion, but they were of lowly status and not officers but NCOs. A gravestone to one of these men is found in Hadrian's Wall and records a tender farewell to this young surgeon of the Tenth Legion.[11] These Roman medical officers had surgical instruments of advanced design and copper salts were used in treatment. Another remarkable find is a stamp used by an army oculist to save time in writing one of his favourite prescriptions.[12] The clear ideas of the Romans on sanitary matters can be seen in Hadrian's and Antonine's Walls, where running water was used together with sedimentation tanks, latrines and hot and cold baths.[13] It was to be almost 1500 years before these sanitary principles were re-introduced into Scotland and only after the loss of a large number of lives.

The missionaries

The next influence on Scotland was the work of the christian missionaries. The first to reach Scotland was St Ninian, a native-born Scot from the Lowlands of Scotland. He is thought to have been descended from one of the scattered christian families settled by the Romans in the Lowlands, and he was possibly educated in Rome.[14] Having established a church in Whithorn in the late 4th century, he pushed north to Strathclyde. The work of conversion north of the Forth was left to the Irish missionaries, first St Oran in 548 and then St Columba in 563, who made his base on Iona and by his travels spread christianity throughout the west and north of Scotland.[15] The missionaries also brought with them a code of non-violence and they had a confident approach to disease and healing. These tough and resourceful men thus could engage successfully in contests of healing skills with the folk healers and medicine men they encountered in their mission. They set up two institutions which were to be major factors in health care in Scotland in centuries to come. The first innovation – the hospital – was intentional. The second – the healing well – was probably unintentional.

St Columba constructed a simple hospital at Iona, the first of many such monastic hospitals scattered through Scotland. These early hospitals were not primarily for the sick, but were refuges for the old, the disabled, and the travelling pilgrim. Nevertheless there is evidence that the Iona hospital was also used for sufferers from disease who travelled to Iona for help. Columba's biographer tells of an ill pilgrim arriving on the shore opposite Iona and shouting over to the island and Columba remarked that the traveller had come for a cure of the body but unless he did penance he would be dead in a week.[16] This role of the Church in providing a cure for the soul, and hence the body, was an unquestioned assumption of early thought since disease was considered to be either a divine affliction for spiritual misconduct, or the work of evil spirits. Hence healing came only to those who repented and were worthy of relief: with these assumptions, physicians were largely unnecessary. The great body of secular medical knowledge and skills built up in ancient Greece had no place in this theory of disease and the early church was therefore responsible for the eclipse of the ancient knowledge. Nevertheless some medical problems were clearly not divinely induced and the missionaries took an interest in the treatment of wounds and fractures and possibly even the problems of childbirth. The extent to which the missionaries used physical methods of healing is difficult to assess. Their biographers record the miracles performed rather than the saint's conventional skills. Nevertheless, there was a herb garden at Iona, and the library doubtless contained medical manuscripts, though none of these texts have survived.[17] It seems likely that medical and surgical help was given together with spiritual help, and since Columba was consulted on conventional problems such as nose bleeds and fractures,[18] it is unlikely that he would scorn all available remedies. Indeed the saints' reputation for immediate cure of blindness may now be explained by their use of surgical couching of cataract, as used by later orthodox and itinerant healers.

In the north and west of Scotland, Columba and the other missionaries may have been the only persons with medical training. But in the Borders, the biography of St Cuthbert shows the existence of other healers, since he was successful in cases

> that leches [healers] before heel ne moght [could not heal]
> with na medecyne that thai brocht.

These 'leches' are the first medical men or women of what was later to become Scotland, and were either folk healers or priests who had taken a special interest in medicine.[19] Nothing else is known of any secular healers in Scotland, though a well developed medical care system existed at this time in Ireland and the Irish Brehon laws regulated their practice and fees.[20]

Another activity of the Scottish missionaries was to promote an extraordinarily durable idea, namely that the water of some wells and springs had healing powers. From St Columba's days onwards, the saints blessed many of the wells and streams they encountered on their travels,[21] and if they did not do so personally, then after their visit or death the wells were named after them. The missionaries probably did not intend to encourage a belief in the healing powers of the water. All the evidence instead suggests that the missionaries were seeking to annul other primitive beliefs in the pagan gods of water, springs and rivers, but that in blessing the water to make it holy, the old belief in healing by water was not given up by the people and instead the saints' own god was established.[22]

Though this explantation is the most likely one, a more practical explanation of the saints' actions has been offered, albeit tentatively, namely that the saints were indulging in some elementary public health education.[23] The sophisticated education of the saints may have given them knowledge of the sanitary principles of personal cleanliness and efficient disposal of waste. They might know of, or might even have seen the public baths of Rome. Since it is likely that Scotland was developing small habitations in which there was pollution of the running water, the missionaries, it is argued, blessed the wells and springs to prevent the people wasting or polluting the water. Certainly, to have lectured the inhabitants of Scotland on public health would have been useless. Whatever the motives, the saints certainly caught the people's imagination in an astonishing way, and belief in the divine healing by water was a prominent part of religious orthodoxy in Scotland for many centuries, as well as forming part of the baptismal transference of blessing or the washing away of sins by immersion.[24]

Health and disease

Doubtless the main threats to health in the later Dark Ages continued to be war or loss of crops or cattle, and personal illness was of lesser concern. The miracles accomplished by the saints had as much to do with ensuring the growth of crops and animal health as with human wellbeing. Scotland continued to be a backward area but this less developed civilisation still made her fortunate in one respect. The poor communications and the rarity of travellers diminished or prevented the spread of epidemics, though Columba's biographer claimed that the saint's work in Scotland had left such a state of grace that epidemics passed her by. Certainly, the early historians suggest that Scotland escaped the worse effects of the European plague epidemic of 550 to 560, and when it returned to Britain in 664, though it killed St Boisil, prior of the abbey of Melrose but spared St Cuthbert in the same abbey, it seems to have made only a sporadic attack on Scotland.[25] The early Scottish historian John of Fordun said of this epidemic, revealing the current view of the causation of disease, that it 'spared the Picts, although great sins were not wanting among these people'.[26] Thereafter, Scotland appears to have been free of the plague until it returned as the Black Death in the autumn of 1349. Wyntoun, Scotland's other historian, could say almost correctly that this was the 'first pestilence' in Scotland, suggesting that the earlier attacks were less serious.[27] Scotland's relative immunity until this time may have been the result of fewer places of pilgrimage and few visits by the pilgrims and monks who may have spread the early epidemics. Moreover, the simple housing of the early inhabitants and slightly cooler climate did not encourage the rats which spread the plague.

2
The middle ages 1100–1600

Of the social life and conditions in medieval Scotland, we have more knowledge than of the preceding period. To the records are now added accounts of Scotland by historians and travellers and glimpses of the social life and the health problems can be obtained from the legislation of the Privy Council, the Provincial Councils of the Church and later from the records of the Burghs.

Scotland developed fairly successful ways of dealing with two troublesome non-epidemic diseases – leprosy, common in early medieval times, and syphilis, which appeared later. With increased travel within Britain and an increasing number of small towns, conditions suitable for the spread of epidemics arose, and the towns had to devise primitive defences against the catastrophic medieval plague epidemics and the many smaller outbreaks of this disease. Typhus was ever present and it regularly followed starvation resulting from failure of the harvest or the theft or burning of crops and stores by passing armies. The change from primitive tribalism to a feudal organisation meant that peasants could be displaced from their land. Many beggars appeared and Poor Laws were enacted.

Under the rule of Malcolm and Saint Margaret starting in 1058, Scotland abandoned her isolationist ways and became a significant influence in Europe. Diplomatic links were opened up with European countries and this exchange brought Scotland into Europe, and Scottish scholars and clerics became frequent travellers and students there. During James IV's peaceful reign, Scotland was a leader in the early European renaissance and under this enlightened King, the study of medicine in Scotland was particularly favoured and the growth of a separate secular profession encouraged. Medical practice outside the monasteries developed, and the surgeons in Edinburgh were first to appear as a corporate body. In the Highlands a separate less feudal society persisted and they maintained a scholarly system of hereditary physicians. In this period no less than three universities were set up, in one of which in Aberdeen, it was clearly intended that medicine be taught, though this plan never flourished. As a result, although Scotland's new universities slowly undertook the education of her own clergy, medical education for the physicians continued to be sought on the continent.

In this period the towns of Scotland began to grow in size, as a result of their markets or trade with Europe. These new small towns were dangerous since their position on rivers made them exposed to floods and their wooden construction led to uncontrollable fires. Both fire and flood could destroy grain stores, and famine and diseases of man and animals followed. However, the simple construction of the homes made reconstruction easy, and when Edinburgh was burnt down in 1385 by Richard II it was quickly rebuilt in three days, requiring 'only three poles and some boughs' to start a new house. The new towns were dangerous in other ways, since they began to harbour the rats and fleas which spread the plague. Other health problems resulted from the increasingly insanitary conditions.

Under the changes made by Malcolm and Margaret, lowland Scotland changed from a tribal to a feudal society. Feudalism was based on the King's power to grant land and expect homage in return. The nobles in turn sublet the land given to them and at the bottom of this organisation was a peasant without the security of land holding he had previously possessed in the tribal society. When the monarch was strong the feudal system was an efficient mechanism not only for waging war, but also for the enforcement of law, through the King's constant travelling in the land and also through his royal burghs. But when the King was weak or too young to govern, as happened in Scotland from 1406 to 1587, the nobles gained power, fought with each other, and national enforcement of law and order failed. Thus social life in medieval Scotland was constantly changing. If there was peace and a good harvest, there was prosperity, but a war or famine could suddenly produce a local or national social crisis. It is little wonder therefore that the descriptions of Scotland by travellers are widely different.[1] Some recorded a fertile land with an industrious healthy peasantry: others disagreed. 'The Scots', said the Spanish ambassador in 1498 'are not industrious and the people are poor. They spend their time in wars, and when there is no war, they fight one another'.

The external wars were against the English and Norwegians: at home the nobles and their followers clashed in the Lowlands and the clans feuded in the Highlands.[2] These encounters were often followed by public hanging and mutilation of prominent captives, while a victorious army would pillage, loot and sack the vanquished leader's land. A dismal sequence of famine and disease followed, and bands of paid-off armed men roamed the land afterwards in semi-legitimate banditry. In 1390 the Wolf of Badenoch – a son of the King – raided the Moray Coast and burnt down the towns of Forres, Elgin and its manses and cathedral. In 1452 the avengers of the murder of the Earl of Douglas burnt down Stirling and in 1455 it was recorded that 'the King byrnt all Douglas Dale and Avondale and all the Lord Hammiltonnis landis, and great pestilence followed'. In 1544 Henry VIII of England told the Earl of Hereford, then invading the Borders, to 'put man women and childe to the fyre and sworde without exception, where any resistence shall be made agaynst you'. The Earl did so, plundered and burnt Edinburgh, Leith, Holyrood and Haddington, and appropriated 10,000 cattle and 12,000 sheep. In 1545 he returned and sacked seven abbeys, sixteen castles, five towns and 243 villages. Though the wooden shacks of the towns and villages were easily rebuilt, famine and disease followed. There was no possibility of relief, not through lack of compassion for these sufferers, since 'God's poor' were highly regarded in medieval times, but simply through the difficulty of obtaining food supplies and moving them to where they were required. These 'mortality crises' of war, famine and disease (usually typhus or dysentery) were all closely interlinked and were to be a prominent feature of Scottish life until the 18th century.[3] Though typhus was always present, only when the person's resistance to disease was low, as after famine, did the disease become epidemic. The horrors of a great famine and mortality crisis are mentioned in Wyntoun's description of the aftermath of the siege of Perth 1340 when 'mony ware in hungyr dede' and he reluctantly reported tales of cannibalism among the survivors.[4] Famines of national importance after failure of crops are hinted at in the legislation of the Scottish Parliaments in 1449, 1452, 1478, 1485 (a 'great famine'), 1535, 1541–51, 1555, 1556, 1571–3 and 1585–7.

Both the Crown and the Church acting through its Provincial

Council in Scotland, sought to regulate the life of the nation, and attempt to prevent starvation. During periods of concern for the food supply the King was prepared to make rules about personal consumption to fix the price of food and to curb gluttony and hoarding. Export of food was also banned from time to time. Warnings in 1436 were issued against gluttons and drunkards who, if they persisted, were to be punished by being 'drowned in ane fresch rever'. Since the grain crops were also used to brew ale, the King even ordered in the same year that 'na man in burghe be fundyn in tavernis at wyne aile or beir eftir the straik of ix houris and the bell that salbe rongyn . . .' or to incur a penalty of imprisonment or a fine of one shilling. In 1551 a limit of eight courses was put on the evening meal of archbishops, while the lords and abbots were limited to six and the burgesses could sit down to three courses only.[5]

The feudal system also meant that people could be displaced from the land and in the problem years of the 14th century many were turned into beggars. In the 15th century parliament had to issue comments on the state of the poor attempting to distinguish for the first, and not the last time, between those who could not work – 'the impotent poor', also known as the 'King's beggars' – and those who wilfully would not work – the 'masterful beggars'. This was to be the basis of the Poor Law for three centuries. The impotent poor were entitled to financial aid and in 1535 each parish was made responsible for its own poor, an arrangement which was to last until the 19th century. In sharp contrast, the masterful beggars were to be outlawed and punished. Another proclamation of the Provincial Council of the Church is of interest, since it forbad mothers and nurses to sleep with their children because of the risk of smothering the baby. Extremely unusual, this statute may represent an attempt to deal with the high infant mortality of the time, or to remove an alibi for infanticide.

The plague

The rise of the small towns, together with better transport resulting from drainage of marshland, cutting of the forest and travel abroad for diplomacy and education, set the stage for the spread of epidemic disease. The Black Death or bubonic plague – the worse epidemic in European history – entered Britain in August 1348 at Weymouth in Dorset.[6] By autumn it had reached London, and one year later it entered Scotland. There was some delay at the border and the Scots considered it to have been a special affliction by God on the English army then at the Border. Its eventual entry into Scotland can be blamed entirely on the Scots army who, encouraged by this evidence of divine assistance, made a foolhardy attack on the English. On withdrawing back into Scotland they brought the plague with them. John of Fordun wrote:

> By God's Will, this evil led to a strange and unwonted kind of death, in so much that the flesh of the sick was somehow puffed out and swollen, and they dragged out their earthly life for barely two days.[7]

Wyntoun also recorded this national disaster and he may not have exaggerated in saying

> . . . it was sayd, off lywand men
> The thyrd part it dystroyid then.[8]

Both historians agreed that the poor were more affected by the epidemic than the rich.

The bubonic plague must have been one of the most terrible diseases ever to affect man.[9] The rapid and usually fatal course, with death between the 4th and 7th day, makes it recognisable in the contemporary records, helped by its characteristic pause in incidence in the winter months when the rats which spread the disease were less active, and when shipping and internal trade was reduced. Another characteristic was that the poor were most at risk and their sensitivity can be explained by two factors. Firstly, their living conditions may have been more favourable to the rats, and hence flea bites more likely: secondly, their poor nutrition left them with poor resistance. Thus the reason for the virulence of the Black Death may be 'not because of its nature, but because of the suffering and servitude in which it surprised its victims',[10] and hence may have been simply a special form of the medieval mortality crisis and no different in its causation from typhus. While no records of the harvests or weather exist for this period of Scottish history, she doubtless shared the series of bad harvests noted elsewhere in Europe at that time. Epidemics returned again in 1362 ('the second pest') 1380 or 1392 ('the third pest') and though none of these epidemics equalled the violence of the first, Wyntoun says that they spread more widely in the country, doubtless as a result of better communications. The early historians give no details of any measures taken against the plague and in other countries quarantine was not introduced until 1403. Certainly there were no laws made in 14th century Scotland against these epidemics, in spite of sensible legislation in force dealing with leprosy.

Later epidemics[11]

The plague or typhus returned in smaller national epidemics in the 15th century, but by the 16th century the diseases were endemic, breaking out at many different times in local attacks and as a national problem in 1511–13, 1529–30, 1538, 1556, 1574, 1584–88, 1600–09. (The final great epidemic came in 1647 and will be described later.) These epidemics were described in Scottish literature and the terror caused by them is reflected in the poetry of Robert Henryson (?1425–1506). In his *Ane Prayer for the Pest* he asks God to

> half mercy of us, indigent and pure;
> That dois no wrang to puniss our offenss:
> o Lord, that is to mankynd haill succure,
> preserve us fra this perrelus pestilens.[12]

William Dunbar's (1465?–1530?) *Lament for the Makeris* also describes the fear of the plague and its sudden and fatal appearance:

> The state of man does change and vary,
> Now sound, now sick, now blyth, now sary,
> Now dansand mirry, now like to die:-
> *Timor Mortis conturbat me.*[13]

Dunbar also noted that even the doctors could not save themselves from the plague:

> In medecyne the most practicianis,
> Lechis, surrigianis, and phisicianis,
> Thame-self fra ded may not supple [defend]
> *Timor Mortis conturbat me.*

During this period an understanding of the mechanism of the spread of the disease was slowly obtained. While the early people of Scotland had recognised that cases of leprosy were worth isolating outside the towns and legislation was produced for this, the plague in its first and even later visitations did not call forth any local or national measures to deal with it. Thus it was probably regarded as a divine punishment rather than a disease. However the later medieval epidemics of plague were looked at in a more hard-headed way, and a contagion theory arose with suspicion rightly falling on goods and baggage, and cloth and clothes in particular: legislation slowly followed.[14] But the main reaction to the plague was to get away from it and in the 15th and 16th centuries repeated efforts were made to avoid it. The simplest remedy for the people in time of epidemic was to move out of town, and those who could depart did so, leaving the business of the town at a standstill. Churches closed, parliament broke up or met elsewhere. The universities moved out of town to continue teaching elsewhere, or sent all the scholars home, as in Edinburgh in 1498. Glasgow University moved to Irvine in 1645 and Aberdeen University decamped to Fraserburgh in 1647.[15] Parliament was first dispersed in 1475 and the Privy Council had to gather outside Edinburgh on numerous occasions.

Quarantine measures were first devised in Venice in 1403. In Scotland, national measures were first taken in 1452 when an Act of Parliament allowed for the burning down of any house affected by the plague. The first national quarantine regulations came in 1456, the year after the King had marched against the Lord Hamilton, and laid waste to his lands. As a result pestilence followed – a disaster probably localised to the Hamilton lands – and Parliament tried to contain the problem by forbidding movement out of the area since those who 'walde steyle away' would 'fyle the cuntre about thame'.[16] The first local quarantine regulations are found in the decision by Peebles in 1468 to close their gates to persons from infected areas. Stronger and stronger measures were recorded during the next 150 years and eventually all the burghs attempted to prevent the spread of the disease to their towns, but the frequency with which these laws appeared suggested that their effect was incomplete.[17] When news of the plague reached a town, all trade and movement in and out of the town was forbidden, guards were posted at the town gates to enforce these regulations and a watch kept for beggars or travelling entertainers and merchants who might attempt to enter. Inside the town, regulations were broadcast by officials accompanied by drummers and were read out in the churches. The east coast ports were particularly at risk from the disease as a result of their trade with Europe. At these ports the vessels and their cargo were put into quarantine, which at Leith, Edinburgh's port, involved taking the vessel and its contents to the rocky islet of Inchcolm, Inchkeith or to the Isle of May for 40 days.

The cargoes were opened to the wind or washed in sea water and the vessel grounded at low tide, the sea-cocks opened and the ship flooded by the tides. Cloth and clothing were particularly suspected of carrying the plague. Within the town, severe sentences were introduced for breaking the regulations, notably in failing to report cases of the plague. In Aberdeen, if plague was imminent, gibbets were erected, one at the Mercat Cross, one at the Bridge of Dee and the third at the harbour mouth. The penalties for breach of the regulations were that the 'men would be hangit, and women drownit' but only one execution under these rules is recorded. For less severe breaches of these quarantine rules, branding on the face or cutting off a hand and banishing from the town could be enforced. Gradually the regulations became more comprehensive and from 1529 the towns started to segregate the plague victims outside the town and maintain them there at the towns expense.[18] In Aberdeen, helped by its narrow trade routes from the south and a lesser volume of trade with the continent, these measures were notably successful and in 1603, the records could say that 'it has pleasit the guidness of God in his infinite mercy to withhauld the plague frae this burgh this 65 years bygone'. Nevertheless, the plague did reach Aberdeen again. In 1644 the armies of Montrose and the Covenanters spread the disease north, and a fifth of the population of Aberdeen died. The plague hardly affected the Highlands. The dispersed population and the difficulty in travel did not favour the spread of the disease. Sir Robert Gordon had another explanation: 'Ther is not a ratt in Sutherland: and if they doe come thither in ships . . . they die presently how soon they doe smell the aire of that Cuntry'. Scotland, however, escaped the last, severe, epidemic of plague in England in 1665.

In spite of early cynicism about the powers of the medical men, by the end of the period their advice on the epidemics was being sought and listened to. The problem of the plague also inspired Scotland's first printed medical work in the vernacular – Gilbert Skeyne's *Ane Breve Descriptioun of the Pest* (1568). Though he did not dismiss the need for repentance of sins and upheld the value of prayer, he considered the disease to come from lack of public health and sanitation – Aberdeen's 'stinkand corruptioun and filth.' Skeyne was mediciner at Kings College Aberdeen, and his short text gives the medieval management of the plague. Cleanliness and good sanitation were necessary and stray animals were to be destroyed. For an established case, treatment by bleeding and purging and some herbs was given.

There is other evidence that the medical practitioners were being consulted more often for advice on epidemics, since in Lanark in 1570 an allowance was made to 'the doctor that the minister brocht'. In 1578 Edinburgh employed a surgeon, Robert Henrysoun, to advise on the problem of the plague, the town having lost one tenth of its population during an epidemic ten years earlier, and news had come of plague in Fife.[19] Thus the appointment arose out of one of the recurring civic panics in the face of threatening epidemics. Henrysoun was first employed to go to Wemyss in Fife to check on a report of an outbreak of the plague, which he confirmed and which, as feared, later reached Edinburgh. He took upon himself the arrangements for dealing with the epidemic and as usual a camp was set up for sufferers outside the town, on this occasion at the edge of Blackford Hill. This proved to be one of the worst epidemics ever in Edinburgh and those who could leave the town did so. Robert Henrysoun nevertheless took up the new and unattractive appointment of Medical Officer to the city at an annual salary of £20. The plague epidemic lasted for a year and when it was over, the gratitude of the returning council was such that his appointment was made permanent and the town recorded its gratitude to him for his work. The death of his own wife of plague was also noted with sorrow. In gratitude for Henrysoun's sacrifice and his civic responsibility, he was made Principal Medical Officer to the town, a salaried post which gave him security, without preventing private practice.

These ravages which in Scotland periodically reduced the medieval population by a third or a quarter were probably part of periodic Malthusian crises caused by the population outgrowing the food supply. There was one possible benefit to the poor, who suffered most from famine and disease. With the periodic reduction in the numbers of working people, they were temporarily, as in war time, in a stronger bargaining position in negotiations with the ruling class over their terms and conditions of work.

Leprosy

In addition to these epidemics, some endemic chronic diseases are well described in Scotland. Individual diseases well documented in medieval times are leprosy in the early period and later syphilis.

Leprosy appears in the earliest records of Scotland.[20] The best known person thought to be infected was Robert the Bruce and his skull shows evidence of the disease. Though the cause of the disease was unknown in medieval times and was often explained as punishment for sin, the communities regarded it as an infectious disease and isolation of cases outside the towns was routine. The disease probably reached Britain with the crusaders returning from the East. The first European regulations on leprosy were made by Charlemagne and in England the first leper house appeared in 936. The first Scottish legislation came in the 12th century and the first recorded leper hospital appeared at Legerwood in Berwickshire in 1177. Robert the Bruce was thought to have founded the leper house at Kingcase near Prestwick as the result of help he received from a holy well nearby, and by 1500 there was a leper house outside every principal burgh in Scotland. In Glasgow the lepers were housed on the south bank of the Clyde and in Edinburgh the leper house was near what is now Waverley Station. Whether or not a leper house existed in Liberton in Edinburgh is controversial.

Legislation anent the lepers was common and is detailed in national and town council records. This legislation compelled the isolation of cases, and the diagnosis was made not by medical men but by the town's officials. Since these lepers could not earn their living, laws were made to help to feed them. Any dead or wounded beasts found in the forest were sent to the lepers and any unsaleable meat or fish from the market was given to them also. Both these regulations were designed to save money for the town, by reducing the local levy. The restrictions on the life of the medieval leper and orders for a tax for their upkeep are seen in this Act of Parliament of 12th century Scotland:

> Gif ony that duellis [dwells] in the kyngis burgh or was borne in it be fallyn in lepyr that is callit mysal gif that he hafe gudis of his awne thruch the quhilk [which] he may be sustenyt and cled he sal be put in the spytaile [hospital] of the burgh. And gif he has nocht of his awne the burges of that toune sal ger be gadderyt amangis thaim a collec to the valure of xx s. of the quhilk he may be sustenyt and cled. And it is to wyt that mysal men sal nocht entre in the toune gangande [going] fra dur to dur bot anerly [only] to pas the heway [highway] thruch the toune and thai sal sit at the toune end and thar ask almons at furth passand men and ingangand.[21]

This Act thus gives the first record of a local levy to aid the sick. It also hints that either qualification by birth or by residence was required for hospital confinement and it is likely that other lepers from outside the town would be expelled. Further legislation in 1427 restricted the entry into the towns of lepers from the leper houses to between the hours of 10am and 2pm on two or three days a week. The lepers could beg outside the town at the gate and they were compelled to announce their approach by wooden clappers. The lepers of Glasgow – the names and occupations of the six confined to hospital in 1589 are recorded[22] – were to walk near the gutter 'and sall haif clapperis and ane claith upoun their mouth and face the sall stand afar of cuihill [those] they resaif almous'. It seems highly likely that some of the 'lepers' did not have leprosy, and that a large group of ulcerating diseases of the skin were included under this diagnosis. Hence these patients would account for the occasional cures reported and the successful return to the community of some sufferers. One such misdiagnosis has been found[23] but it also emphasised the care normally taken in examining such a case, and the diagnosis, made by town officials, was based on criteria which had a precision not to be seen in clinical practice for centuries. Thus the stigmata of leprosy were accurately recorded by Henryson when his heroine Cresseid is inflicted with leprosy:

> Thy cristall ene minglit with blud I mak,
> Thy voice sa cleir unplesand, hoir [aged] and hace [hoarse]
> Thy lustie lyre [skin] ouirspred with spottis blak,
> And lumpis haw [livid] appeirand in they face;

She asks to be taken to the 'hospitall at the townis end' and her father knew that

> . . . thair was na succour
> To hir seiknes, and that dowblit his pane;[24]

The disease lasted in Scotland until the 1700's when it slowly disappeared from south to north in Britain, the last case being in Orkney.

Syphilis

Another endemic disease of the late middle ages was syphilis.[25] It first appeared as an epidemic in 1497, possibly brought to Scotland by Perkin Warbeck's motley and cosmopolitan army. It was known then under a number of names usually the 'grandgore' or 'glengore'.

The spread of syphilis at that time was undoubtedly aided by the sexual permissiveness of the day, and it spread quickly through Europe. Many commentators consider that its European origin was in Naples in 1494, having been brought there from the New World by Columbus. The Town Council of the city of Aberdeen (reached by Warbeck's army in 1495) were among the first to realise that it was a sexually transmitted disease. An entry in the Town Council Minutes for 1497 shows that the Council knew that the disease was spread by sexual contact and implies that prostitutes were the cause:

> 21st April 1497
>
> The said day, it was statut ordanit be the aldermen and consale for the vin [avoidance] of the infirmitey cumm out of Franche and strang [foreign] partis, that all licht weman be chargit and ordanit to decist fra thar vicis and syne of venerie . . . under the payne of ane key of het yrne [iron] one thar chekis, and banysene [banishing] of the toune.[26]

The problem in Edinburgh must have been as great. Five months after the Aberdeen measures were announced, James IV persuaded the Edinburgh Town Council to issue 'Ane Grandgore Act' to protect the citizens from the disease. This plan was an attempt by the inventive King to free Edinburgh from the disease, since those infected as well as those who claimed to be able to cure it, were to gather on the sands of Leith at an appointed time. From there they were to be taken to the island of Inchkeith and the treatment was to be started. Any sufferers who did not appear were to be branded on the cheek, and thus be recognised in future. The simple and apparently workable plan doubtless failed in its objective. The King maintained this interest in syphilis and other health problems and on his travels and pilgrimages in 1497 and 1498 he noted sufferers from the grandgore at Dalry, Glasgow and Linlithgow, to whom he gave alms.

Thus the spread of the disease through Scotland was rapid and the number of persons infected was considerable. Though Aberdeen had acted in 1497 to stem the spread of the disease, further regulations in 1507 show that the disease was still a problem. These proposed that 'diligent inquisitiuon be takin of ale infect personis with this strange seiknes of Napillis' and added that the 'infect personis' should not visit the butchers, bakers, brewers or launderers: instead they were to 'keip quyat in ther houssis'.[27] There was a period of acute concern in Glasgow in 1600 and a special hospital existed there for those with the disease. All the doctors and officials of the town were summoned to discuss the increasing problem of the disease in that year.

The medieval doctors obtained an undeserved reputation for successfully treating syphilis by mercury since the natural course of the disease is of a skin phase which passes away spontaneously only to appear later as a diffuse disease of the internal organs. Treatment with mercury was not without risks to the user and this may be the reason why Thomas Lyn was imprisoned in Edinburgh in 1509 for 'ye slauchtir of . . . Sir Lancelote Patonsoun . . . be negligent cure of ye infimitie of ye grantgor'.[28]

Medieval hospitals[29]

The hospitals constructed by the early missionaries and attached to the early religious houses of Scotland may not have survived into medieval times. Thereafter some hospitals were built in response to the decree of Pope Innocent III setting up hospitals in all sees. In addition a considerable number of smaller institutions were founded by benefactors often after survival of some personal crisis. Records of about 150 of these hospitals have been traced in Scotland and many more may have existed. Place names containing 'spital' are common and may suggest either the earlier presence of a hospital or that the revenue of the lands went to the upkeep of such an establishment.

The hospitals were a mixed group of institutions offering a wide range of social services. Firstly, hospitals of abbeys in such remote spots as Inchcolm – the best preserved building of this time – were clearly designed for the sick among the staff. Secondly, hospitals found at bridges, fords and ferries or at the remotest part of a route – e.g. Soutra on the edge of the Lammermuirs – served the medieval travellers most of whom were pilgrims, though ill or injured travellers would also be looked after. The most distinguished such visitor was Edward I who was nursed to health in Torphichen Priory after his injury at the battle of Falkirk (1298). Doubtless noble travellers would be relieved of a subscription to the hospital after their stay. Thirdly, hospitals in the towns sheltered the old or feeble, the stronger of whom were encouraged to beg in the town, and such long term incumbents of these hospitals (the bedesmen) had to pray for the soul of the benefactor. Only one such town building survives, that of St Nicholas' Hospital in Glasgow, later known as Provand's Lordship, though the original accommodation for the four poor inhabitants may have been adjacent to the existing building. Lastly, the only medieval hospitals in the modern sense were for the isolation of infectious disease and the permanent or temporary accommodation of cases of leprosy, syphilis and the plague, as discussed earlier, together with the occasional hospital set aside for the treatment of erysipelas. Thus the evidence suggests that in early medieval times Scotland had a network of institutions caring for the disabilities of life, notably old age, disease, and even unemployment, but how far this met the need is not known.

One problem with the hospital system was that the financial support came from a multitude of personal and private foundations, administered by the noble families or the Church or the King. In those turbulent times the frequent changes of land ownership and the decline in the Church meant that the pious intentions of the original founders were easily lost. Also as a particular institution gained in wealth, its social function became easily paid for without need to remember the terms of the original foundation. The masters of these rich hospitals had status and power and they also became part of the political power struggle. These men came to regard themselves as having little or no obligation to continue the work of the institution and often became non-resident, holding the post as a mere benefice or sinecure. Thus the original aims of the hospitals became obscured.

This problem with the hospitals became a political issue when they proved insufficient to meet the needs of poverty in late medieval times. The matter of the original intention and foundations of the hospitals was a splendid issue for the Kings to raise in their struggle with the nobles on the question of 'who governs'. James I made the hospitals question the first item on the agenda of his first Parliament and successfully passed a statute anent the hospitals calling for steps to 'reduce and reforme thame to the effect of their original fundations'. Little action followed however and James II and III again attempted to clear up the uncertainties. In 1457 orders were laid for the 'reformation of the hospitalys' and a commission composed of the Chancellor, one cleric from each diocese and 'twa persons of gude conscience' were to search locally for the original intentions of the founder. If this could not be found, then a new charter was to be written. In the end, little was achieved and right up to the Reformation, the Church itself was calling ineffectually for the return of the revenues to the original purposes. Though most of the smaller hospitals were destroyed in the violence of the Reformation or suffered withdrawal of income, a small number survived particularly in north-east Scotland.

The healers

It would be a mistake to look for an organised medical profession in medieval times. In one sense there were no doctors, except for the small but growing number of physician-clerics who had studied medicine abroad and the barber-surgeons of the towns. Yet in another way, everyone was a doctor. Self-care by prayer, pilgrimage, charms, herbs, magic stones, visits to holy wells and simple surgery was widely practised by rich and poor. Even in times of epidemic disease, no trace of the summoning of professional healers is found, nor much evidence of their advice, until late medieval times. Thus people doctored themselves and there was little alternative in a land with so many obstacles to travel. In the 12th century towns, the diagnosis of leprosy was made by the community and not by the medical men.

Thus healing skills and advice were available from at least three sources. The first and commonest was self-help or the advice of a local folk healer. The next was the advice of the local nobleman whose knowledge of disease and therapy, if not superior to the folk-healers, was obtained in a different way through his formal education. The nobles probably treated themselves, each other, their servants, their tenants and their animals. Lastly, there were the professional healers – not only the clerics who were beginning to extend their general education in medicine into a more full-time interest – but also the lowly surgeons and barbers of the towns who in medieval times grew in importance and formed their powerful craft guilds. Of these various healers and their methods we have only scraps of information and since most of these come from the records of government, the church and the court, it is inevitable that we know most about the educated class of medical men and little of the folk healers.

It was from the Church that the physicians had their origins. In England some monasteries had a reputation for medical knowledge and skills but it is not known if any in Scotland took a similar interest.

About the year 1100 two changes occurred almost simultaneously which were to encourage the emergence of a separate cadre of professional healers throughout Europe and in Scotland.[30] The first was that the Church began to allow and encourage the education of its trainees outside the monasteries, studying instead at the secular universities: in Scotland this meant travel in Europe. The second change was that medical practice by the monks on the staff was discouraged.

The encouragement by the Church of the secular education of their clergy brought with it two problems. The first was that the increasing rediscovery of the previously forgotten corpus of Greek medicine and the teaching of it at the universities was an unwelcome trend for the Church. The new emphasis on natural explanations of disease, and the use of physical healing methods, and even the concept of the healing power of nature – the *vis naturae medicatrix* – contrasted with the Church's teaching of disease as a divine affliction and the relief or prevention being achieved by faith and freedom from sin. Greek medicine in the eyes of the church was a pagan belief, and its reappearance via Moslem sources seemed to confirm this. The second problem was that some priests were beginning to make money from their medical practice and the successful treatment of distinguished patients. A series of papal decrees from 1130–1215 sought to prevent monks from studying medicine for financial gain and to remove medical practice from the monasteries. In addition the monks were discouraged from performing surgical operations. The best known of these decrees, the 1163 edict of Pope Innocent III, included the phrase '*Ecclesia abhorret a sanguine*'. This is considered to be not so much a prohibition on moral grounds against spilling of blood by surgical operations, dissection or blood letting but rather an attempt to limit the medical practice by the priests. These regulations seem to have been enforced. An example that the Church could act in Scotland was seen in 1445 when the Vicar of Haddington was found guilty of 'simony, perjury and irregularity, through exercising publically the art of medicine without canonical dispensation'.

The effect of the Church's attitude in England has been carefully analysed. Whereas in early medieval times the court employed monk-physicians, after the regulations of the Church discouraging medical practice by monks the English court only employed priests who had left the monasteries. This gave an impetus to the establishment of a class of lay medical professionals and the practice of medicine slowly separated itself from the Church. In Scotland it is likely that similar changes were occurring and the charter signatories of some official documents show that medical specialists had appeared. Thus in the late 12th and early 13th centuries a number of charters to Glasgow and Arbroath were witnessed by Henry 'the Physician' or Nicholas 'Medico Meo' or by Mr Martin 'the Physician'.[31] These practitioners at the court had trained in the Church and then left the monasteries for the court, to return to the Church later. The records of the royal household also make it easy to identify some of the later priest-physicians attached to or consulted by the court. In 1282 Alexander, Prince of Scotland, wrote recommending his own priest-physician, Mr Adam de Kirkcudbright, to Edward I, the recommendation being that the doctor had cured the Prince of a disorder, contrary to the opinion of the other physicians. In time some of the practitioners took on the name of 'leich' and some may have formed families of hereditary physicians in the Lowlands, since in 1443 Christine Leche successfully treated one of the King's servants, and was noted to belong to a hereditary family of physicians in Bute. Having moved medical practice out of the monasteries, but not out of the Church, the Church occasionally attempted to control the standards of care outside. 'We forbid', said the Provincial Council of the Church in 1200, 'anyone ignorant of medicine to administer . . . potions of poisonous herbs to a sick person and to practise any divination'.[32]

At about the time when the Church was discouraging the practice of medicine by the monks it also adopted the change in policy in the education of its trainees. While the early Church taught their own students, from about 1100 onwards they looked with favour on higher education obtained at a secular university. For Scottish students this meant travel to Europe. Thus, until the foundation of St Andrew's University in 1411, Scotland's young clerics were to be found throughout Europe seeking the university education that would ensure success and promotion on return home. Few went to Oxford and Cambridge, since only during the short military truces between Scotland and England could a passport be obtained. Hence the continental universities were favoured by the Scots students. The Italian universities were favoured in the 13th century, the French in the 14th and the German and Italian in the 15th. Of the 230 Scottish graduates prior to 1410 whose European university faculty has been identified five took a medical degree, including practice and theory, after their Arts degree and all five then continued their career in the Church.[34] The salary offered to holders of medical degrees was less than those holding doctorates in Theology or Law.

One such graduate did sustain a lifelong interest in medicine, but did not settle in Scotland. John Gray was the illegitimate son of a Scottish nun, graduated MA at Paris in 1392 and stayed on to study medicine there. It had a separate medical faculty, though one with a low status in the University. He returned to Scotland to the church of Kirkandrews, but later returned to teach in Paris and to hold the office of Dean in the Faculty of Medicine. Returning to Scotland, for which journey a safe conduct pass through England was required, he became 'counsellor and physician' to James I.

Europe was an exciting place for these students, particularly those with an interest in medicine.[35] The revival of interest in the original texts of Hippocrates and other Greek physicians showed that the early Church had used some corrupt latin versions of the Greek originals. These versions lacked any anatomical basis or physiological insight and had added a belief in the divine infliction of disease and relief by magic or spiritual means. The revived and sensible Greek medicine reached Europe by a tortuous route. Arab scholars had translated Hippocrates, and their manuscripts passed by way of North Africa to reach Spain and Sicily where the renaissance scholars eagerly reconstructed the Greek knowledge from the Arab texts. From Spain these new manuscripts spread to the rest of Europe and became available to the universities.

One of the best known of these scholar-translators was a wandering Scotsman – Michael Scot – and his colourful life has attracted considerable study and debate.[36] Legend has it that he was born in the Borders about 1175 and that he returned later to live in Balwearie in Fife until his death about 1232. His education was at Oxford before the troubles between Scotland and England. He then moved to Paris and Padua, and is described in the works of Dante (himself a licensed apothecary) and Boccacio. But it was in Toledo in Spain that his crucial contribution to the new European intellectual life was made by his translations into Latin of the Hebrew and Arabic texts of Aristotle. From Spain, he moved to Sicily in 1277. He had been brought there under the patronage of the Holy Roman Emperor Frederick II, and Scot made the necessary and crucial translations of the Hippocratic medical and scientific texts of Avicenna and Averröes. In Sicily he also wrote a popular work on medicine and physiology, his *Liber Physionomiae* which was widely circulated in manuscript form, and after the invention of printing it went through fifty editions in various languages. His own medical practice used the orthodoxy of the day – divination and astrology, but his success with these occult methods exposed him to rumour and gossip, in much the same way as Roger Bacon was persecuted in England, and it was easy for his rivals to suggest that his success came from his contact with evil forces. On his return home to Scotland he continued to be credited with supernatural power and to have contact with powerful spirits. In the Borders it was said that he was followed about by a demon and Scot had to set tasks for this restless spirit, one of which was to split the Eildon Hills into the three peaks seen today. The last, endless task given to the spirit was to make a rope from the sand of a Fife beach, apparently leading to the old saying that 'the Devil is buried in Kirkcaldy beach'. Sir Walter Scott used the legend of Michael Scot's powers in *The Lay of the Last Minstrel*.

Unlike Scot, many Scots scholars returned home after education in Europe. The Church provided a secure income and allowed a career in teaching or an appointment at the court. Many of the churchmen continued with an interest in medicine. The monasteries still had the ancient and irreplaceable manuscripts and soon acquired the new printed books, and their interest in medicine continued to the Reformation. Analysis of the books held by clerics in Glasgow in the 16th century suggests a continuing interest in medicine.[37] The career of William Schevez (?1428–1497) also shows the easy inter-relationship between the Church and medicine since, having studied at the University of St Andrews and then at the medical faculty of Louvain, he practised in Scotland and became a physician to the court.[38] In 1478 he became Archbishop of St Andrews and later Primate of Scotland. John Damian, James IV's French physician and unsuccessful alchemist, had a similar career and was appointed Abbot of Tungland in 1504 though he may not have taken up this post. The close links with Europe also meant that European practitioners were regularly employed by the court or the hierarchy of the church in Scotland. Thus in 1552, the rich asthmatic Archbishop Hamilton of

St Andrews instructed his personal physician, the Spaniard William Cassanate, to seek a second opinion. Cassanate managed to induce the famous Milan physician Jerome Cardan to travel to Scotland, and after studying the Archbishop for 70 days his advice apparently restored Hamilton to health. The successful treatment used Hippocratic methods of change in diet, attention to sleep and exercise: the Archbishop also had to regulate his sexual exertions.[39]

Other medical visitors had less straightforward motives.[40] From England in 1536 came Andrew Borde. 'I am now in skotland, in a lytle unyversyte or study namyd Glasco' he wrote, but under the guise of a travelling physician he was reporting on the political situation in Scotland to the rulers of England. A Dr Gorleth had been made welcome in Glasgow earlier in 1469, but an unfortunate physician Paul Crawar, who had arrived in Scotland with excellent testimonials in 1433 was burnt to death at the stake at St Andrews since it was suspected that he had been sent by the heretics of Prague to spread their views. Doctors at the Scottish court were well treated, though the rapid changes in these appointments suggest that they preferred to move on, or that they merely served a period before returning to the Church or that they fell in and out of favour. Nevertheless, practice at court could be risky, and their counterparts in Europe could put their lives at risk by unsuccessfully treating a noble patron.[41] In the early 14th century Pope John XXII had his physician flayed to death after suspecting him of a poisoning attempt and burnt to death another medical man suspected of being a sorcerer. About the same time, King John of Bohemia had his surgeon thrown into the river after failing to cure an eye problem, and it is little wonder that Leopold, Duke of Austria, could find no surgeon willing to carry out the necessary amputation of his gangrenous leg. In Scotland, such unpleasantness is not recorded, and instead gifts of money and clothes to physicians regularly appear. In 1386 Robert II generously rewarded his physician Ferchard Leche with the island of Jura and the Sutherland lands of Hope and Melness.

As the Scottish physician was emerging as a specialist trained at European universities, the surgeons craft had a separate development. A number of factors resulted in this gulf between these two practitioners. Firstly, in a feudal society, the surgeon's manual work was not highly regarded. Secondly, the medieval physician's theory and practice was based on scholastic argument and required a university education, whereas the surgeons skills were acquired by apprenticeship in the towns. Lastly, the shedding of blood – and hence bloodletting – by the priest-physicians had been prohibited. The barbers working in or visiting the monasteries to attend to the monks tonsure seem to have taken on the surgical work possibly as a result of their familiarity with the use and care of sharp, rust-prone instruments. That monastic barbers with these skills existed is noted in 1503 when a barber was summoned from Cambuskenneth Abbey to pull the teeth of King James IV.[42]

Whatever the origins of the barber-surgeons, the surgeons and barbers of Edinburgh were the first of the Scottish practitioners to develop an organisation of their own. In 1505 they obtained a Seal of Cause which gave them control of the practice of their craft in Edinburgh and laid down regulations for an apprenticeship. At that time they had only a lowly status among the other crafts of the town.

The organisation of the Aberdeen surgeons took place almost as early in the medieval period. Indeed, the 'barbours' are mentioned in an early Council Register in 1494 in a way that suggests that they were an organised body. In the same year as the Edinburgh surgeons obtained their Seal of Cause the Aberdeen barbers are noted as taking part in a pageant, and in a procession for Corpus Christi Day in 1531 they took sixteenth place among the seventeen crafts. By 1674 they were called 'barbers chirurgeons and periwigmakers'. The Glasgow surgeons organised themselves in 1599 into a joint Faculty of Physicians and Surgeons, but there is no trace of any other surgical craft guilds in other Scottish towns, though Dundee was larger than Glasgow.

Medical science

Scotland kept a sharp eye on developments in medieval European science and medicine. The establishment of no less than three Scottish universities in this period indicates the advancing status of Scottish scholarship. In the reign of James IV (1473–1513) this achievement was at its height and, like the later Enlightenment of the 18th century, this early enlightenment was helped by the peace and prosperity in the land. The King was powerful and an interested patron of the orthodox medicine and science of the day: medieval scholarship could only prosper when such support was given.[43]

The interest of the Scottish crown in medicine had been an ancient one. Like other nobles the King received medical training as part of his general education, but many seem to have taken this interest further. Thus when George Buchanan, the Scottish historian, constructed his colourful (and largely imaginary) history of Scotland, he said that Josina, supposedly the ninth King of Scotland, obtained his education in Ireland and wrote a thesis during this time on 'the virtue and power of herbs'. The historian commented thus that 'the rest of the Scottish nobility, complying with the humour of the King, it came to pass that for many ages there was scarce a nobleman or gentleman in Scotland which had not the skill to heal wounds'. The tradition continued for centuries and James IV in particular patronised the lowly practice of surgery, since he was 'weill learned in the airt of medicine and ane singular guid surgeon'. His skills included blood-letting, treatment of wounds and the pulling of teeth and he showed an interest in patients recently operated on for bladder stones or for hernias.[44] James also encouraged the fight against the plague and the sensible regulations in Scotland against its spread made during his reign certainly arose from his interest, as did probably the regulations against syphilis and the bold attempt to abolish this disease in Edinburgh in 1497. James also encouraged the establishment of King's College in Aberdeen and the provision for the 'mediciner' to teach medicine may have been at his prompting: the King's interest in medicine is mentioned in Aberdeen's Papal Bull. James' view that natural phenomena could be analysed and explained marks him out as one of the new thinkers of the Renaissance. This assumption is most clearly demonstrated in his own rather bizarre experiment in which two children were put on Inchkeith, an island in the Forth, with a dumb nurse, in order to establish the language that the children would speak without human tuition. The result of this experiment is not known.

The development of alchemy was also patronised by the King. He established a French (or Italian) alchemist, John Damian, in a laboratory in Stirling Castle where the futile, but necessary hunt for the *quinta essentia* and the methods for the production of gold was carried on, work necessary to keep abreast of the orthodoxy of the day.[45] Scotland's alchemists were highly regarded and from them and their techniques came a fine tradition of chemistry which flourished strongly later. Another of Damian's endeavours should be mentioned, that of his attempt to fly. Bishop Lesley records that:

> This abbott tuik it in hand to flie with wingis . . . quhilkis beand fessinit apoun him, he flew of the castell wall of Striveling, bot shortlie he fell to the ground and brak his thee [thigh] bane;[46]

Though it is easy to ridicule this attempt, its assumption that technological innovation was possible was a major innovation in an age that had only just escaped from the shackles of a static intellectual and spiritual environment. Damian had other contemporary critics. Dunbar said of his medical skill:

> In pottingry he wrocht gryt pyne,
> He murdreist mony in medecyne,
> In leichcraft he was homicyd.[47]

Though the universities had taken no part in this early enlightenment, the establishment of three universities in Scotland in the 15th century reduced the number of students seeking higher education abroad. In copying the continental universities, the Scottish founders also had in mind the need to provide for the small but growing number of students interested in medicine, but in the end they were not successful in establishing medical teaching. In Aberdeen a specialist teacher of medicine – the mediciner – was allowed for and this was the first such specialist teaching post in medicine in Britain. Though the job attracted distinguished scholars, notably Gilbert Skeyne author of the previously mentioned classic text on the plague, the teaching of medicine was not a success and did not produce specialist physicians in any quanitity, though whether through lack of students or poor teaching is not known. Though formal teaching of medicine at Aberdeen failed to emerge as a recognisable medical school, a small output of medical men resulted and the shrewd public health measures in Aberdeen and their insight into infectious disease suggests that medical thought was advanced in that town. The number of Aberdonians who achieved fame in medical practice in Britain or on the continent in this period is striking.[48] Gilbert Skeyne had studied medicine at Aberdeen and Duncan Liddel (1561–1613) left Aberdeen to wander the continent, eventually becoming professor of physic and Dean of the Faculty of Philosophy in Helmstadt, returning to Scotland, as many others had done before him, at the height of his fame. Also leaving Aberdeen was Gilbert Jack (1578–1628) to become professor of philosophy in Leyden and teach medicine and metaphysics there, Thomas Forbes went to the chair of Medicine at Pisa and James Leith to fame and fortune in medical practice in Paris. Hence by the 16th and even the 17th century, while many Scottish students intent on the Church or a career in law were content to have a Scottish university education, those wishing to be physicians still had to seek their education abroad, often staying for a career on the continent. Their presence there was noted and they were useful to visiting Scottish dignitaries, such as Queen Mary of Guise in 1551:

> During the time that the Queen douarier and the nobilitie of Scotlande was in France, thair come ane doctour phisitiane, callit Ramsay, Scottisman, furth of Turing in Pyedmount to France, being of gret aige and guid lerning and experience, quha served all the nobillmen of Scotland and thair haill cumpanye, with sic things as was necessary for thame, frelie apoun his awn charges, moved onely for the zeill he buir toward his cuntrey; swa that he wald not suffer thame to cum under the cuir and medicine of strangers, in case they mycht haif happenit in sum onrecoverabile inconvenient, ather be evill drogges or onlerned mixtour thairof.[49]

Other Scottish medical travellers were Henry Blackwood of Dumfries who became regent at the University of Paris in 1551 and Mark Duncan from Roxburghshire who was physician and regent at Saumur in 1598. Peter Lowe, the Scottish surgeon, became distinguished in France before returning in 1598. In addition, a number of Scots achieved fame in Europe for their skill in alchemy. Alexander Seton reached the continent in 1602 and conducted public demonstrations of the transmutation of base metals into gold. Hounded by jealous and greedy rivals, he was eventually imprisoned by the Elector of Saxony and tortured in an attempt to extort his secret. He escaped but died of his injuries. His book *A New Light of Alchymie* was a 17th century bestseller. Another physician who travelled dangerously was Dundee's David Kinloch (1599–1617), M.A. (St Andrews) M.D. (Paris), a writer in obstetrics and a poet. When travelling in Spain he was seized by the Inquisition, but his execution was delayed by the illness of the Inquisitor. Kinloch, the legend goes, sent a message (via a black cat) successfully offering his services and advice, and on the recovery of the Inquisitor, he was allowed to go free.[50]

Even when the East India Company first reached Persia in 1620 there was a Scottish doctor waiting to greet them. The Company, impressed by Strachan's local knowledge and his contacts with local rulers, took him onto the payroll and initial reports back to London were enthusiastic. Later they turned sour. 'Strachan, our antichristian physician . . . flattering, lying, dissimulation, continually despizeth his owne country and yts church'. After the discovery of his industrial espionage he was dismissed, having it was realised, obtained a year's salary in advance.[51]

Medical practice

We know little of day-to-day medical practice in medieval Scotland, but it is certain that the methods of the orthodox practitioners were only available to a small section of society. In the Lowlands, the rich nobles, the Court or the churchmen might consult with or write to a physician or surgeon and the few surviving Lowland Scottish medieval texts on medicine all suggest that Hippocratic methods of therapy were in use, namely change of diet, change of climate and regulated exercise and sleep, together with the herbal methods of treatment and bloodletting as taught at the Salerno medical school. These methods are mentioned in some of Henryson's poems which incorporate them in the preservation of health:

> Use mesurable rest with sobir eiting,
> Use bissines but sair sweiting,
> Be nevir crabbit for no kin thing.

and

> Cleir air and walking makes guid degestioun.[52]

There is evidence, however, of a less admirable trend in medical practice. The materials for the physicians' prescriptions and the dispensing of them was carried out by the apothecaries, who had evolved from the grocers and spicers to supply the physicians' needs. Since medical knowledge and methods of therapy were possessed by all educated men, the only way open for the physicians was to make the healing arts more complex, and the apothecaries, who also did some treatment as well as dispensing, clearly welcomed any sophistication of medical treatment. It increased the volume of their work and their hunt for rare materials from overseas was also very profitable. Though this trend was to reach its ludicrous peak in the late 17th century, there were already complaints about the complex mixtures and exotic materials in the 16th century prescriptions methods which were satirised by the Scottish medieval poets.[53]

We know little more about day-to-day surgical practice. The records of James IV describe alms given to survivors of surgery for bladder stones, couching for cataract and relief of obstructed hernias, but as these operations were shunned by the orthodox surgeons of the towns, it is likely that the patients had been treated by itinerants. Certainly the Bishop of Ross had to travel to Paris in 1564 for a lithotomy. He died after the operation causing John Knox to remark unkindly that 'God strake him according to his deservings.'

One procedure that the town surgeons certainly took on was embalming the dead; after the death of Bishop Kennedy, his heart was removed by expert division of the bones of the chest.[54] The day-to-day practice of the town surgeon was therefore healing wounds, treating ulcers and fractures, embalming and bloodletting both as a treatment and as a regular tonic. There are a number of instances of salaries being offered to surgeons to settle in the towns, and it may be that even the orthodox medical men were itinerant at times. Town surgeons might expect to be given a fee for regular work among the poor or to be paid for each item of service to the town. Thomas Mylne was rewarded by Glasgow in 1580 for 'curing Thomas Muir hurt in the towns besynes' as was Allester McCaslan in 1596 for 'curing sindry puir anes in the toune'. The surgeons in early medieval Scotland might be expected to join the armies or to help in the aftermath of war, as when four Edinburgh surgeons were paid £12 each for 'passand to the bourdouris for curing of all personis that hapint to be hurt be the Inglis menne.'[55]

Lastly, there are some fragments from the records of the Burgh and Head Courts in Dundee that record the litigation in which local surgeons were involved, thus giving some insight into medical practice of the time.[56] The records show that a patient consulting a medical man could demand that the fee for treatment be agreed ahead and that the fee could be withheld if treatment was not successful. Records also show that in cases of assault, the guilty party was liable for the doctor's fee and even to pay compensation for loss of earnings. Thus in March 1556 the Dundee Court records that:

> the quhilk day Jhone esak is conuict [convicted] in strublance of yis gud towne in hurting of thomas duff in ye heid to ye gryt effusion of ye said thomas blude And yare for ye Jugis decernis ye said Jhone Esak to pay . . . s for curing & helyng of ye said

> thomas duffis heid & satisfaccion of ye faile [injury] maid by hym . . .

In 1523 Robert Dawson was ordered to pay Willy Dougal 12 pence for 'ilk day that the leich will depone that he may not guidly labor thro the hurt'. The records also show the fees of the time for treating injuries – £5 Scots for a broken leg, £10 for treating a wound and up to £20 for a broken thigh.

From this same source comes a poignant tale of lost confidence and professional discord in 1614:

> 2nd. Feb. Qlk day anent the actioun and clame p'suit at the inst. of Alex. Smyt in Overyeards agains John Fordyce chirurgian, makand mentione that the space of nyn yeiris syne Mart. Chalmeris spous to the said Alex. being hurt and woundet in the left arme and the said Jon being than imployit be him to undertak the curing and heilling of the said Mart. and he for the sowne [sum] of fourtie lib. monie wt. ane boll of quhet [wheat] and tua bollis meill [meal] payit and delyverit be the said Alex. to him enterit to the curing of the said wound and promittit undr God to heall the said Mart. yroff [therof] and to warrand hir fra mitilacun [free of mutilation] and impotence yr in and urwayis [otherwise] to refund the sowne and uthir feis ressavit be him fra the said Alex. yrfore. Notwithstanding it is of veritie that qn. [when] the said Jon had endit his curing of the said hurt, the said Mart. was so impotent and mutilate in the said arme that the samen commonellie hang doun and was not habile to lift the samen to hir head and that yrfore I past wt. the said Mart. to Edr. [Edinburgh] qr. [where] James Kaitmure [Skaithmure], prinnll. chirurgiane thr. and uthirs in that burt. [burgh] haillit and curit the said airme and declaryit that the said Jon haed not rytlie understuid the said hurt and haed putt the same in corss [worse] estate nor [than] at his entre yron [thereon] . . . And albeit of veritie the said Jon be haldane to refound to the said Alex. the said sown and urs. [others] aboues peit bot lykewayis the haill chairges and expenss debursit be me in Edr. upone the said cuir, extending to the sowne of 1^{c}lib. nothwithstanding he refusit wt. out he be compellit . . .

These Dundee regulations have an ancient lineage. The Brehon Laws of Ireland contain similar provisions, which in turn are reminiscent of the very early (18th century BC) Code Hammurabi in the

Babylonian empire, which laid down statutory fees and allowed for the punishment of unsuccessful practitioners.[57]

There is more than a hint that surgery was regarded more highly in Scotland than in England and in this Scotland took a more European view. Certainly James IV held surgical skills in high regard and in 1505 as a mark of his favour the King waived the usual fee for the ratification of the Seal of Cause of the Edinburgh Surgeons and Barbers. This attitude was to be crucial in future developments in Scotland and the early organisation of the surgeons and the delay in the appearance of a physicians college had important effects later.

Self-treatment

The first impulse of the great mass of the people during illness was probably to attempt some personal therapy, rather than consult a trained or untrained healer. Nor would their first choice always be the widely known herbal remedies, since the power of the healing stones and wells were highly regarded as was prayer or pilgrimage to the holy places in Scotland, such as the relics of St Ninian at Whithorn or the chapel of the Virgin on the island of Scarba.

The best known of the healing stones was the Lee Penny, still held by the family of Lockhart of Lee and Carnwath. It was brought back from the East after a crusade in the 14th century and is a gem of dark colour set in a coin – a groat of 1422–1483. The stone was put into water with 'twa dips and a swirl' and the water drunk by the patient or used as a lotion. It was used for fevers, stopping haemorrhage and curing hydrophobia. No words were spoken or the cure would be ineffective. This charm and others like it – the crystal held by the Stewarts of Ardvorlich – were in regular use until the 18th century.[58]

Also much used were the holy healing wells and their popularity in medieval times is suggested by the large number of wells in Scotland named after the early saints and missionaries.[59] There are a dozen or so 'St Columba's' wells and almost as many named after St Ninian. The extent to which they were used and the ritual involved are revealed as a result of the prohibitions on their use by the Kirk Sessions after the Reformation. In the north east of Scotland (the best researched area) there were ten major holy wells which attracted large numbers of pilgrims and sufferers, some coming even from the Western Islands. The wells were thought to have powers in different diseases, notably skin diseases and mental illness: details of their use are given later.

Lastly, there must have been a network of local folk healers, bone-setters and charmers plus travelling honest or dishonest healers. We know of these healers and their works only indirectly. There is a painting held in Arras of the gypsy who cured 'King James of Scotland' but which James is not revealed.[60] Other evidence comes from the 1599 Charter to the Faculty of Physicians and Surgeons in Glasgow which complained of 'ignorant unskillit and unlernit personis quha . . . abusis the people' and an Aberdeen doctor complained in 1615 of a local problem with 'highland leeches, imposters mountebanks, mercurial mediciners . . .'.[61]

Health and health care in the Highlands

The Highlands had a separate series of changes in medieval times.[62] Iona had been the base for Columba's mission and though he travelled widely on the west coast and founded more monastic institutions, they then faded in importance in that area and were not replaced. The clan feuds, the Norse invasion and inhospitable land prevented the further development of monastic institutions. Nevertheless, the clergy and the clan chiefs were well educated and travelled in Europe and their physicians were well read and talented.

Indeed, the surviving gaelic medical manuscripts outnumber the handful of latin medical manuscripts rescued from the Lowland monasteries after the Reformation. The Highland physicians had a high place in the hierarchy of the clan, taking second place to the bard at the banqueting table. The most distinguished of these hereditary families was that of the Beatons – the latin form of the Gaelic MacBheathadh, MacBeath, or Bethune – who served the MacLeods and the Lord of the Isles. Some legends say that the first Beaton came from Ulster with Angus Og's bride about 1303 but others assert that the name is a corruption of the pictish 'Bede', in which case the family was the one shown in the Book of Deer to have gifted land to Columba for his monastery. Whatever the explanation, the Beatons' medical knowledge came originally from Ireland. The family continued to be distinguished until the 17th century and held extensive land in the west coast. For 200 years the office of principal physician of the Isles existed and in 1609 James VI confirmed to Fergus McBeath the land he held given to him by the Lordship of the Isles. Later,

Martin Martin in 1699 found Beatons practising in South and North Uist and heard of a Beaton physician who happened to be on the Spanish treasure ship *Florida* when it was blown up by the islanders in Tobermory Bay in 1588, and who survived to practise for many more years. Martin also found a Beaton in Skye who, although he was an 'illiterate Empiric . . . extracts the Juice of plants and roots after a Chymical way peculiar to himfelf'. Of the other medical families the best known were O'Connachers who served the Argyles and held land in Lovat. The McDonalds employed a family of McLeans as hereditary physicians.

The fame of these healers extended beyond the west coast and their skills were repeatedly employed and rewarded by the Kings of Scotland and a Beaton – 'a skilled empiricist' – travelled with James VI's court to London. Gaelic legends enjoy to tell how the metropolitan physicians substituted a sample of bull's urine for that from the King, but having spotted the trick, Beaton confounded these doctors and went on to cure the King. Health care methods in the Highlands are well described since the hereditary physicians' Gaelic translations of the famous continental texts of medical practice have survived in reasonable numbers. Some of these volumes suggest by their small size that they were carried by the physician while at work and during visits, much as the monks carried a missal as a *vade mecum*. This is also suggested by the tale of a Skye physician's visit to a patient which involved a journey across a sea loch. So precious was his copy of the famous Montpellier medical text *Lilium Medicinae* (1303) that, risking nothing, he sent the text round by land to meet him on the other side. These rare Gaelic texts are preserved and consist partly of a pharmacopoeia and partly of instructions for bloodletting and dieting.[63] The medieval emphasis on astrology and the best seasons for treatment is shown by the medical calendars at the back of the book. In addition to transcribing the ancient texts into Gaelic, some texts are synopses of the classic works, in which the authors took the best of Aristotle, Galen, Rhazes and Vesalius and to which the physicians added their own experiences. The most interesting of these works is the *Regimen Sanitatis* of a John MacBeath, probably written in the 16th century and based on the text of the same name from Salerno, which in turn was based on Greek medicine. The text is comprehensive and follows orthodox lines, dealing with anatomy, botany, disease, therapy and the fees to be charged. The text is remarkable for an emphasis on prevention of disease – 'keep a firm grip on health' says the text, 'eat not too much' and 'spare the wine'. On rising in the morning exercises are recommended and walking is regarded as beneficial. Extracts of simple herbs are prescribed – violet (for headache and catarrh), nettle, mustard, hyssop, saffron, shepherds purse for bleeding wounds, fennel and parsley to increase the urine flow, celery for diseases of mouth and stomach, mercury for lice and tannin for wounds.

To herbal cures, healing wells and healing stones are added magic charms, probably at their most powerful when spoken by highly regarded folk healers. In Highland folklore some of these charms are clearly medieval in origin since they use pre-Reformation mysticism in invoking the Trinity or call on the Scottish Saints' names. St Bride, for example, was often in charms for toothache.

Reformation

Towards the end of this period, religious life in Scotland was convulsed by the overthrow of the Roman Catholic Church with the Reformation of 1559. Though great change in social welfare seemed likely, little emerged. One of the abuses which had led to the Reformation was the decline in the care of the poor by the Church. The medieval Church had grown steadily richer, more secular and more corrupt, and its clergy degenerate. Among many abuses was the alienation of revenues originally intended for the upkeep of the hospitals and the support of the poor. As noted earlier, attempts were made without success to restore the original intentions of the foundations of the hospitals and this and other failures left a way open for the revolution led by John Knox and his followers. Indeed the first blow struck for the Reformation was the nailing of the 'Beggars Summonds' to the doors of the friars houses in the towns which called on them to surrender their possessions to the poor 'to whom it rightly belongs'. It was therefore appropriate that on gaining power, Knox and the new Church should place emphasis on the well-being and sustenance of the working people of Scotland. In the new Church's manifesto, as laid out in the *First Book of Discipline*, there was a remarkable plan for social welfare and education, including medical education. Though Knox's campaign against moral weakness was to be rigorously pursued and came to characterise the new Church the plans for social welfare were later laid aside, when the interests of the ruling class were restored. What little remained of the plans gave Scotland only a moderate programme of welfare, and it has been commented that

> the Scottish provision for the poor in the 17th century was weak and mean and the very opposite from what was intended by the reformers in that first flush of excitement and idealism.[64]

The best that can be said is that the Church at the parish level preferred to put their limited funds into schools rather than poor relief.

On reading Knox's and his co-reformers plan, as laid out in the *First Book of Discipline*, their simplicity and comprehensive nature are striking.[65] Education was always the keystone of Knox's programme and he urged that:

> The riche and potent may not be permitted to suffer thair children to spend thair youth in vane idilnes, as heirtofore thei have done. But thei must be exhorted, and by the censure of the Churche compelled to dedicat thair sones, by goode exercise, to the proffit of the Churche and to the Common-wealth; and that thei must do of thair awin expenses, becaus thei ar able. The children of the poore must be supported and sustenit on the charge of the Churche, till tryell be tackin, whethir the spirit of docilitie be fund in them or not. Yf thei be fund apt to letteris and learnyng, then may thei not (we meane, neathir the sonis of the riche, nor yit the sonis of the poore), be permittit to reject learnyng; but must be chargeit to continew thair studie, sa that the Commoun-wealthe may have some confort by them.[66]

Not only were all children to receive education, but reorganisation of the universities was also planned, with emphasis on educating the youth of the land for the professions. An introductory 3–4 year course of general studies was proposed following which the student could proceed to study law, medicine or divinity. A total of five to six years study for medicine was thus suggested, to be conducted by a specialist medical teacher with a salary of £133.6.8, a figure slightly less than that for the professors of divinity and the classics. Only St Andrews University was to teach medicine, probably because the demand for physicians in Scotland at that time made only one medical school necessary.

These plans were never introduced and it was over one hundred years before regular medical teaching appeared in Scotland, and almost two hundred years before a statutory medical course with graduation examinations was introduced. In choosing St Andrews, Knox and his colleagues may have erred, since a non-clinical medical school would have emerged there, as at Oxford. A medical school of this kind without a hospital, though appropriate to the 17th century, might later have inhibited other medical teaching in Scotland and could have prevented the success of the hospital-based Edinburgh school, just as Oxford held back the rise of London medical schools.

There were some attempts to set up medical teaching, but these were half-hearted. It is clear from the reports of the inspections of the universities by the new Church that the teaching of medicine, though mentioned and recommended, was not seriously supported. No bursaries were set up to help poor students and no lists of medical texts were recommended, as had been done for other faculties.[67] Certainly Buchanan in his plan for St Andrews repeated the earlier proposals of the *First Book of Discipline*, and the Visitation by the General Assembly of the Church of Scotland in 1578 recommended that the Principal of St Andrews should be the professor of medicine and teach four times in the week, but when the Visitation returned four years later they found that the plan had failed. While the Principal protested that he had taught the Aphorisms of Hippocrates twice each week, other members of the staff confided uncharitably to the Visitors that 'he nevir teichis, skantlie anis in the month'.

Knox's plan for the relief of destitution was to use the revenue of the overthrown Church to aid those in need:

> We ar nott patronis for stubburne and idell beggaris quho rynning from place to place mak a craft of thair beggyng . . . but for the wedow and fatherless the aiged impotent or laymed . . . also for personis of honestie fallin into decay and penuritie . . . The ministers and the Pure [poor] togidder with the Schollis . . . must be sustened upoun the chargeis of the Churche: we must crave of your Honouris that ye have respect to your pure brethern the lauboraris and manuraris of the ground; who by these creuell beastis the Papists have been so oppressit that thair life to thame have been dolorous and bitter.

In other writings he gave details of his financial plans, and implied that the revenues of the old Church were to be split in three ways – one third to the schools, one third to the ministers and one third for the relief of the poor. Had Knox's scheme come to pass, social welfare in Scotland would have been the most advanced in Europe, and would have equalled the new Scottish educational system in its radicalism. 'Even Mohammed never had such . . . licence in promising . . . the dividing of the goods of the Church among the poor', it was said of Knox.[68] Expectation ran high. In 1561 the Town Council of Edinburgh resolved that the

> landis, annuellis and utheris emolimentis quhilikis [which] of befor war payit furth of landis and tenementis within this burgh to papistis preistis freris monkis nonis . . . for manteinying of idolatrie seeing it hes plesit the Almychti to oppin the eis of all pepill . . . thairfoir that the saidiss rentis and emolimentis by applyit to mair proffitable and godlie usiss sic as for sustenying of the trew ministeris of Goddis word, founding the biging [building] of hospitals for the pure [poor] and collegis for leirnyng and upbring of the youth . . .[69]

Knox's schemes were, however, thwarted by the landowners who prevented the new reformed Church from reclaiming the lands and benefits belonging to the pre-Reformation Church. So confused was the legal ownership of land that Knox's schemes were easily prevented by those in possession. Instead therefore of a guaranteed and automatic income for the relief of poverty and starvation, the old voluntary system continued in each parish depending on special collections and donations for the poor or the sick, the fines collected after Kirk Session convictions, hiring charges for mortcloths, plus an occasional levy on the parishioners and heritors. This system continued until the 19th century when the increased mobility of the population and the growth of towns destroyed the parish as an administrative unit and a new Poor Law was passed in 1845.

After these hopes for a new social order were dashed, Scotland entered a century of civil strife and intellectual stagnation, a period all the more regrettable in view of the progress in science and medicine in England and elsewhere.

3
The troubled years 17th century

Though Scotland's population grew little in the 17th century, the changes in agriculture forced many off the land and the number of homeless beggars rose. These changes and the 17th century warfare made the conditions for famine and the spread of epidemics more likely than before. Though the Reformation had promised much for the poor and new proposals were made for the relief of famine and the control of food supplies, in the end little was done.

During the 17th century, life in Scotland was almost continually disturbed by feuds and war, both internal and external. While in England and the continent considerable intellectual progress was made, Scotland lagged behind. The Reformation resulted in a new and advanced school system for the nation, but the reformers' plan for medical education never appeared, lost in the buffeting of the universities by the various interested factions. Thus university education for the physicians continued abroad in the European medical schools. However a College of Physicians appeared in Edinburgh and this was the first of a series of events which led eventually to the remarkable success of Scottish medicine in the 18th century. In rural Scotland the three traditional levels of health care continued – self-help, folk-healing and professional advice but the folk healers of the 17th century ran the danger of being accused of witchcraft. In the towns the fourth type of healer appeared – the itinerant quack, who clashed with the doctor's organisations.

Social life and the people[1]

The majority of the people of 17th century Scotland worked in agriculture, living in loose collections of dwellings called farmtouns, or kirktouns if a parish church was present or milltouns if a mill existed. Agriculture was primitive, even at a time when it was improving in England and the bankrupt feudal system could not encourage improvement in the land. Crops were repeatedly wrung out of unfertilised and unrotated land and the 'black' house was the standard habitation. The diet was simple: oatmeal, kale, fish, ale and milk. The grain fed the people, paid the rent and was next year's seed. 'Ane to sow, ane to gnaw and ane to pay the laird witha' was the fate of the grain crop. The dress of the farming community was of coarse woollen cloth and shoes were uncommon. Personal hygiene was low – 'the clartier the cosier'. The small landowners were not well off and many travellers commented on the austerity and lack of comfort in the lairds' houses and in the inns for travellers. Only a few of the great barons and the Highland chiefs lived in great style. The drink of the time was claret for the rich and ale for the peasants – whisky was to be favoured later – with all evidence pointing to drunkenness and excess as being a problem. It seems likely that the health of Scotland was deteriorating relative to England and was perhaps worse than in the preceeding 16th century. Expectation of life did not exceed 30 years and life was cheap: it was not necessary to record the interment of paupers or children in burial records. Infanticide and the concealment of illegitimate births were both common, possibly a result of the reformed church's obsession with sexual offences.

The population could not be regularly supported at all times and after famine or war, displaced persons wandered throughout Scotland, begging and stealing: many emigrated to Ulster or Europe. Fletcher of Saltoun estimated that 1 in 5 persons was a beggar in the late 17th century. Begging was of two kinds. The official type was sanctioned by the Kirk Session and was signalled by the possession of a badge. These beggars were well known to the parish and probably served a useful function as messengers and spreaders of news. The other was the 'strong and masterful beggars' who, having either failed to win official approval or despairing of it, had left their homes and wandered the land. Begging could be quite successful, as the nobles regarded it as their christian duty to give alms to the poor they encountered each day and the diaries of the period show a steady disbursement. The nobles were therefore a magnet for beggars, as were funerals and weddings, and it was estimated that 1,000 beggars attended the Earl of Eglinton's funeral to fight for the £30 distributed.[2] Thus if the masterful poor kept moving and searching there was always the chance of something turning up.

The great hazards to life were famine, epidemics, natural disasters, war, fires and floods: each problem could lead in turn to the others.[3] The towns of 17th century Scotland were expanding and this growth made more likely the spread of epidemics. With greater ease of travel and the constant movement of armies and armed bands around the land, disease was easily spread through Scotland, helped by the billeting of soldiers in the towns. The appropriation or burning of the crops by the troops also helped increase disease by causing famine and starvation: war killed more civilians than soldiers. Civil warfare in 17th century Scotland was particularly vicious. General Leslie's army defeated the Covenanters at Philiphaugh in 1645 and then massacred all the prisoners, women and children included. Torture of prisoners was routine and new methods were devised. Affleck of Cumlachie was tortured by the 'boot' applied to his legs and 'wes maid impotent of baith his leggis and deit theireftir within a few days of extreme payne'.[4]

The growing towns were largely of wood and disastrous fires occurred. In 1623 fire destroyed three-quarters of Dunfermline, and most of Kelso was made homeless after a fire in 1645: Glasgow also suffered fires in 1652 and 1677. The successful towns had expanded beside the lower stretches of the large rivers and hence damage by floods were also likely. In 1621 the Tay flooded the centre of Perth and 'all the peipill in the castell gavill and west port were wat in their beddis, and wakened with water to the waist in their floores'.[5] The newer substantial town houses also harboured the rats which spread the plague, and the squalor of the towns provided the overcrowding, lack of sanitation and deficient personal cleanliness which ensured the rapid spread of typhus and other diseases. The inadequate nutrition of the new poor gave them little resistance to disease. In times of dearth in rural areas, cattle were not fed, leading to the death of the animals, thus removing the ultimate source of food. Domestic animals also were not fed during hard times and house rats could further multiply when cats and dogs were ailing. The relative immunity of the ruling class to disease – a result of their good housing and better nutrition – was repeatedly remarked on and regarded as a divine dispensation.

Of the 17th century Scottish towns, Edinburgh was the largest, Dundee came second, with Glasgow one of a number of smaller towns. Travellers through Edinburgh describe the tightly packed wooden dwellings of the town within the old city wall and record that the town totally lacked sanitation and running water. Drinking water was supplied by water sellers using the water from the many wells of the town, a system which spread disease easily. Washing and bathing were difficult in view of the restrictions on water supply and only the well-off might, with great difficulty, arrange for a bath to be taken, on the rare occasions when this was considered necessary. The rest of the community simply lived and died in their rotting clothes and the rich used more and more perfume to disguise the smells. An English traveller to Edinburgh in 1634 commented that:

> the city is placed in a dainty, healthful, pure air and doubtless was a most healthful place to live in, were not the habitants most sluttish, nasty and slothful people. I could not pass through the hall but I was constrained to hold my nose or use wormwood.[6]

In the country things were little better. The less densely packed villages and towns were probably safer, since in times of epidemic they were less likely to be reached or be badly affected and the other blessing was that the primitive housing in the country was less likely to harbour rats. The country areas therefore were a sanctuary during epidemics and the well-to-do fled there to escape the epidemics of the town. Housing continued to be primitive and in Kirkintilloch a traveller could report:

> the poorest houses and people that I have seen inhabit here: the houses have not more light than the light of the door: no windows, the houses covered with clods, the women only neat and handsome about the feet, which comes to pass by their often washing by their feet.[7]

Disease and famine

The sources of information on disease in 17th century Scotland are slightly better than in the earlier period and come from better literary and official sources. The attacks of the plague are easily identified when typical – a link with the march of armies or trade routes plus the arrest of its progress in winter – but a lesser or localised outbreak of 'pest' or 'fever' may have been typhus or other disease and not the plague. Under the term 'flux' was grouped the dysentery group of diseases. A number of other diseases are named more precisely – 'chin cough' (whooping cough), the 'pox' (smallpox) and ague (probably malaria). The significant disasters of the 17th century in

Scotland were the great famines of 1623 and the 1690's and the bubonic plague of 1644 onwards. Famine devastated the countryside: plague hit the towns.

Though the famines of the 1690's gave in total the longest period of starvation recorded in Scotland, historians consider that the famine of 1623 was the worst single year of starvation. Parish records in towns like Dumfries showed a twenty-fold increase in burials in that year and the town lost 10–15% of its own inhabitants, plus a large number of the wandering poor who came into the towns in their last desperate days hoping that some food remained in the town's stores. Two-fifths of the burials were of children.[8]

The problem was foreshadowed in 1621 when a very dry summer was followed by torrential rains and flooding which spoiled the harvest. Prices rose and grain imports from the Baltic increased. It was recorded that never

> in this countrie, in so short a time suche inequalitie of prices of victuall; never greatter feare of famine nor scarstie of seeds to sow the ground . . . Everie man was careful to ease himself of suche persones as he might spaire, and to live als retiredlie as possible he might. Pitiful was the lamentation not onlie of vaging beggars, but also of honest persons.[9]

The Privy Council, now politically stronger, issued warnings against the hoarding of food, particularly by those merchants deliberately seeking a price rise – 'unmerciful forestallers and regraitteris'. Export of food was also banned. Imports were encouraged and fasts and prayer were ordered by the Church to help obtain better weather and harvests. There appears to have been little loss of life in 1621 and a good harvest in 1622 would have restored normality. But bad weather destroyed this harvest as well and Scotland entered into a second winter with little food and starvation reappeared. After the starvation came disease, probably typhus. Disease among the ill-fed cattle also appeared. The *Chronicle of Perth* in 1622 recorded that

> about the harvest and efter, their wes suche ane universall seikness in all the countrie as the ellyke has net bene hard of . . . Thair wes also grat mortalitie amongs the poore.[10]

The Poor Law broke down entirely: in Midlothian by summer 1623 the Privy Council could report that

> the haill pure are impotent, opprest and overrun . . . sua miserable and waik that they can hardlie transport thame selffes

> fra ane parochin to ane uther . . . the pur is so enfeiblit thair is no constable nor uther persone that can be movit in the parochins to put the said Act in executioun.[11]

There were many accounts of deaths in the streets and highways of those desperately trying to reach food in their last moments. A heroic import of grain from the Baltic and the good harvest of 1623 overcame the crisis.

Famine returned briefly in 1674–6 and in the north in 1693–5, and the century ended with the famines of King William's 'Ill Years' 1695–1700. Though national mechanisms for the relief of famine were still primitive, the mortality in these last years of the century was less striking, possibly because of a huge exodus of the population to Ulster. An insight into the interrelated problems of disease and poverty is found in the writings of the physician Sir Robert Sibbald later in the century:

> God Almight . . . requireth of us, a due Care for the Relief of the Poor; This is one of the Tributes we owe to Him, and he hath Dispersed the Poor amongst us, as his Substitutes and Receivers to whom it is to be payed . . . For Poverty and Want Emasculate the Mindes of many, and make those who are of dull Natures, Stupid and Indisciplinable, and unfit for the Service of their Countrey: these that are of a firy and active Temperament, it maketh them unquiet, Rapacious, Frantick or Desperate. Thus, where there are many Poor, the Rich cannot be secure in the Possession of what they have . . . And such Considerations ought now to be la'id to heart, when the Bad Seasons these several Years past, hath made so much Scarcity and so great Dearth, that for Want, some Die by the Way-side, some drop down in the Streets, the poor sucking Babs are starving for want of Milk, which the empty Breasts of their Mothers cannot furnish them: Every one may see Death in the Face of the Poor, that abound everywhere; the Thinness of their Visage, their Ghostly Looks, their Febbleness, their Agues and their Fluxes threaten them with sudden Death, if Care be not taken of them.[12]

Thus the relief of poverty was seen primarily as a christian duty, but also as a reasonable political precaution and a sensible economic measure.

Bubonic plagues

Scotland suffered her last and catastrophic epidemic of plague in the middle of the 17th century. She had been relatively free of the plague in the earlier part of the century and after this 1644 epidemic, Scotland was to be entirely free of the disease, in spite of severe epidemics in England.[13]

The origin of this last great plague starting in 1644 came when camp followers of the Covenanters army started trickling back from the siege of Newcastle. When cases of plague were heard of at the Scottish border, a public fast was held at Tyninghame in an attempt to avert disaster, but seaborne disease reached Bo'ness on the Firth of Forth on 17 December in spite of quarantine regulations against shipping visiting the east coast and other measures, including instructions to guards to shoot infected persons leaving affected areas. The erection of gallows outside Linlithgow to hang any visitors from neighbouring towns seems to have had the required effect and the winter months, which caused hibernation of the disease-carrying rats and reduced trade and travel, brought a temporary end to the spread of the disease. With the warmth of spring 1645, the disease broke out in Edinburgh and Leith and the usual civil arrangements seen in earlier centuries were once more put into effect. Cleaners of the houses and the streets were appointed, plague huts were erected – this time at the Meadows or Burghmuir in Edinburgh – and mass burial of the dead was arranged. In Perth the plague huts were erected at Kinnoul. Disinfection of the houses was attempted by burning rubbish or heather inside and this was the cause of a disastrous fire in Kelso. Often the people were unwilling to touch the bodies of those who died and the house was sometimes burnt or pulled down over the dead bodies. There arose an abiding supersition that not only the bodies but the graves of plague victims should not be disturbed or an infective 'miasma' would escape and the disease would once more break out. Another fear was of direct infection. It was recorded in Paisley that all the money necessary for trade was placed on a brass ladle and boiled in a pot before being handed over to merchants from neighbouring towns. In the towns the usual life was suspended and those who could leave fled to the country.[14] The schools were closed and the churches did not open. Large gatherings of people were banned, notably at weddings and funerals.

The victorious army of Montrose appeared at the outside of Edinburgh but wisely turned away from the plague. David Leslie's army took the plague to Argyll and produced severe devastations in Kintyre as did General Middleton's forces in Glasgow. The plague left Edinburgh in 1646 and the councillors were ordered to return to the town. A special tax was levied to pay the costs of the epidemic, in spite of the damage to the prosperity of the town.

The plague however continued elsewhere. An army spread the plague to Brechin in 1647 and 600 people, one third of the population, were buried in a mass grave in the churchyard. In Aberdeen the approach of the epidemic was watched with alarm and a 24 hour watch was set at the entrance to the town. Orders were given to clean the town and prevent entry of visitors: beggars were expelled. Of great interest were the new Aberdeen regulations to kill all cats and dogs and to lay poison for mice and rats, which if successful, would have dealt with the plague vector.[15] Nevertheless the plague appeared and a plague hospital had to be built on the links together with a gibbet for those who tried to escape. Mass graves were dug in the sands. The cost to the town was put together after the epidemic had passed:

9th December 1647

	Scots £	s	d
To James Graham, cleanger, for his services and attendance on the people	1,086	10	0
To James Campbell, ditto	121	6	0
To John Barclay, ditto	26	13	4
To George Watt, ditto	80	0	0
To Expense of burying the dead and for 37,000 turfs to cover the graves and carriage	153	6	8
To Expense of wood, for huts, in the Links, Castlehill, etc	378	10	0
To Expense of constructing a Court de Guard in the Links	2	4	0
ditto, of a double tree for a gibbet, and for erecting it	2	15	0
ditto, of a pair of joggis upon it, and ten fathoms of ropes	2	9	4
To Captain John Duff, and the military, for guards	820	11	0
To Expense of rosin, vinegar and medicines	125	2	4
ditto, for meal, and baking it into bread for the poor people	181	6	4
To Sir William Forbes of Craigievar, for 300 bolls of meal, at £5 the boll	1,500	0	0
To Lady Marischal, for meal	1,366	16	6
	£6,847	10	6

Source: G. A. G. Mitchell[16]

By 1649 the plague lifted from the last remaining places on the east coast, and on the 1st February 1649, the church at Montrose opened, having been shut for nine months.

The plague never returned to Scotland in epidemic form, though England was still to have its worst attack.[17] Certainly, the quarantine measures in Scotland had become stronger and stronger and the advice of the Privy Council had been increasingly respected and obeyed. It may be that Scotland had favourable factors in defence against the disease, notably that the cooler Scottish climate discouraged the already diminishing number of black rats and that internal trade in Scotland may have halted more completely in winter. Nevertheless the vigour of the measures taken against the plague in Scotland may have played a part.[18]

Poor Law

The provision for a primitive Poor Law in Scotland had been made in statutes of 1574 and 1579. Attempts were made from time to time in the 17th century to levy a poor rate but in practice little was done, since the landowners stoutly resisted any compulsory taxation. Even in 1623, at a time of severe famine, the Privy Council's request to the East Lothian authorities to raise a levy could be answered in these famous terms:

> Every contribution is odious and smellis of ane taxatioun . . . We think it ane hard matter to be employit in ane service toylsome and trublesome unto us importing nathair credeit ner benefeit but ane schadowing appeirance of ane common weil.[19]

A more subtle reply from Selkirk to an earlier Privy Council request to step up poor relief came from an unknown but skilful negotiator:

> as concerning the ordour appointit be your Lordships for suppressing of the sturdie and idell beggaris and supporting off the trewlie puir and indigent, we both allow off it and sall gladlie follow it in so far as the present estate of this puir shireffdome will permit; which being for the most pairt off his Hienes propertie . . . hes bene subject to the yeirlie payment off feu dewties, deir maillis [rents] and continwall taxations, whairwith they be so exhausted and impoverished that they be scarselie abell to interteine [support] themselffis, for les to help otheris; it were better therefor to be wishit that your Lordships wold appoint some commoun work in everie paroche, as the mending of hiewayis or suchlyk, whairby the idell may be forcit, the willing imployit, both interteined and the countrie disburdened.[20]

The Poor Law funds were therefore raised without a local assessment and continued to come from church collections, Kirk Session fines, occasional bequests and the hiring of mortcloths for funerals. Since church collections were the biggest contribution, the funds collected for the poor declined just at the time they were required. In times of famine or epidemic the churches were badly attended or might even shut. Hence the parish had to try to keep a reserve of money, but if this ran out, it might appeal to the Privy Council. Conversely, in prosperous times the poor box might be full and was used to give loans to local heritors. Payments to the poor were organised by the Church and were based on the assessment by the minister and Kirk Session of the circumstances of each case. To obtain poor relief in the larger towns, application to or entry into an alms-house might be required and in for instance Aberdeen in the 1640s, 50 paupers were housed in five such hospitals.[21] Glasgow Town's Hospital had a similar role. These were not the equivalent of English workhouses, possibly because the new Scottish merchant class opposed any cheap manufacturing that would threaten their emerging market.

For those who were sick, the main aid given under the Poor Law was help with money or food, which was in any case the most effective therapy available. The minister's knowledge also helped him recommend other measures in special cases. It is estimated that about half of the money paid out under the old Poor Law was for temporary relief, including medical assistance, food or money, the other half going to the permanently destitute – the paupers. Medical relief under the old Poor Law has not been systematically surveyed but in one study of the parish records of the north east of Scotland, payment for operations on cancers of lip, breast or elsewhere, removal of bladder stones, amputations of limbs and treatment of cataract (by an oculist at Glamis who had a reputation for this procedure) are reported. The money given to pay for these operations was in the range of £2–£8 Scots. Money for drugs was also occasionally granted – for mercury, ointments and alcoholic stimulants. The Kirk Sessions were also prepared to raise money for particular patients by special collections. The Poor Law funds were also used to help the sick travel to the Scottish mineral wells at Peterhead, Pencaitland, Strathpeffer and Pannanich.[22] The Session could also act in a different way in health matters since the Kirk Session of Largo in Fife in 1650 were suspicious of the medical skills of an Englishman called Hollande 'who gave him selfe foourth to be a phesitian, he being onlie ane imposter . . .' He was expelled.[23] How far these medical arrangements went towards meeting the total need is not clear, and the distinction between the deserving and undeserving poor meant that many sick poor may have been unsupported. Historians have usually regarded the old Scottish Poor Law as being mean and grudging with its funds.

There were, however, alternative sources of help for the poor in the 17th century and at least in the towns these may have partly subsidised the parish effort. The burghs of Scotland in the 17th century fairly regularly made part-time appointments of medical practitioners to help with the treatment of the poor. These were always surgeons or surgeon-apothecaries and the earlier appointments in Edinburgh and Aberdeen in the 16th century have been described previously. Glasgow in 1599 employed Peter Lowe, founder of the Faculty of Physicians and Surgeons, for a short time and later the town had no less than three part-time employees – a physician, a surgeon and a 'cutter for the stone' (i.e. bladder stones), though in the hard times of 1685 the town had to give up the services of the physician and surgeon. From time to time individual doctors might be consulted by Glasgow and in 1652 it agreed a £30 Scots payment for the treatment over ten weeks of 'ane burgess bairne wha had the knap of her elbow strucken frae her by aine of the sojers wha cam frae air [Ayr]'.[24] In Inverness, a Dr MacKenzie was taken on as their first municipal doctor in 1680.

In Glasgow and Edinburgh there was yet another source of help for the poor. An obligation to provide attention to the poor was written into the charters given to the Faculty of Physicians and Surgeons of Glasgow in 1599 and the College of Physicians of Edinburgh in 1681, probably at the insistence of the Crown during the negotiations. In Glasgow a free clinic was held once a month and in Edinburgh the poor were seen three times a week. This work was done faithfully for a century or more until other ways of treating the poor appeared. This obligation was more onerous than it seems, for whilst it was easy for the doctors to give of their time, there was no way of paying for the drugs used other than from their own pockets. The similar service given by the College of Physicians of London had foundered after squabbles about who should pay for the drugs. This pressure towards simpler and cheaper drug therapy for the poor must also have impressed the Scottish doctors that the complex prescribing for their private patients may have had no extra value.

The healers

The three levels of health care noted in the medieval period are seen even more clearly in the 17th century since there are more sources describing the orthodox physicians and surgeons, more information on the self-treatment by the rich and poor and better details of the quacks and folk healers methods. The 17th century Scottish medical men were now more clearly divided into the various crafts, changes best seen in the towns. Rural districts and the Highlands and Islands were badly served with conventional medical help and relied more heavily on other kinds of healers.

The trained medical men in Scotland showed only brief signs of the eminence to be attained in the 18th century. Much of their energies were devoted to the political and religious feuds of the time and they were also diverted to join the numerous armies and bands raised in Scotland. It is hardly surprising that while England was experiencing a great surge of new thought and discovery, intellectual life in Scotland was at a low ebb, though scientists like James Gregory in the relative peace of Aberdeen and later at St Andrews devised the reflecting telescope and John Napier, from a family distinguished for alchemy, invented logarithms.

Physicians and medical treatment

The most prestigious and rare of the healers was the physician. He was distinguished by a medical education abroad and the large fees charged. While the 17th century saw one advance in their practice, namely the dropping of astrology, this progress was marred by the unnecessary and deliberate increase in complexity of the methods of treatment by medicines and drugs. Medical education for the physician still hardly existed in Scotland in the 17th century.[25] Though King's College in Aberdeen had the post of 'mediciner' set up in 1497 there was little separate teaching of medical practice. The St Andrews medical school planned at the Reformation had never developed, and though there was intense interest in the universities after the Reformation in 1559, nothing was done which allowed the appearance of permanent teaching of medicine.

In the 17th century, the Scottish universities became a pawn in the struggle between church and state. Each claimed authority over the universities and each visited them in turn. In general the Crown favoured the teaching of medicine, but the Church was lukewarm towards it. The Crown visitation to Glasgow of 1637 set up a chair of medicine and Robert Mayne was appointed, but the Church's inspection in 1642 abolished the chair, though Mayne was allowed to continue in post until his death. Only in Aberdeen are there traces of a reasonable continuity of the teaching of medicine to small numbers of interested students from the 16th century onwards, after they had taken a degree in Arts. This poor performance of the Scottish universities, so ineffectual compared with the later success of the 18th century, may not necessarily be attributed to organisational failure: if few students appeared to study medicine, then teaching was not worth while.[26]

Thus the tradition of the Scottish physicians travelling to train on the continent continued and was much admired. Because of the expense involved in this venture, the 'students of physic' came only from rich families. In Europe the medical curriculum for physicians consisted of lectures on the various theories of disease and therapy by chemicals, plants, and animal extracts, but Leyden University was gaining a reputation for teaching not only theoretical knowledge but the new clinical skills based on practical problems, and many Scots students were attracted to that centre.

The best known of the 17th century Scottish physicians were Archibald Pitcairne (1652–1713) and Sir Robert Sibbald (1641–1722). While Sibbald was a conservative figure who helped revive the Hippocratic methods of treatment, Pitcairne combined the restless life of a medieval scholar with advocacy of new thinking in the understanding of the working of the body.[27]

Pitcairne graduated M.A. at Edinburgh in 1671, then studied medicine at Paris. He returned to Scotland and helped set up the Royal College of Physicians in Edinburgh. He was involved in Scottish politics and lived dangerously by jesting about the new presbyterian Church and openly supporting the Jacobites. As a scholar he has a secure reputation and left Scotland to be appointed professor of medicine at Leyden in 1692 where he had the great Boerhaave as a pupil. He left Leyden after only one year's highly successful tenure having treated the authorities shabbily by failing to give any notice of his departure. Returning to Edinburgh, he was again involved in feuds with his colleagues, but began the systematic teaching in the town that was to prepare the way for the later rise of the Edinburgh Medical School.

Though a less swashbuckling figure, it was Sibbald's careful planning which gained the Charter for the Royal College of Physicians in Edinburgh.[28] Like his rival Pitcairne, he had intended to enter the Church, but after studying theology, the religious feuding in Scotland repelled him and he took up medicine instead, training at Leyden and Paris. He returned to Scotland, flirted with Roman Catholicism and then settled as a respected physician and polymath. His valuable autobiography, admired by Dr Johnson, gives a picture of 17th century Scotland and the events in Edinburgh of the time.

In their clinical practice the physicians methods were changing. Some used the old Hippocratic advice on life style, diet and change of climate for health, but others were adding complex new therapy by plant or animal extracts and occasionally chemical drugs. The patient was also concerned to obtain a prognosis from the doctors and though the physicians had abandoned astrology for this purpose they now used uroscopy to do so and specimens of the patient's urine were solemnly inspected and the outcome predicted.[29] Professional life was thus eased by the lack of a need to examine the patient and the physicians were prepared to treat and prognosticate by post. Because of this, the Highland lairds were not as remote from conventional advice as might seem.[30]

In attempting to establish themselves as a superior caste, the physicians had to distance themselves from the other healers, but they also had to convince their educated patrons that they had something to offer that the gentry had not picked up in their general education. To do this, the physicians of the 17th century took the widely known medical recipes and made them even more complex. The Edinburgh *Pharmacopoeia* of the late 17th century shows the efforts of the physicians in this direction.[31] The first edition had substances ranging from the exotic to the disgusting – spiders webs, ant eggs and snakes skin. Powders made from Egyptian mummies (alleged to contain the 'essence of health') were advocated as were extracts of the skulls of humans dying a violent death. Human faeces – an ancient method of driving out demons by offending them – also appeared in the prescriptions as did extracts of woodlice. Elaborate combinations of these materials were also prescribed and the remedies could contain 30 to 40 constituents prepared with extensive boiling, extraction, mixing and decanting. A serious prescription of the day had one ounce each of nine roots and half an ounce of four others, a handful of seventeen different herbs and a half ounce of each of ten seeds. We have the comic and pathetic sight of the physicians of the day devising preparations of more and more complexity to establish their status.[32] The cost of obtaining the materials, many of which came from abroad, would be passed on to the patient, who doubtless considered, like all patients before and since, that the more expensive, unpalatable, and rare the remedy, the more chance of a cure. The scientific aspects of these methods were also deplorable, since even if an effective drug were included, its dosage would vary with each batch and its effectiveness within the mixture would be hidden.

The physicians claim for benefit from these remedies and their insistence on such rituals while at the same time deploring folk medicine and the quacks is remarkable. Indeed closer inspection shows that many of these remedies were merely folk methods legitimised with some pseudo-scientific chemical manipulation and over-elaboration by mixture of numerous ingredients. One such remedy however was to be a lasting success. Dr Patrick Anderson in 1635 put together a pill which contained 40 ingredients and took four days to prepare. Anderson's Scots Pills, later known as Grana Angelica, moved reluctant bowels and were still on sale in Edinburgh in 1910 in a simple form.[33] Another complex mixture found in the Edinburgh *Pharmacopoeia* was a number of forms of a nostrum known as Orvietan. This was also widely sold by the travelling quacks but who was copying whom is not clear. The *Pharmacopoeia* also shows evidence of the argumentative factions in Edinburgh in the 17th century, since the failure to issue the book in 1683 as planned was blamed on an internal squabble in the College probably between Sibbald and Pitcairne. The Edinburgh opponents are described in the preface to the first edition as 'malevolent, heedless, yelping men' which indicates the tensions within the College and the antagonisms based on the Scottish problems of religion and Jacobitism. These disagreements led to a riot in the College in 1695. The early editions of the *Pharmacopoeia* were also used by the physicians to assert their authority to control drugs in Edinburgh and to attempt to limit the growing power of the local apothecaries.

Hard things are said in the Introduction about the dangers of leaving the preparation of drugs to the apothecaries alone. Even so, the physicians' joint effort was a remarkable one, since their rivalry for prestige naturally led to secrecy in prescribing, a secrecy which was relinquished to write the *Pharmacopoeia*, though the use of latin restricted its intelligibility.[34] The physicians however did not deliver or administer the therapy they recommended: their role as educated men was to understand disease, prognosticate and to advise. The rest of the work was done by others and surgeons carried out the necessary bleeding or dressings and an apothecary made up and delivered the drugs prescribed. As the work of the apothecary became more sophisticated and as their work became essential to the physicians, the apothecaries became rich and troublesome.

Apothecaries

The apothecaries are first mentioned in early medieval records but the rise of the towns and the methods of the physicians in the 17th century give them a new importance.[35] This was in spite of their lowly place in the town's hierarchy: unlike the surgeons, they did not have a craft guild. Relations between the physicians and the apothecaries were not cordial and the tension between the two groups became important in medical politics in Edinburgh as it did also in London. The reason was simple. The physician's code did not allow them to make up their own medicines or lower their considerable fees. As the apothecary's skills and knowledge increased as a result of the physicians complex prescriptions, the patients started to consult directly with an apothecary and were treated by them. This was a constant source of outrage to the physicians. In London, the College of Physicians had legal power to control the apothecaries, and they were constantly brought before the College for treating patients. The apothecaries in defence devised a simple expedient in which they ostensibly charged only for their drugs, though the bill included their considerable fee.[36] In Edinburgh the apothecaries were not under the control of the new College. Hence they had more freedom and were even more likely to charge extravagantly for their drugs and services. The wealth of the 17th century Scottish apothecary is made clear by the returns for poll taxes taken in 1696 which have survived in Aberdeen and Edinburgh.[37] In Aberdeen, the three active physicians and the four surgeon-apothecaries were in the highest professional tax group – £12 Scots p.a. Only some of the Aberdeen merchants reached this level of tax. In the Edinburgh Poll Tax of 1694 – the earliest in Scotland – a similar picture of the affluence of the physicians and apothecaries appears. There were four physicians and three pure apothecaries and the apothecaries appeared to be as well-off as the physicians: both groups had large houses and averaged 2–3 servants in their houses. It is easy to understand the tension between the two kinds of practitioner. This provocation was increased by a justifiable suspicion that the apothecaries adulterated the medicines supplied and hence increased their profits. Since virtually none of the therapy used had any potency, the situation was a difficult one, and the physicians could only attempt to get legal power to inspect the apothecaries shops and the materials used.

In the 17th century physicians treatments there was still the use of magic on occasions. Though astrology had almost disappeared from medical practice and the patient's prognosis and drug therapy and its timing no longer depended on the position of the heavenly bodies, the physician's weakness for magical methods remained. There was printed in Glasgow in 1658 a treatise on *Sympathiae et Antipathiae* written by a physician Sylvester Rattray, an M.D. of St Andrews, but whose place of medical training is unknown.[38] He worked in Edinburgh, was active there in the early moves to found the College of Physicians, and then moved to Glasgow. His book was reprinted on the continent at Tübingen and Nürnberg. The metaphysical reasoning involved in his argument led to a simple enough practical application. In the treatment of wounds the therapy or drugs need not be applied to the wound but to the weapon causing the injury or even to a dressing from the wound. This involved the principle of 'sympathetic' medicine and a search started in the 17th century, supported by the Royal Society in London, for a single powder which would accomplish this sympathetic cure. Nor was the 17th century doctrine of 'signatures' more soundly based: the drug was matched to the patient's condition, yellow medicine for jaundice and so on.[39] Even Pitcairne, who led Scottish medicine towards more rational methods, when faced with a difficult case, suggested the application of live doves to the feet of patients who had not responded to his initial treatment.

Surgeon-apothecaries and surgery

The Scottish surgeons occupied a lower rank than the physicians, but not as low as in England. The training of the surgeon for these manual skills was one acquired by apprenticeship and the surgeons took their place among the craftsmen of the towns. The day's work of the surgeon largely involved the healing of wounds, setting of fractures, occasional amputations, embalming the dead, removal of teeth, the treatment of skin disease, and bloodletting, often at the instructions of a physician. Blood letting involved the removal of about 100 ml of blood into a dish and the wound was sealed by pressure. Next day a servant of the surgeon would call to remove the pressure dressing and it was customary to tip this messenger with 'drink money'. In the healing of wounds – common enough in the civil and military violence of the times – they used elaborate plasters and applications almost in the same way as the physicians had obfuscated their methods.[40] The surgeons were much in demand for the army and had the rank of lieutenant. The surgical apprentices often left for a spell in one of the many Scottish armies in the land, then returning to their training on half pay. Paradoxically, the 17th century surgeons shunned the operations which were to be their routine practice later – couching for cataracts, cutting for bladder stone and release of hernias. Bladder stones were extremely common in Scotland.[41] Their removal, the one procedure which resembles surgery as practised later, was avoided by the surgeons probably because the high death rate and the frequent complications would ruin their reputation. The diagnosis was easy to make since the stones produced severe pain and a prolonged obstruction of the flow of urine. The removal of the stone could produce a cure and this was accomplished by the specialised 'cutters for the stone' who by rapid cutting upwards beside the rectum reached and removed the stones. Operating without anaesthetic or pain killing drugs was a formidable task and the post-operative complications of leakage, infection and death were common: the patients postponed the operation for as long as possible. A number of early references to surgery for bladder stones in Scotland are available and we know that a fostered son of Lord Lovat who had 'used too much of the milk diet, and turned dull under a complex of maladies' was cut for the stone by Gillean-dris Beatton in 1612, somewhere in Ross-shire.[42]

The only details we have of a lithotomist in early Scotland is of Evir MacNeill, appointed in Glasgow in 1656 as lithotomist to the town.[43] He was a Highland man, probably speaking only the gaelic, who made a cross instead of his signature on the minute of his appointment. Despite these handicaps he was admitted after ten years work in the town as a colleague by the Faculty of Physicians and Surgeons. The need for his work is shown by his continuing in this employment for nineteen years until his death, when a second lithotomist was promptly appointed in his stead.

More details of the possible effects of the operation are found later in Ridpath's 18th century Diary:

> Friday Oct. 3, 1755: . . . saw Somervail who seems to be in a low dangerous way. He was cut for the stone about three weeks ago. Saw two stones of considerable weight (betwixt two and three ounces) that were taken out of the bladder. He has sad piles on which the urine dripping through the wound gives great torment.[44]

His piles (probably a prolapsed rectum) might have occurred before surgery, as a result of intense straining to pass urine against the chronic blockage. The diary records that Somervail died two weeks later.

Even surgery for hernias and cataracts was avoided by the trained surgeons and descriptions of some of these operations are missing from the standard texts on surgery of the day, though Peter Lowe's Glasgow text included hernia surgery, but not cutting for the stone.[45] Hernia surgery was therefore rare and was considered to be dangerous. Even though a bold surgeon did save the life of the Earl of Morton in 1578 who 'lay deidle seik of rumburssanes [hernia]', in 1756. Ridpath could record the slow death of a boy with a strangulated hernia, which was not operated on in spite of frequent visits by the Kelso surgeon – 'a man not very ignorant in his business.'

The apprenticeship of the surgeon lasted from three to five years and entry was restricted.[46] It was formalised by a written agreement and the likelihood of the apprentices disorderly conduct is suggested by the numerous prohibitions on drunkenness, fornication and haunting of taverns which appear in these indentures. The apprentices lived in their master's house and at the end of the training they were submitted to a test of their work. In the case of the surgeon this was an oral examination and perhaps a practical test on dealing with a wound or similar problem in a patient. The candidate then had to entertain the examiners to dinner whether they passed or not, but if successful he joined the craft by paying a substantial fee. One such apprentice in Glasgow in the early 18th century was the novelist

Tobias Smollett who used his Glasgow master John Gordon in *Humphrey Clinker*.[47] The pragmatic surgeon teases his apprentice's fancy new ideas:

> You can already account for muscular motion, I warrant, and explain the mystery of the brain and nerves – ha! You are too learned for me, damn me. But let's hear no more of this stuff. Can you bleed and give a clyster, spread a plaister and prepare a potion?

The apprenticeship scheme lasted till the 1800s, when the increasing amount of university instruction involved in the training allowed surgery to be easily converted to a university or college degree, and the apprenticeships disappeared.

There is some evidence that the craft of surgery was more highly regarded in Scotland than in England and in this Scotland resembled many of the nations of Europe, notably France. At the end of the 17th century some Scottish surgeons were studying at the European universities.[48] In Scotland, the surgeons also had an organisational advantage. In London the College of Physicians not only had legal control of the apothecaries, but also had power over the surgeons and their activities, whereas in Scotland the surgeons were free of interference from the physicians. Hence the surgeons in Scotland had the confidence that this freedom gave and the close links with France encouraged the idea of a higher status of surgery. There had also been an ancient royal interest in surgery in Scotland, originating from the interest taken by the Stuart Kings. Whatever the reasons, the craft of surgery in Scotland was esteemed and it is of interest that at the beginning of the 17th century a number of distinguished surgeons found their way back from abroad to Scotland while at the height of their powers – Peter Lowe to Glasgow, and Andro Scott and Robert Auchmowtie to Edinburgh. All three had been in Paris and shared the attitudes of the French school, namely that surgery was a worthy calling and that it could be taught by universities. This assumption meant that the surgeons played a crucial role in the great era of Scottish medicine in the 18th century.

Relations between the surgeons and the apothecaries in Scotland were usually more cordial than between the physicians and the apothecaries. Indeed, the physicians' attitude to the apothecaries and their later attempts to bring them under the physicians control, made the Edinburgh apothecaries look elsewhere for political alliances. In

1657 their chance came when the Incorporation of Barber-Surgeons membership had fallen to 8 persons and the apothecaries were invited to join them.[49] For 130 years almost without interruption the two types of practitioner were joined together in Edinburgh, and though this union had its origins in a short-term organisational expedient, it was in practice a sensible arrangement and created an attitude to medicine and a new kind of training from which the apprentice emerged with a knowledge of both surgery and medicine. In the Glasgow Faculty a similar union existed and these surgeon-apothecaries were the early 'general' practitioners who spread widely to settle in the small towns of Scotland.

It is crucial to the understanding of the success of Scottish medicine in later times to note this fusing of surgery and pharmacy. In London the College of Physicians was in firm control of the apothecaries, and the English physicians rigid attitude that medicine and surgery could not be practised together made no union possible. Thus a general medical education and the emergence of the general practitioner was long delayed in England. Only after the flood of broadly trained Scottish graduates into England occurred in the 18th century was reform conceded.

Barbers

The last of the organised groups involved in the provision of healing were the barbers. As discussed earlier, the barbers entry into surgery may have come when the monks in early medieval times were discouraged from practising medicine in general and surgery in particular. These skills may have then naturally devolved onto the monastic barbers, who were accustomed to the use and maintenance of metal instruments and the shaving of heads for the application of cold water to the scalp, a treatment favoured in some diseases. The town barbers also took on some of the operations of surgery and indeed the barbers were often organised as a town craft prior to the surgeons. Thus the barbers had appeared first in the Town Council statutes of Aberdeen.

In Edinburgh there are hints that the barbers had an earlier independent existence, but they and the surgeons emerged as a craft in 1505 when they obtained their privileges in Edinburgh in a joint Seal of Cause in 1505. In Glasgow, the barbers were treated less well. The founders of the Faculty of Physicians and Surgeons had clear ideas on the high status of surgery and the barbers were not included in the charter and thereafter were only allowed in as members under strict conditions. Thus Robert Haries, barbour, was admitted in 1645 and allowed 'onlie to medell wt simple wounds' and not to 'medell wt physic, tumours, ulsors, dislocations fractors'.[51] The Charter for Glasgow also allowed for the barbers craft to be removed from the Faculty without appeal or discussion, and this was done in 1722.

In Edinburgh the barbers were earlier removed from the Incorporation of Surgeons in 1648, but the resulting shortage of shops for hair cutting and beard trimming compelled the surgeons to bring back some individual barbers into their corporation. They were allowed strictly defined activities within Edinburgh. The barbers fought back strongly in 1718 with an attempt to restore their equal rights under the original Seal of Cause, and almost won their case, but had to settle for a diminished status within the Incorporation. The surgeons and barbers remained legally joined until 1845. The end for the Edinburgh barbers came when restricted trading was abolished in 1847 and anyone could set up as a barber. Thereafter, the Society of Barbers lingered on in Edinburgh since a small income still came from their Widows Fund, but in 1892 the last meeting was held, attended only by a father and son. One was elected president, the other as box-master. Shortly after, the father died and his son left the country.[52]

Colleges of Physicians and Surgeons

The activities of the physicians' and surgeons' corporations have already been referred to above, but can now be looked at more closely. The three Scottish corporations still vigorously exist and are now called the Royal College of Surgeons of Edinburgh, the Royal College of Physicians and Surgeons of Glasgow and the Royal College of Physicians of Edinburgh. The names have changed slightly over the centuries since their origins in the 16th and 17th centuries.[53]

The motives for the organisation of any medieval craft were primarily the protection of the members' interests by the limitation of the number of practitioners. The maintenance of standards to protect the public was usually mentioned also. The first of the medical men's corporations to appear was the Incorporation of

Surgeons and Barbers in Edinburgh.[54] The terms of the Seal of Cause given in 1505 to the Edinburgh surgeons and barbers were similar to those of any of the crafts of the town, namely that they alone could give a licence to practise in the burgh of Edinburgh. The normal method of gaining this was by apprenticeship to a surgeon in the town followed by an examination by the guild on anatomy, on the ability to read and write and on the signs of the zodiac, necessary for the prognosis of disease by astrology. Entry to apprenticeship was limited to the sons and sons-in-law of the craftsmen or the sons of the nobility or those marrying the daughter of a surgeon, provided she was a 'clene virgine'.

The fee to join the Incorporation was £5 plus the cost of a dinner given by the applicant to the established members. Curiously, the Edinburgh surgeons were given the monopoly to sell aqua vitae, the earlier form of whisky, a drink which had not yet become popular and which was considered only to be a therapeutic agent. The funds of the Incorporation came from the entry money and fines on members for offences such as slandering other members, moral failings or drunkenness at meetings. The surgeons were an organisation linked closely with the town's crafts and hence with the Town Council, a link which was retained until 1851, prior to which they had risen in status to be the first in precedence in the town crafts.

The next group to organise themselves formally were the Glasgow physicians and surgeons.[55] This move, in 1599, was unusual in two respects. Firstly, Glasgow was not then a major town, ranking only about fifth in Scotland, and secondly the link between the physicians and surgeons, though sensible later, was an innovation in those days. Since in Glasgow in 1599 there was only one physician, six surgeons, one apothecary and two midwives in the town, one Faculty made sense. Perhaps to increase its potential membership, the new Faculty of Physicians and Surgeons was also given control of a huge area in west central Scotland, well beyond the Glasgow area.

Much can be explained by study of the founder's background.[56] Peter Lowe was a Scot, whose birthplace is unknown, but may have been Errol, near Perth. He travelled abroad for his education, and like many others, chose France, whose close political ties with Scotland allowed common citizenship at that time. The place of Lowe's first degree is unknown, but may have been Orleans, and his degree was certainly *magister artium* (Lowe seldom omitted the "Mr" or "Maister" before his name). He then proceeded to Paris where he obtained training in surgery at the College of St Côme, a body of surgeons who claimed to be the 'Faculty of Surgery' in Paris and to have equal status with the Faculty of Physcians there – a claim persistently denied by the physicians. Thus Lowe could claim to be a 'gown surgeon' – a university trained surgeon – rather than one simply taught as an apprentice. After thirty years of successful civilian and military surgical practice and political intrigue in Europe, he arrived in Glasgow.

That he should move, in middle age and at the height of his powers, to a small town with only a handful of doctors is perhaps odd but may have been the old medieval scholars habit of continuous travel from place to place, or as a return to the land of his birth. As suggested above, Scotland, for some unknown reason, attracted back some of her sons at that time. Perhaps they were attracted back as a result of the Reformation, but Lowe was an adherent of the Catholic faction in France. In spite of conversion to protestantism, he must have found post-Reformation Scotland a sombre place. Indeed, he was brought before the Kirk Session of Glasgow on an unspecified charge. The main atraction of Glasgow may have been that it gave him unhindered scope for his clinical and political activities, and he was probably useful to the King as a result of his travels and knowledge of Europe. He may have been involved in political intrigue and in 1601 he travelled back to France in the ambassador's entourage.

He arrived in Glasgow in 1598 and his presence was quickly felt. Within a year, James VI could describe him as 'our chirurgiane, and chief chirurgiane to our dearest sone the Prince'. In Glasgow Lowe doubtless was the moving spirit behind the protest made by the church and magistrates in 1598 over the number of unskilled practitioners in Glasgow. Armed with this protest from the town, and using his royal connections, he obtained a charter for the establishment of a Faculty of Physicians and Surgeons in Glasgow. The vernacular of these extracts from the charter make splendid reading:

> The King . . . understanding . . . the grit abuisis quhilk [which] hes bene comitted in time bigane, and zit daylie continuis be [by] ignorant, unskillit and unlernit personis, quha, [who] under the collour of Chirurgeanis, abuisis the people to their

plesure, passing away but [without] tryel or punishment, and theirby destroyis infinite number of oure subjectis, quhairwith [wherewith] na ordour hes bene tane in tyme bigane, specially within oure burgh and baronie of Glasgow, Renfrew, Dumbartane, and oure Sheriffdomes of Cliddisdale, Renfrew, Lanark, Kyile, Carrick, Air and Cunninghame; FOR avoiding of sik inconvenientis, and for gude ordoure to be tane in tyme cuming, to have made, constitutit and ordanit . . . Maister Peter Low . . . with the assistance of Mr Robert Hamiltone, professoure of medecine, and their successouris, indwelleris of our Citie of Glasgow, GEVAND and GRANTAND to thaime and their successoures, full power to call, sumonnd, and convene before thame . . . all personis professing or using the said airt of Chirurgie, to examine thame upon thair literature, knawledge and practize: gif they be fund wordie, to admit, allow, and approve thame . . . Nixt, that the saidis visitouris sall visit everie hurt, murtherit, poisonit, or onie other persoun tane awa extraordinarly, and to report to the Magistrate of the fact as it is: Thirdlie, That is sall be leisum [lawful] to the said visitouris, with the advice of their bretheren, to mak statutis for the comoun weill of our subjects, anent the saidis artis, and using thairof faithfullie, and the braikeris thairof to be punshit and unlawit be the visitoures according to their falt: Fordlie, It sall not be leisum to onie mannir of personis within the foresaidis boundis to exercise medicine without ane testimonial of ane famous universitie quhair medecine be taught . . . Fythlie, That na manir of personis sell onie droggis within the citie of Glasgow except the sam be sichtit be [inspected by] the saidis visitouris, and be William Spang, apothecar. Sextlie, That nane sell retoun poison arsenick or sublemate . . . excep onlie the apothecaris quha [who] sall be bund to tak cautioun of the byaris for coist, skaith [injury] and damage. Seventhlie, Yat the saidis visitouris . . . sall convene every first Mononday of ilk moneth at sum convenient place to visit and give counsell to pure [poor] diaisit folkis gratis'.

This Charter gave more privileges to Glasgow than had been given to the Edinburgh surgeons, since the Glasgow medical men had a stronger medico-legal role and had power to inspect drug sellers. Unlike Edinburgh, the Glasgow Faculty was not formally connected to the Town Council. The Charter conceded that the physicians were a superior group and could be admitted without examination, whereas the surgeons were to be examined closely.

While the Edinburgh College controlled Edinburgh, the new Glasgow Faculty not only had territorial rights in Glasgow, but also in the whole of the West of Scotland. An attempt was later made to extend this influence even further to Ayrshire but this proved to be unworkable and the scheme was abandoned. Later, both Cullen and Smellie practised near Glasgow without a licence. The power given to the Faculty to inspect and control the drugs sold in Glasgow was unique, and similar authority in Edinburgh was only given to the College of Physicians decades later. Lastly the obligation on the Faculty to visit the sick was probably a request made by the King as a condition of the power given to the Faculty. As noted before, the barbers were nowhere mentioned as members, though an approved apothecary, William Spang was included. The barbers were allowed in individually from time to time.

There were only seven members in the original Faculty, and the physicians played little part in the early days, since they disliked the association with the barbers and they had no concern with training of apprentices. When the physicians did come into the affairs of the Faculty later they were automatically allowed to elect the President from among themselves, the surgeons taking the lesser post of Visitor. Though the Charter may appear only relevant to medieval times, its terms were subject to minute legal scrutiny in the 19th century when the Faculty held that their Charter gave them the sole right to license practitioners in surgery in Glasgow, whereas the University of Glasgow held that a university degree permitted their graduates to practise in Glasgow. This led to a bitter, expensive, and in the end, futile confrontation in the 19th century.

The third and last college to be founded was that of the physicians of Edinburgh in 1681.[57,58] While the other corporations had been born peacefully the physicians had considerable difficulties in obtaining a charter. There had been little need for the Scottish physicians to become organised until this time since their numbers had been small, largely through the scarcity of rich patients and the difficulty in obtaining a continental university degree. The Union of the Crowns of Scotland and England doubtless took away a large number of rich patrons and patients. The physicians skills were not learnt by apprenticeship in the town and hence local associations and regulations were not necessary. Nevertheless, they were growing in number and doubtless were envious of the London College of Physicians' power and their control of the London surgeons and apothecaries.

Early in the 17th century, the Scottish physicians made their first move towards a college in Edinburgh and although the declared motive was the need to control unqualified practitioners and quacks and to inspect the drugs sold, it seems more likley that the motives were to limit the numbers of physicians, curb the practice and wealth of the apothecaries and give themselves a powerful political organisation in Edinburgh. Doubtless also they were apprehensive of the increasing power of the surgeons in Edinburgh. Four attempts to obtain a charter were made.[59] Of the unsuccessful attempts to set up a college in 1621 and 1633, little need be said, but the third application to Cromwell in 1656 is of interest. The physicians argued plausibly from the patients' interests. A college was required in view of

> the frequent murders committed universallie in all parts . . . by quacks, women, gardiners and others grossly ignorant . . .

and

> the unlimited and unaccountable practices of Chirurgeons Apothecaries and Empiricks pretenting to medicines . . . all these undertaking the cure of all diseases without the advice and assistance of Physitanes.

The powers claimed were considerable, but were not unreasonable and the suggestion that the physicians should have power over the surgeons and apothecaries would merely have given the Edinburgh doctors the powers already held by the London physicians. A less strident complaint made in the application was that the absence of medical education in Edinburgh forced students to travel abroad for both elementary medical education and further experience. This application by the physicians lacked tact and political skill, and Cromwell's reply to them was even less realistic. It proposed, doubtless at the physicians' prompting, even greater powers for the Edinburgh physicians to control medical practice not only in Edinburgh, but throughout Scotland as well as local control of the surgeons and apothecaries by the physicians in Edinburgh. The surgeons' territory was to be further invaded by a proposal that human bodies for dissection were to be granted to the new College of Physicians.

The proposals caused trouble. The surgeons were particularly annoyed and made a 'buzzling and a stour' at the idea of being subjugated to the physicians, and that anatomical study should be encouraged in the physicians' college. The other Scottish medical organisations were also understandably outraged: the Faculty in Glasgow rightly felt their power would be reduced. King's College Aberdeen, who alone had been teaching medicine in a small way, stated plainly that the proposals for the physicians to license practice in Scotland were contrary to the Aberdeen charter, which allowed their graduates to practise throughout the world, an argument which was to be a key issue in the later conflict between the University and Faculty in Glasgow. Even the physicians of Dundee and Montrose opposed the College, fearing control from Edinburgh. But the most effective opposition came from a less obvious source. The Town Council of Edinburgh, acting through the Convention of the Royal Burghs in Scotland, strongly opposed the plan. In June 1657 they studied the details of the physicians' application and rejected most of the powers claimed. The Town Council's vital interest in containing the power of the physicians arose from two considerations. Firstly, the Edinburgh surgeons were closely linked to the Town Council as a craft guild, and hence the Council always had the surgeons' interests at heart: indeed the Council contained some surgeons as members. But the Edinburgh Council's second interest was probably more important – they controlled the University in Edinburgh, known then as the Town's College. Set up in 1583, this University was constitutionally quite different from the earlier foundations at St Andrews, Aberdeen and Glasgow in being under the control of the Town Council, while the others were independent bodies. Though the teaching of medicine had never become fully established in Edinburgh in the 17th century, there were continual hopes and plans that it might be, and the Town Council feared that a college of physicians might be a move towards the teaching of medicine outside the Town's College. Thus via the Convention of Royal Burghs they determined to thwart the physicians.

The Convention first asked the physicians to explain what they were planning, and in October 1657 the physicians sent in a long and breathless reply to the Convention:

> Whairas of late wee haveing obteaned a patent for erecting of ane colledge of phisicians in this natione, have notwithstanding met with great oppositione from severall interests beyond all that could have bein expectit in prosecuting so just ane intendment, and whairas wee have bein misrepresentit to the honorabill burrowis [burghs] as men of dangerous designs not onlie as to the fortuns but to the verie lyves of the people, and especiallie as to the jurisdiction of magistratis in the respective places, and in all those wee find the former oppositionis have bein so stronglie directit and fomentit from privat interestis wndir the pretence of publict concernment as on these grounds hath moved the burrowis in thair last particular meiting at Edinburgh to give in ane paper to the counsall of estait against the present establischment, in vindication of ourselves frome such groundles misrepresentationis wee had resolwed to have givin in ane humble remonstrance to the former meitingis. . . .[60]

The physicians went on to disclaim that they wanted to be totally in charge of Edinburgh medical practice:

> . . . and, that wee may farder tak of all suspicion of intending anie arbitrarie jurisdictione over chyrurgianis and appothecarris, wee have offered that what ever inspectione the patent trustis ws with as to the foresaidis professionis salbe regulat by and don in presence and with concurrence of the magistrat of the place . . .

Such devious arguments appear to have made no impact on the hard-headed councillors, who insisted that a new and watered-down constitution be produced by the physicians for the inspection by the Burghs. At the meeting to discuss these proposals, the physicians failed to produce the modified document and the suspicious Convention minuted that the physicians

> did ingeniously declare that they continuewed still cleir in thair judgementis in adheiring to all the promissis but that they found severall of thair colegues both in this and wther burghis and schyres auers and indifferent beyound expectatioune, so that they had not resaued [received] from thame thair comissionis nor satisfactorie ansueris, and that thairfoir they had not trubled themselues with the making up of any new draught of ane patent.

The Convention was not charitable in their attitude to the physicians' excuses and prevarication and concluded that the physicians were intent on evasion. It was therefore recorded that the Burghs

> haue just reasone to suspect that some of the doctoris doe wait for ane opportunitie to pas the said patent or some wther of the lyk natur without consent of the burrowis and wtheris interessed, to thair manifest prejudice in thair liberties, and doe thairfoir find themselues oblidged by all just and lawfull meanes to secur themselues from any such patent, wndir the name of ane colledg of phisitianes, may prove a dangerous monopolie.

The Burghs instructed their agent in London to watch for the appearance of any charter for the physicians and to oppose it totally. In any case, this application for a constitution for the College failed when Cromwell died.

By 1670 the physicians had regrouped. Sibbald and Balfour set up a comprehensive herbal collection in a new Physic Garden though the surgeon-apothecaries, ever watchful, had unsuccessfully opposed this on the grounds that they had already such a garden and that this move might 'usher in a Coledge of Physitians'. In this they were right. The final, and successful, bid for a physicians college in Edinburgh was made in 1681.

This success was the result of the skill of Sir Robert Sibbald's new and more moderate proposals and the help of friends at court, namely the Duke of York and Sir Charles Scarborough, the King's physician. The opposition failed on this occasion as the Town Council at that time was weakened in its opposition by a temporary feud with the surgeons. The apothecaries had also temporarily abandoned their pact with the surgeons and the College proposals went through. The College of Physicians under the new proposals was to control practice in Edinburgh only and the surgeons and apothecaries were not to be under their control provided the surgeons limited their practice to 'wounds, contusions, practices, dislocations, tumours and ulcers'. On one other point the physicians were clear: the Town Council was to have no part in the control of their new College. The apprehension of the physicians over municipal control was because the Town Council contained surgeons and apothecaries, and they stated

> it was inconsistent with reason that the physicians, who are a superior order, should be brought before them [i.e. the surgeons and apothecaries] in a Town Council.[61]

The Town Council agreed to the proposal for a new College but only after obtaining major concessions in return, notably that the

College could only test the contents of an apothecary's shop in company with representatives of the surgeons and apothecaries and that the College would not teach medicine. This concession was of crucial importance to Edinburgh medicine in later years, as it prevented the College of Physicians from blocking the development of the University medical faculty.

The College plan went through and they, like the Glasgow Faculty, took on responsibilities for treating the poor, setting up a thrice weekly consultation. The College also went to work in establishing a monopoly of the practice of medicine in Edinburgh, but left the surgeons and apothecaries relatively unmolested. One entry in the minutes of 1696 shows that a Doctor of Divinity was

> found to be treating the sick and enquyered at by the president if he intended to doe so without any license from the College. He answered that he was not weell resolved and could give no positive answer.

He was given one week to 'resolve in'. The College had no jurisdiction in rural areas and took little interest in practice there. As a result the ministers and landowners continued up to the 19th century to give medical aid outside the towns.

Quacks

In addition to the orthodox practitioners and the folk healers, there were numerous travelling healers.[62] These irregular practitioners were noted in the Kirk Session minutes in Glasgow in 1598 when the Town Council resolved to examine those 'mediciners and chyrurgianes quha dayele resortis and remanis within this towne . . . in respect thai have not cunyng nor skill'. The quacks or 'mountebanks' were characterised by their itinerant habits, their lack of formal training (but this was not invariably absent) and particularly their use of publicity, self-advertisement, and showy dress. They also made a lot of money, which irritated the local orthodox practitioners. They sold medicines, antidotes to poisons, operated on the eye and elsewhere and offered cures for ageing and impotence. Though the cutters for the stone were not considered as quacks, there were itinerants who claimed to be able to dissolve these stones. In 1615 in Aberdeen, Dr W. Barclay complained about 'the Highland imposter which is lately come to Inverness and made a false rumour that he can dissolve any stone in the bladder, were it ever so great'.[63] The doctor recommends the public to consult 'only learned physicians' and avoid 'barberous apothecaries, highland-leeches, imposters and mountebanks, Mercurial mediciners, that is to say rubbers with quicksilver, and all they which can give no reason for their calling'.

This definition of a quack is an appealing one but is useless in separating out the claimants to healing skills in the 17th century. Since a faulty theoretical basis for medical methods was used by trained practitioners, the abuse of the empirics was unjustified. The only useful distinction that can be made in retrospect is between those healers who were dangerous and those who were not, and it is far from clear into which category the quacks and the orthodox practitioners each fell. To the patient it was results that counted and the pragmatic Town Councils and Kirk Sessions were prepared to employ anyone whom they trusted, casting aside the objections by the physicians and surgeons. Thus the quack John Pontius and his entourage of ten were made welcome in Edinburgh in 1633 and allowed to set up a stage and act a play, provided they acted 'no obscene thing'. The highlight of the show was a dancer

> upon a single tow or rop, when the actor danced Seven Scour tymes at one tyme without intermission lifting himself and volting six quarters high above his ain head, and lichting down upon the tow as punctuallie as gif he had been dancing upon the plane stanes.[64]

He had previously visited Scotland in 1633 and 1643, putting out printed leaflets on his drugs in advance. His itinerary included Edinburgh, Stirling, Glasgow, Cupar and St Andrews. Another such mountebank was John Baptista, whom the surgeons of Edinburgh unsuccessfully tried to prevent practising in Edinburgh in 1676. Another quack was Cornelius Tilbourne who visited Edinburgh, Aberdeen and Dundee in 1684, using an act with rope dancing to pull in the crowds. The new College of Physicians tried to prevent him setting up in Edinburgh but the Privy Council overruled them. Another quack who gave satisfaction was Joannes Philo who, among other things, cured thirteen blind people in Edinburgh and 'cut several cancers'. The quacks usually managed to prolong their stay by telling the authorities that they had several difficult patients still under treatment. Philo used this method with success and was still highly regarded by the authorities in spite of this. He left Edinburgh with a recommendation from the Privy Council to other burghs in Scotland.

Self-treatment

At the same time as the towns were developing a primitive form of a medical profession and were visited by travelling healers, the rural areas had few practitioners of any sort, though surgeon-apothecaries had begun settling in the smaller towns of Scotland. Thus the bulk of the people of Scotland either treated themselves or sought the special advice and powers of a folk-healer, or visited the healing wells. Self-treatment was practised at all levels of society. The gentry recorded their medical methods in their diaries and day-books and the medical methods of the ordinary people were recorded by travellers. The popular almanacs also had some medical methods in their pages, and astrology was still used in judging prognosis and treatment. These almanacs often contained diagrams showing the best veins to use in blood-letting.[65]

Of the diaries, that of the Rev. Robert Landess of Robroyston, and formerly minister in Blantyre, written in 1670, is of medical interest.[66] It is perhaps not surprising that the prescriptions found in it are rather similar to the methods of the town physicians, since the ministers basic education was similar to that of the physician. Many of the Scottish ministers had made extra study of medicine and some had even travelled to Leyden for this purpose.[67] The ministers were also familiar with the standard popular works on medicine of the day. Thus these remedies used by Landess are the familiar mixtures of exotic and unlikely materials reminiscent of the Edinburgh *Pharmacopoeia*:

> *A Singular Remedie for gout or cramp*
>
> Take a fatt young whelp, scald him like a pige, take out ye gutts at ye side therof Then take Netles and stamp them with 2 unces of Brimston with 4 yoks of eggs and 4 unces of Turpentine, Incorporat all togither and put it in the whelps bellie, so sowd up that nothing of this composition come out, Then Rost the whelp at a soft fire, keep the Dropings that comes from him and anoint the grived place therwith: and in the mean time Rub the paind place softlie befor you anoint it.

To ease any payn of ye head
Take violet oyl and woman's milk of each a like quantitie, and mix in them ye yoke of a hen's egg; when wrought togither, and lay it on cadass or tow plaister wise, warm to ye place wher the payn is.

For payns in ye ears
Take ground worms and boyl them in gooss grease, and when they are well mixt take and strayn them and then pour in a little of that liquor in the ear that is paynd.

For the falling of ye Uvula or palat of ye throat
Boyl hysop in vinager and gargaziz [gargle] the throat therwith. Or shave the croun of ye head and sett a ventese thereon. Or salt made verie hott and tyed to ye Nap of ye Neck in a cloath. or the pith of a wheat Loaff mixt wh salt and applyed hott.

For ye Squinacie [quinsy]
Dry mans dung or dogs dung and bray it to pouder, then mix it with honey and when it is warm apply it to ye patients craig. Or take the pouder of amber or dogs dung and Blow it in the throat of the patient wh a pen or pype.

While these prescriptions can at least be said to be free of magic and superstition, this method of treating gout is not:

> Apply the Skin of ye right heel of the big vultur to ye right heel of the patient and the Skin of the left heel of ye same foul unto ye left heel of the patient.

Though Landess does not include any prescriptions for sufferers from bladder stones, the later *Estate Journal of MacNeill of Carskey* in Argyll about 1720 does so:

> Take ane quart of white wine and take into ane Glass yrof for nine mornings nine slaters [woodlice] being dryed and bruised into powder wt the juice of three . . . onions being strained through a clean cloath, also put ane ordinary Dram of brandy into the Glass of white wine qch quantity drink for the sd space of Nine mornings and itt will cure yow.[68]

Comparison of these remedies with those of the Edinburgh *Pharmacopoeia* shows considerable similarity.

One landowner's personal collections of prescriptions was published in the early 18th century and achieved fame as a popular text of medicine. The author was John Moncrief of Tippermalloch in Perthshire and the title was *The Poor Man's Physician*. Published in 1712, it was eventually eclipsed by Buchan's *Domestic Medicine* of 1769, but in the interim was widely read.[69]

A more personal account of self-medication is found in the *Diary of Alexander Brodie of Brodie* (1672) of Moray who suffered from stones in the kidney and bladder and recorded his numerous attacks of colic:

> About 9 of the clock I sensibli found the stones plump doun through the uriter to the bladder . . . The ston fell . . . and the water stopd. I prest but no water. The Lord stopd the passages of natur and opened them again . . . and ther cam one ston of a great bigness, and 3 less, and 40 small stones.[70]

Earlier in the year he recorded a 'great stop in water passages and the beli . . .' for which he took 'spirit of salt . . . urin of a hee goat killed . . . blood of the goat distilld. Ther cam away smal stons and shells.'

It was this *post hoc, ergo propter hoc* argument that was to give support to all forms of therapy in the 17th century, as it did for long before and long after. It was perhaps fortunate that the bulk of the population lacked the higher education to know of these sophisticated remedies. For healing, the mass of the people relied on traditional methods, recourse to folk-healers for more powerful methods and the use of healing wells.

A good description of folk-medicine as practised in the Highlands of Scotland in the 17th century comes from Martin Martin, one of the earliest travellers in Scotland and the interest in his account is that he was a physician himself.[71] The diary was written in 1695 and shows great curiosity about the healing methods used. Indeed his tour may have been at Sibbald's suggestion, and the gathering of folk-methods may have been one of its objects, confirming the suggestion that the sophisticated town practitioners kept a sharp eye on folk healing in their quest for effective therapy.

Martin noted that few physicians were to be found in the Western Isles and that superstitions prevailed and resort to healing wells was made. He noticed that major epidemics were absent, which confirms that rural Scotland did not share the sufferings of the towns. The main diseases, he noted, were 'chin-cough [whooping-cough], diarrhoea, fever, the falling down of the uvula, jaundice and stitches'. The cures he found being used were the letting of blood (for fever and pleurisy), and a range of prescriptions of great simplicity – black mulacca beans (for diarrhoea and dysentery), oatmeal and boiled water or nettles and roots for cough, ointments of herbs mixed in fresh butter for wounds. In cases of jaundice, red hot tongs were applied to the lower spine. For constipation, the red seaweed (dulse) boiled in fresh water and butter reliably produced 'a passage both ways'. Wild garlic was prescribed for stones in the kidney, violets for fevers, chickweed for insomnia, tansy for worms and oatmeal for colic. For toothache a green turf was heated and applied to the cheek. For the 'falling down of the uvula' Martin noted a neat local surgical cure in which a loop of hair was threaded through a quill, the uvula caught in the loop, the loop tightened and the uvula avulsed with this snare. Martin Martin also travelled to St Kilda and described that when strangers arrived, a cough broke out in the inhabitants of the island. This observation was the first record of the susceptibility of this isolated population to disease brought by visitors. Magic was much in use in the areas visited by Martin Martin, since he noted the use of magic stones which imparted their healing powers to water, and resort to healing wells. Though Martin does not describe any of the healing spells and charms used, they were probably favoured in the Highlands, and have been well described by others later.

In comparing the self-treatment methods described by Martin with the conventional practice of the towns, a marked contrast is easily detected. The materials used in the traditional folk remedies were simple with only one ingredient used at a time. Thus, alone of the healing methods in 17th century Scotland, these traditional methods could be called scientific, since if the method used was toxic or ineffective it was easy to stop or alter the method. With the complex methods of the professionals, tracing the ingredient responsible for success or failure was impossible. However progress was prevented in the folk methods by a rigid distinction made between healing herbs and poisons. Only when it was realised later that useful drugs could be poisonous in higher dosage and helpful in lower amounts could progress be made. The primitive methods used to make extracts from plants also compounded this problem, since a variable amount of the active drug was obtained with each extraction.

Of the folk methods and the plants and herbs described by Martin, many have effects on the body, though none have survived to the present day as an extract of the original plant. Though the use of foxglove is recorded by Martin, it was only used externally. Another feature in comparing the amateur folk healer and professional is the dislike of the town physicians for surgery. Their treatment of the 'falling down of the uvula' mentioned earlier was medical, but the Highlanders simply chopped it off neatly with a snare. For 'faintness of the spirits' – another disease difficult to identify today – the inhabitants of Skye took the patient to the blacksmith, laid the sufferer's head on the anvil, and the blacksmith then took an apparently serious swing at the patient's head with a hammer.

Folk healers

It is probable that self-help was the standard treatment for the mass of the people, using the methods described by Martin Martin.[72] The reasons for consulting a folk healer were probably that self-treatment had failed, and that more powerful methods were required. The methods of the folk healer were sought, not only for their superior knowledge of herbs and other therapy, but because the folk healers had a reputation for supernatural powers to heal. Doubtless many of these healers acquired a local reputation for this skill after a spectacular cure of some kind. The healers also provided other services to the community, notably foretelling the future and the preparation of love potions. One other power was to cause them problems in the 17th century: it was thought that they could not only help but could also harm humans and animals by magic.

The charmers and folk healers used mostly spoken charms. The charms used for erysipelas often invoked the Trinity or St Columba: charms for toothache invoked St Bride. There were magic numbers, and 3 was particularly powerful since it used the Trinity. Healing plants were pulled three at a time, healing bracelets were used with three-ply cord, or had three knots in them. Some of the charms could be worn in a locket or silk bag round the neck. Often threads were employed for healing, usually a thick black thread with nine knots tied round a limb. Recourse to healing stones and 'dead' water was common in the Highlands, namely the use of water from a stream over which the dead were taken to or from the church. The addition of metal – lead or silver – to ordinary water could give curative powers as could healing stones put into water, such as the Lee Penny, the crystal of the Stewarts of Ardvorlich, the curing stone of the Campbells of Glen Lyon, and others.

Folk healers generally accepted no payment and no ostentatious show of skills were made, unlike the quack and the mountebank. Some members of the community had been regarded as possessing healing powers from birth, and in Scotland a posthumous child – a child born after the death of the father – traditionally had these powers, as did those born inside intact foetal sacs.[73] A seventh son, particularly the seventh son of a seventh son, was also blessed with healing gifts. Both the posthumous child and the seventh sons exercised their healing powers simply by looking at the ill patient or by rubbing, stroking or touching the affected part. Children born by a breech delivery – feet first – traditionally had powers to heal rheumatism.

Throughout Scotland's history these folk healers played a valuable role, particularly in places far distant from more conventional advice. The reformed Church struggled mightily to abolish such 'unwarrantable healing' and those who resorted to the healers were even brought before the Kirk Session. One form of healing, however, still won the approval of the Church. The King continued to be regarded as having healing powers in his touch, particularly in curing scrofula – tuberculosis of the skin and glands – and up to the time of the Hanoverian succession touching sessions were part of court ritual.[74] It is estimated that Charles I touched 100,000 persons for the disease and at Holyrood in 1633 'after offringe, healit 100 persons of the cruelles or Kingis eivell'. Coins touched by the King had similar powers.

Some details are available of patients treated by these methods. On 24th June 1633 Marjorie Gray of Banffshire obtained a church certificate from the Grange session allowing her to seek the King's touch in London for her disease and declaring her 'free of church censure and public scandal'. In 1660 Lady Wemyss took her daughter from Fife to London to be touched by Charles II for the 'cruells in hir arme'.

The use of these magical methods of cure were regarded with suspicion in the 17th century. Not that the success was doubted, but there was concern that the power of Satan was being used. Though the King was above suspicion, some practitioners and folk healers were put under scrutiny. Martin Martin found an illiterate member of the Beaton family of physicians practising in Skye, and records that it was thought locally that his

> performances have proceeded . . . rather from a Compact with the Devil, than from the Virtue of Simples. To obviate this, Mr Beaton pretends to have had some Education from his father, tho he died when he himfelf was but a Boy.[75]

Other persons to come under suspicion were the aristocratic owners of the stones with healing powers. These healers were usually excused: not so lucky were humble folk healers who came under suspicion of witchcraft. In Rothesay, Bute, one such woman had a close brush with authority. The Kirk Session of the parish finding in 1661 that Jeane Campbell was

> undertaking to heal desperate diseases by herbs and such like, the session did discharge the said Janet in time coming to use the giving of any physic or herbs to anyone under certification that she shall be esteemed a witch if she do so.[76]

Doubtless a successful folk healer operating successfully was safe but when the remedies failed or a credible story of doing harm to individuals got about, the authorities might act. Even then, a stable and popular member of the community might escape, but if he or she was old, solitary or confused, then a trial and prosecution with the death sentence might result during the time of the witch-hunts.

Witchcraft

Witchcraft was a criminal offence, and was processed through the usual legal channels in a formal matter-of-fact way. Though much of the evidence to back up the charge of witchcraft came from the demonstration of supernatural healing and harming powers, the essential evidence necessary for a conviction was to prove that a compact with the Devil had been made. Supernatural power alone was not thought unusual, and much disease, notably the epidemics, was thought to be inflicted by God in this way. It was *bad* magic that had to be punished.

Until about 1200 belief in witchcraft was largely absent, though a lively belief in the Devil existed. The increased descriptions of witchcraft, and the persecution of witches which followed it, resulted from the Bull of Pope Innocent VIII in 1484, announcing that some European Christians:

> were entering into alliances with the Devil and by charms and incantations were causing harm to other human beings, animals and produce of the earth.

This was followed by the lamentable document *Malleus Maleficarum* which gave guidance to judges in the inquisition of witches, and a systematic persecution then followed. In 1563 the Scottish Parliament passed a statute against 'Witchcraftis, Sorcarie and Necromancie' and thus came into line with the Church on the continent. Even King James VI, who was later to publish a treatise on witchcraft, considered that the winds and storm on his hourney home in 1590 were caused by a conspiracy of witches, and the group was brought before him and tortured. From then on the prosecution of witches proceeded rapidly and the methods were notoriously reliable in producing proof that the suspects used supernatural powers to cause disease, famine or natural disasters.

The prosecution of witches in Scotland came in waves, and there were bursts of trials in different areas at different times.[77] The Highlands were almost free of such prosecutions and executions, largely as a result of the decision about 1600 that all charges of witchcraft had to be reviewed first in Edinburgh, and the legal papers sent to the capital first. This was a disincentive to the authorities in the Highlands to proceed. Moreover there was also the problem of the need for gaelic translation in the legal proceedings, and the Kirk Session was less powerful in the Highlands. In the Lowlands those brought to trial were often solitary women, sometimes tough and resourceful rather than demented: of all the prosecutions only 20% were of men. The peak years for prosecutions were 1589–97, 1629–30 and the period 1640–70, when 200 to 300 executions were carried out. The total number dispatched in this way is controversial. Certainly the legal papers for 1159 such executions have been traced but other women were prosecuted locally and killed in the early period and no details of their cases remain.

There may also have been citizens' trials. One (possibly exaggerated) description of mob rule and violence was recorded in Elgin:

> The whilk day, ane gret multitude rushings through the Pannis port [of Elgin] surroundit ye order [ordeal] pool, and hither

wis draggit through ye stoure ye said Marjory Byssetth, in sore plight, wid her grey haires hanging loose, and crying 'Pitie! Pitie!' Now Maister Wiseman, the samin clerk, who had stode up at her tryal, stepped forward, and saide, 'I kno this womyan to have been ane peacable and unoffendynge ane, living in ye privacy of her widowhoode, and skaithing or gainsaying no ane. Quhat have ye furthir to say again her?' Then did ye Friaries agen repeate how that she had muttered her Aves backward, and othirs that ye maukin [hare] started at Bareflet, had been traced to her dwellinge, and how that the aforesaid cattal had died by her connivance. Bot she hearing this cried the more 'Pitie! Pitie! I am guiltless of ye fausse crymes, never sae much as thought of be mie'. Then suddenlie there was ane motion in ye crowd, and ye peopel parting on ilk syde, ane Leper cam doun frae ye Hous, [the leper house] and in ye face of ye peopel bared his hand and his haill airm, ye which was wythered and covered over with scurfs, most pyteous to behold, and he said; 'At ye day of Pentecost last past, thys womyan did give unto me ane shell of oyntment, with ye which I annoynted my hand to cure ane imposthume which had cum over it, and beholde, from that day furthe untyll thys, it hath shrunk and wythered as you see it now'.

Whereupon ye crowde closed rounde and becam clamorous; but ye said Marjory Bysseth cried pyteously, that God had forsaken her – that she had meanyed gude only and not evil – that the oyntment was ane gift of her husband, who had been beyond seas, and that it was ane gift to him from ane holy man, and true, and that she had given it free of reward or hyre, wishing only that it mote be of gude; but that, gif gude was to be payed back with evil, sorrow and gif Sathan mot not have his owin. Whereupon the peopel did presse roun and becam clamorous; and they tak ye womyan and drag her amid mony tears and cryes, to ye pool and crie, 'To tryal! to tryal!' and soe they plonge her in ye water. And quhen as she went down in ye water, there was ane gret shoute; bot as she rose agayne and raised up her arms, as gif she wod have com up, there was silence for ane space, when agane she gaed doune with ane bubblinge noise, and they shouted finallie – 'to Sathan's kyngdome she hath gane', and forthwith went their wayes.[78]

A Lowland trial which was more typical of the period was that of

John Brugh of Fossway near Dollar, in 1643. It may be taken as an example where the powers of healing and harming were prominent in the charges and where the powers of the accused had been highly regarded. The charges mentioned the causing of disease first and his compact with the Devil second, beginning thus:

> the said John Brughe shaiking off all feir of the Omnipotent and Almytie God, reverence or regaird to his blessed word, and to the lawis and acts of parliament of this Kingdome groundit thereupon, and geiving himself haillielie over to the service of Sathan, the enemie of mane's salvations, for thir threttie sax zeirs by gane practeized, used, and exerced the devellishe charmes of witchcraft and sorcerie upon dyverse persones, alsweill men as women, be onlaying of seikness, and deseass, and apptaking thereof upon ther personnes, and guids and geir, hantit and frequentit the ungodlie and damnable meittings of witches, and kepit companie and trystis with the devill and thame at dyverse his appoyntit trystis; in sua far as the said John hes been ane continuall ressaver of sarkis, coller boddis, beltis, and uther abuilziementis perteneing alsweill to men as women for cureing them of their seikness, urgeing thame to bring the samyn unto him, declaring himself thereby to have a mediate paktione with the devill, and, in sua doing, abuseing his Maj. leidges maist abominablie in makeing thame to beleive that he was able to give thame health of bodies for the quhilk he tuik from thame dyverse great sowmes of money, victualls, butter, cheise, and uther commodeteis, impoverishing thame thereby. And be his causing thame likewayes for their cure and healthes to weishe thame selfis in southe ryning wateris, involving therthrow the ignorant peaple consulters with him in a second giltines qlk was auqheable to baptisme in the name of Sathan the devill playing the ape in all God's workis, and be sua doing to draw away the heartis of God's peaple fra ther blissed creator to be cured and helped be Sathan and his infernal instrumentis . . .[79]

In detail he was charged with using 'ane enchanted stane as of the bignes of a dow' to cure a patient, and after his advice had been sought during a cattle epidemic, he recommended the use of 'tua enchantit stanes', and sprinkled over the animals the water into which the stones had been put. He was also confronted with the confession of a condemned witch who alleged he had met the Devil at Rumbling Bridge, and that he had raised bodies from the dead in the Kirk of Muckhart. Brugh was tried, found guilty, then strangled and burned on the Castle Hill in Edinburgh.

The attitude of the medical men to the witches and the trials is difficult to assess, since they seldom appear at the trials and doubtless they accepted the orthodoxy of the day that compacts with the Devil could be made. Dr Matthew Brisbane, a respected Glasgow physician, gave evidence in the Renfrewshire witchcraft trial and concluded that witchcraft had caused the illness of the child involved.[80] In England, though some doctors declared themselves against the belief in witchcraft, even members of the new Royal Society were believers.[81]

The movement against the witches in Scotland continued through the 17th century though the use of torture to get a confession was forbidden in 1662. The trials declined in the early 18th century, after acquittal had became common. The penultimate witch-burning was in Ross-shire in 1726, the accused confessing that she had taken away the sight of the eyes of one of the ministers. The last burning was in Dornoch in 1727: repeal of the statutes against witches came in 1734.

Healing wells

As noted before, when St Columba and the early missionaries travelled the land they encountered pagan belief in gods and spirits of water and springs. To exorcise these views they blessed the springs and wells which they encountered and, perhaps inadvertently laid the basis for a new belief in the healing power of the wells.[82] There grew up a new, christian, faith in the power of the wells and many were given the name of the saint associated with them. Before the Reformation the number of wells was considerable and some attracted pilgrims from far, who often travelled barefoot on the last part of the journey, going down even on their knees as they neared the healing wells. The wells had fame in healing individual diseases – mental illness, eye disease, asthma and skin disease were the commonest ailments cured. Whooping cough was also a reason for resorting to wells where the water was allowed to drip into the patients mouths while lying on their backs.

The ritual associated with the use of the well often had pagan associations and involved a visit at a particular time of the year or day, usually before sunset or at sunrise. Sunrise on May Day was a particularly propitious time for healing. A small votive offering was often left at the well, either by throwing a coin into the water or leaving a rag or strip of clothing on a bush near the well. Other rituals might include the patient being left at the well, sometimes bound and gagged, which was preceded by a ritual such as walking round the well a number of times, usually in silence. It was often considered that the wells, notably that of St Columba in Eigg, could not heal local people. Associated with this faith in water were a number of related faiths, notably that of hydromancy, namely that the water of the wells could be used to foretell the outcome of disease. Thus at St Andrew's Well at Shadar in Lewis the direction of flotation of a wooden plate could foretell the future.

The attitude of the early Church to these practices with stones and charm had been ambivalent. On the one hand there was St Cuthbert's rebuke of those who used these methods, since he said it was impossible that 'by any magical art they were able to avert a stroke inflicted by the Lord', and Anselm tried to stop the recourse to healing wells. On the other hand St Columba himself used a magic stone and the water in which it was dipped in his contest with the power of the Magi. It thus seems likely that the Church was prepared in Scotland at least unofficially to claim the credit for healing and it may be that there was always a tendency to return to heathen beliefs if the powers of the Christian faith were not shown to be as effective. The persistence of these pagan beliefs was recorded by Martin Martin in his visit to the Hebrides, when he found that worship of the sea god Shony still existed in the middle of the 17th century.

A major attempt was made in Scotland at the Reformation to destroy the credibility of these holy wells, as part of the systematic extermination of the Roman Catholic faith. An Act of Parliament in 1581 makes clear the new Church's attitude to this

> pervers inclination of mannis ingyne [imagination] to superstitioun through which the dregges of idolatrie yit remainis in divers pairtis of the realme be using of pilgrimage to sum chappellis wells . . .[83]

Kirk Sessions all over the land made attempts to stamp out pilgrimages to the wells. People in Falkirk were accused of resorting to the Christ's Well, some in Perth of going to the Huntingtower

Well and others in Nigg, Kincardineshire, of resorting to St Fittack's Well. Many other convictions were made elsewhere in Scotland, and the Kirk Session records of north east Scotland have frequent references to attempts to deal with the large numbers of persons using the holy wells in Speyside and Aberdeenshire. Not only the common people were involved. Lady Aboyne had walked 30 miles each year to the Well of Spey, going barefoot for the last two miles.

In trying to end the well-worship and the use of magic stones, the reformed Church was only partially successful. The old beliefs proved to be so popular that they were not easily abolished. Nevertheless, a change in attitudes to the wells did occur, perhaps on account of the Reformation, and the old belief in the healing power of water obstinately appeared in a new form – a belief in the chemical healing power of wells. Throughout Scotland, and indeed Europe, it was held that some newly discovered wells healed, not by divine force, but by physical means through some component in the water itself. This switch in belief from spiritual to chemical healing is easily seen in the diary of Alexander Brodie when, at a time that he was encouraging the Elgin Kirk Session in their prosecution of those who used the holy wells of Speyside, he himself was resorting to other wells at Burgie and Rhives nearby to treat his bladder stones. He was irritated at the complaints from the people over his use of the water as he saw no confusion in the different powers of the wells.[84]

This new type of well was used differently. The water was not pure and contained chemicals which had effects on the body, usually purgative or diuretic. The water was drunk in quantity over a period of weeks, rather than a small amount of holy water taken on one occasion. Many of these secular wells of Scotland have been described individually and some appear in the earliest medical literature of Scotland as a result of the medical men's great interest in the reports of healing powers in the well water.[85] The earliest of these works came in 1580 as an anonymous pamphlet on the *Qualities and Effects of the Well of the Woman Hill besyde Aberdene*. The author was probably Gilbert Skeyne, the mediciner, and although he claimed that the well was the gift of God, the healing power is ascribed to the constituents of the water. These waters had effects on the patient, causing diarrhoea, vomiting and increased urine flow, a desirable outcome in the medical practice of the day. The writer suspected that iron was present in the water from the taste of the water and discolouration it produced on the stones and ground round the spring. The water was considered to be a cure for a large number of illnesses, notably congestive heart failure, obstruction of the bowels and paralysis of limbs. The writer prudently commended the users of the water not to use it indiscriminately but to seek the advice of a local doctor in the best use of the water. Nevertheless, the writer was prepared to reveal some of the secrets of the well: the months of June, July and August were the best, and after the 20th September the well was ineffective. During the day, the water was to be drunk in the morning and three-hourly thereafter, together with medicine prescribed by the local doctor.

In 1615 another tract appeared in Aberdeen written by a Dr Barclay in praise of another well in Aberdeen called the Well of Spa. The claims for this well were similar to those made for the Well of Woman Hill and the amount recommended to be drunk is again considerable. Barclay attempted analysis of this well water, suspecting from the taste and colour that iron and copper sulphate were present. Interestingly, he used one of the earliest forms of analytical chemistry, taking a crushed nut-gall and putting it into a glass of the water. A red colour appeared proving that the water contained a 'vitriolic virtue' and hence iron. Dr Barclay had his own theory that the water worked by removing obstruction of every kind. Obstruction of the bowel or kidney gave colic and this block could be removed by the water together with any ulcers or stones in the parts. Among other diseases, he also advised it for gonorrhoea since the flushing effect would give a cure. For sterility, the water was also good, since he considered that the mouth of the womb was obstructed and flushing out would unblock it. He recommended that the water should be used under medical supervision and that drinking should start with one session a day, two hours after the rising of the sun, gradually increasing the amount drunk daily to four or five pounds weight.

Other wells which achieved fame were at Peterhead and that at Kinghorn in Fife. Both were discovered just at the time of the attempts to stop the use of the holy wells. Kinghorn had a laudatory mention from Dr Barclay again, and was also supported by a pamphlet by Patrick Anderson (of Anderson Pills). He noted correctly that the mineral wells had only recently been discovered in Scotland, and he distinguished sharply between them and the holy wells:

> These waters are not lyk the superstitious mud-earth wells of Menteith or Ladywell or Strathearn and our Ladie Well of Ruthven all tapestried about with old rags as certaine signes and sacraments . . .

Anderson then gave details of how to use the well's water and added that its efficacy was increased by taking nine of his Grana Angelica pills in a poached egg.

Healing stones

Healing stones were still highly regarded in the 17th century, and the Reformation made little impact on their use.[86] But there is a suggestion that after the Reformation it was thought that some chemical escaped from the healing stones, thus explaining their success in secular terms. The Lee Penny was still popular and about 1630 during the reign of Charles I the town of Newcastle-upon-Tyne sought it out and took it to aid the fight against a cattle plague. The borrowers had to give a bond of £6,000 to the Lee family for the safe return of the stone and it is said that the city were so pleased with its use that they would happily have forfeited the money to keep the stone. To use the stone it was dipped three times into water and the water then either drunk or used as a lotion.

The Kirk Sessions having outlawed the holy wells, also considered the problem of the healing stones. In Glasgow a complaint was made to them against the use of the Lee Penny, and the Synod were put in an acutely uncomfortable position, since the stone was owned by a nobleman, and they also believed that it worked. They escaped from this dilemma by a memorable and rather moving judgement.

> Quhilk daye, amongest the referries of the brethren of the ministrie of Lanerk, it was propondit to the Synode, that Gawen Hammiltoune of Raplocke had perferit an complaint before them against Sir James Lockart of Lie, anent the superstitious vsing of an stene set in selver for the curing of diseased cattell, qlk, the said Gawen affirmit, coud not be lawfully vsed . . . The Assemblie having inquirit of the maner of vsing thereof, and particularlie vnderstoode, by examinatioune of the said Laird of Lie, and otherwise, that the custome is onlie to cast the stene in sume water, and give the diseasit cattil thereof to drink, and yt the sam is dene wtout vsing onie words, such as charmers and sorcerers vse in their unlawfull practicess; and considering that

> in nature they are mony thinges seen to work strange effects, qr of no humane witt can give a reason, it having pleasit God to give vnto stones and herbes special virtues for the healing of mony infirmities in man and beast, – advises the bretheren to surcease thir proces, as q'rin they perceive no ground of offence; and admonishes the said Laird of Lie, in the vsing of the said stone, to take heed that it be vsit heirafter wt the least scandal that possiblie maye bie.[87]

So the Synod were prepared to sanction the use of the stone, provided no idolatrous rituals were used: they also clearly believed in its power.

Thus the confusion in the healing arts in the 17th century was total. The physicians, the best educated practitioners, were not the most effective and their attempts to create a monopoly for themselves through a college with wide powers were successfully modified by their opponents. Nor were the apothecaries to be admired. They had used the physicians bizarre prescribing habits to make themselves rich and having taken up medical practice themselves, pushed the physicians into more extreme therapeutic complexity. Probably more effective in healing than the physicians were the surgeons, barber-surgeons and simple surgeon-apothecaries who served the small towns since they used more pragmatic skills in healing wounds and fractures and prescribed the simpler, cheaper drugs. It is also far from clear that the travelling quacks were as dangerous or unskilled as they have been made out to be when the methods of the orthodox are considered. Lastly, it is likely that the folk methods were safer than the orthodox medicine, and these simple methods may have been refined by centuries of experience into effective therapy. All the evidence suggests that the professionals unobtrusively kept a close eye on the folk methods and the physicians methods changed to incorporate these ideas. The attitude to magic was also ambivalent. In spite of official disapproval, the use of healing stones was believed in and their use could be allowed. Serious medical men approved of magical weapon salves, the use of live doves applied to the feet, the power of the King's touch and the power of 'sympathy'. Yet the law was fiercely enforced on witches using methods no different from these which were approved in other hands.

The end of the 17th century also marked the beginning of the Scottish Enlightenment – a period of Scottish achievement which was to be admired by the rest of the world not only for its intellectual distinction, but also for the advancement of the useful arts. The practice of medicine and medical education, after an undistinguished start in the 17th century was to be prominent in the Enlightenment and played a crucial role in amplifying intellectual endeavour in other fields.

4
The rise of the professional 18th century

The 18th century in Scotland was a time of progress, both material and intellectual, made possible by the new peace and prosperity which resulted eventually from the Union of Parliaments between England and Scotland. Although reliable health statistics did not appear until the end of this period, many commentators consider that the people of Scotland had an improvement in health in the 18th century though this halted at the onset of the industrial revolution at the end of the century. Certainly, major epidemics temporarily disappeared, the primitive methods of famine relief became permanent, and the population of Scotland increased from about 1 million to 1.6 million at the end of the century.[1] The rise of the towns and their industries created a new middle class and this, together with a modest increase in medical knowledge, increased the demands for trained doctors. The rigours of the post-Reformation period were slowly abandoned and were replaced by a new spirit of rationalism. This together with a national effort of self–improvement, led to the remarkable flowering of the intellect in Scotland, in which medical research and medical education played a central role.

This was a particularly successful period for Edinburgh medicine where the common effort made by talented medical men and politicians produced a new medical school based on the university and the hospital. The new practitioners, trained in a novel way in both surgery and medicine, were produced in increasing numbers and they spread to all parts of the world, taking with them these new attitudes. In England, and particularly in London, these medical men met with difficulties but their numbers and the success of their education overcame this opposition. With the rise of the professional doctors in the towns, other healers were less used. However, the country parish minister continued his treatment of the sick, and self-help by traditional folk methods and the use of mineral wells was common. The itinerant healers found the authorities to be less helpful in letting them practise but even their methods changed with the new knowledge: the quacks became enlightened.

Social life

Early 17th century Scotland was still regarded, with good reason, as a backward part of Europe and travellers did not expect to be comfortable during their stay.[2] Many recorded that the Scots suffered from an itch, but there is evidence that some Scots had a weekly bath. Edinburgh was still notable for the squalor of its rat-infested, closely-packed, flimsy tenements which however, housed all types of person in an unusually homogeneous society. The smell inside the houses was a constant problem. One way of dealing with it was to burn brown paper in the room, thus as Edward Burt was later to remark 'mixing one smell with another'.

The other great sanitary problem in the towns was the removal of human waste. In Edinburgh it was simply thrown out on to the streets, usually at 10 o'clock at night. Primitive toilets existed in some houses, but they too opened directly onto the streets. The appointed hour for clearing the houses was signalled by the 10 o'clock chimes of St Giles, a signal for the inhabitants to shout the warning 'gardy loo'. Any pedestrians who wished to escape the shower shouted back 'haud yer haun'. The American medical students studying in Edinburgh described this as being 'naturalised' and in 1767, even when the town was improving in cleanliness, Benjamin Rush wrote home to say that though he had escaped the shower so far, 'my unfortunate friend Potts had gained the honour before me'.[3] The clearing of the resulting problem in the streets was carried out in a sporadic manner by city officials or later by entrepreneurs who sold the newly valuable waste for fertiliser. Such was the value of the dung, that these cleaners formed a powerful lobby against sanitary reform.

Edinburgh, which was to be a dominant force in European intellectual life, was also remarkably isolated, and as late as 1763 there was only one stage coach per week between London and Edinburgh, making an uncomfortable journey which took some days. Even at this time there were occasions when the mail bag between these two cities might contain only one letter. For the foreign medical students, the journey to reach Edinburgh could be a tedious one and the Americans complained of the journey through the barren Border countryside and the primitive inns they encountered. There could be other problems for the students. Jonathan Potts, a young American student travelling to Edinburgh in 1766, was nearly shipwrecked off Ireland. Samuel Bard, another student making the same journey in 1761, had been captured by the French, and after his release from prison, was four months late in reaching Edinburgh.[4] For this reason, the start to the winter medical teaching always had a preliminary two weeks of introductory lectures, thus allowing time for the stragglers to reach Edinburgh.

Edinburgh was isolated in another way. The Union of the Parliaments of Scotland and England had removed the legislature and aristocracy to London leaving the ancient capital in the hands of upper middle class intellectuals. Moreover, there were no national laws of much consequence in education or health matters and hence the London government had little significance in day-to-day events. Indeed the main initial effect of the Union was to cause dismay, since the loss of status in Edinburgh was felt acutely and the disappearance of many of the nobility and the administration to London created civic concern.[5] The royal palaces fell into disrepair, the military installations were abandoned and the east coast trade with the continent also declined. Edinburgh actively sought to prevent the decline of the town, and one of the Town Council's schemes, the expansion of the University, was highly successful in restoring the fortunes of the town.

After a delay, the Union did result in economic growth in Scotland, notably in the tobacco, linen and cotton trades. These new industries of the towns attracted the migrant labour from the country to the towns and this led later to overcrowding, squalor and disease. This shift in population was most marked to west central Scotland, and Glasgow grew from having about half the population of Edinburgh to be the biggest town in Scotland. In 1727 Glasgow had won compliments from Defoe as the 'most beautiful, and cleanest and best built city in Great Britain', but by the end of the century it was beginning to earn its reputation as the least clean city in Britain.[6] Edinburgh had an early reputation for squalor, but the new commercial, rather than industrial success and the confidence of the planners allowed the great New Town of Edinburgh to be built in the later part of the century.

The increased well-being of the population and its growth was a feature of the 18th century. Though this improvement was credited at the time to the advances in medicine that were thought to take place in that century, it seems more likely now that the improved health was the result of other factors. The appearance of more useful and cheaper foods like the potato, the better clothing and housing, the early sanitary reform which resulted from the improved economy, better education and increased understanding of disease mechanisms, all these helped to improve health. Starvation was no longer a cause of numerous deaths and there was a notable reduction in early childhood mortality. This improved well-being was remarked on by commentators and visitors to Scotland in the late 18th century.

Though famine occurred occasionally, notably in 1740, the consequences were not so severe as in the previous century and the early part of the 18th century was notable for a long run of good harvests. The great mortality crises resulting from the famine had gone, though periods of high death rates from under-nutrition continued into the 19th century. The reasons for the improvement in the 18th century were that the community accepted an obligation to relieve famine and developed mechanisms for this, helped by the better communications and new methods of food storage.[7] In the 1740 famine, a charitable heritor like Sir John Clerk of Penicuik could buy grain and sell it cheaply to his tenants. Also appearing were greater surpluses of food in good years and hence better and bigger stores of food were kept ready for any dearths. Better transport enabled stricken areas to be relieved. By the end of the century the 'odious taxatione' feared by the 17th century landowners was accepted in times of famine, and a voluntary assessment for the poor was responded to during the famine of 1782. Gone also was the mortality crisis following war and feuding, and the rebellions of 1715 and 1745 gave hardly any of the problems suffered by civilians in earlier centuries as a result of war.

In the 18th century came the first entry of government into famine relief. To meet the Highland famine of 1783, £17,000 of surplus military food was moved north and arrived in most places in time. This increasing concern was partly the result of compassion, and partly reaction to the increasing political power of the working class manifested firstly by the riots during the famines of 1740. There existed a new realisation of the military and economic value of a healthy work force in the increasingly sophisticated manufacturing sector and in the armed forces. Nor did the causes of the French Revolution go unnoticed by the ruling class.

Health

After the plague epidemic of 1644–49 it never returned to Scotland in a serious form. The improved agriculture and the draining of marshland in the 18th century may have been responsible for the rapid disappearance of another disease – the 'ague' – almost certainly malaria. In the middle of the century it had been so common in the rural areas that farmers always planned to lose the labour of a third of their helpers during the summer.[8] By the end of the century it had gone. Also disappearing during this century was the disease known as sibbens (probably yaws) and typhus may also have been temporarily less important. Cholera, a spectacular killer in the 19th century, was yet to appear.

While these diseases became rare, others became more important, and these changes were noted by the first primitive recording of disease.[9] Descriptions of some 18th century diseases can be accepted as accurate, notably of smallpox, measles and chincough (whooping cough), but 'consumption' included not only cases of tuberculosis, but many other chronic wasting diseases also. Of these diseases, the early Bills of Mortality drawn up by the town officials or by interested individuals show that the major killer was 'consumption', second was 'fever' (mostly typhus) and third was smallpox. Of these, smallpox was clearly increasing, and by the end of the century it was a major killer and was studied carefully. Having previously existed in epidemic form, smallpox became endemic particularly in the towns, breaking out from time to time, usually in the summer and killing children with a death rate of 15% to 20% of those affected.[10] By the end of the century it caused 19% of all deaths and 30% of deaths of children under the age of five. It was noted that a second attack of smallpox was unlikely and hence it was common in some places in Scotland to attempt to prevent the disease by inoculation with the fluid from smallpox pustules. This practice may have been part of ancient folklore in the Highlands and this area, like the rest of the United Kingdom, may have copied the ancient practice of the

East, brought to England by Lady Mary Wortley Montagu. There are early references to inoculation in Scotland in 1715, and Monro, writing in 1765 to a European correspondent, described these rural methods of deliberately infecting normal people with smallpox:

> I am assured that in some of the remote Highland parts of this country it has been an old practice of parents whose children have not had the smallpox to watch for an opportunity of some child of having a good mild smallpox that they may communicate the disease to their children by making them bedfellows to those in it and by tying worsted threads with the pocking material around their wrists.[11]

There was opposition to extension of inoculation to the rest of Lowland Scotland for a number of reasons. Firstly it was held that it thwarted God's will. A more secular argument was that the method could cause death from smallpox and that inoculation could re-introduce the disease into an area from which it might be absent for a time. Hence enthusiasm for inoculation varied throughout Scotland and it was more highly regarded in the country than in the town. This may be understandable since the rural epidemics were rarer, but met a population with low immunity so the epidemic would be serious. Inoculation was therefore welcome. The town dwellers' poor nutrition may have led to a higher mortality from inoculation and made it regarded with suspicion. In rural Scotland inoculation was carried out by the parish ministers or lay inoculators. In mid-Yell, Shetland, the blacksmith inoculated several thousand persons, having doubtless acquired skills in picking the appropriate donor, in storing the material, and applying the material at the right time and place. Samuel Johnson noted in 1774 during his tour of the Western Islands that the laird of the island of Muck had inoculated almost half the population at a cost of two shillings and sixpence per head, but the inoculator is not stated.[12]

Medical men

The rewards of medical practice in Scotland and Edinburgh in particular may have declined immediately after the Union as a result of the loss of the Parliament and the migration of the aristocracy to London. Indeed the medical men may have turned to teaching to make up for the loss of income from private practice. But the later 18th century was a time of expansion and success. The steady growth of towns and the rise of a new middle class of merchants and professional men ensured an expanding market for healing skills and a modest expansion in medical knowledge allowed a new confidence to appear. Added to the many old useless remedies there were a few drugs which were effective. Iron, cinchona bark (containing quinine), and digitalis were being cautiously used and opium was available for pain relief. The disappearance of the plague and the control of smallpox by inoculation also contributed to the hopes for progress. The towns could afford to employ more doctors for the poor, and the British army, navy, merchant fleets and companies all required surgeons. Progress in surgery was steady, notably the acceptance of operations like cutting for bladder stones as a part of the routine practice of a trained surgeon, and the Edinburgh Incorporation of Surgeons in 1741 proposed that a Chair of Lithotomy should be set up.[13] This proposal was later turned down by the surgeons, since they felt it would mark out one of their number as having special skills in the operation and hence demean the rest. But occasional cynicism about the powers of the 18th century medical men is encountered. It was said in 1746 of the doctors of Dundee that they

> wore large muffs, dangled gold-headed canes, hummed loud and looked wise: and according to the strength or weakness of their natural constitution, the patient survived or died.[14]

Robert Burns satirised the physicians exotic prescriptions in his poem *Death and Dr Hornbook*. Davie Hume, an intimate of the leading Edinburgh physicians, could nevertheless say in a serious letter to an ill Edinburgh friend,

> I entreat you, if you tender your own Health . . . pay no regard to Physicians . . . You cannot pay a moderate Regard to them: your only Safety is in neglecting them altogether.[15]

Fees charged, particularly by physicians, were substantial. When Foulis of Ravelston's wife was ill in 1702, he called a doctor, who then called in two more, each with an attendant, and the three medical men each charged £14.4 Scots (a guinea) plus £6 for each of their attendants.[16] The town doctors consulted in taverns or set up their own 'shops' and, since examination of the patient was now occasionally thought to be wise, they were prepared to make journeys, at a price, to see a patient. Postal consultations were still common, and Cullen had about one such request per day, which he dealt with promptly using Watt's invention of a copying machine to keep a record of his opinion.[17] His fee for this written advice was one guinea. The management of a case by the physicians was elaborate, and used changes of diet and climate as well as medicine. In the management of scrofula (tuberculosis) they advised, among other things, a house facing in a particular direction, a fixed amount of sleep, a change of diet, particular clothes, the absence of excitement and so on.

The physicians were found only in the towns with a reasonable number of rich potential patients. The surgeon-apothecaries were found more widely in Scotland and these, the first 'general practitioners', provided a wide range of services. There they hoped to obtain the patronage of the local gentry or merchants and obtain parish work with the poor. Many of the surgeon – apothecaries accounts have survived and these bills, though ostensibly only for drugs, include a surcharge for their fee.[18] It is difficult to assess the distribution of medical men in Scotland in the 18th century, but a study of medical practice in Roxburghshire suggests that about the year 1760 there was a doctor-patient ratio of 1:1,840 and by 1795 it was 1:1,390, possibly the most favourable figure ever in the area. This figure should be treated with caution since a full service to the whole community was never provided. The large number of practitioners in this area was probably the result of the wealth of the county in the 18th century, reflecting the large number of wealthy landowners.

Self-help

Apart from the increasing confidence of the trained practitioners and the travelling healers, medical care was still widely obtained by using the traditional remedies of the people and the folk healers. The persecution of witches disappeared in the early 18th century and the rural population went back to their traditional methods without fear. Probably these methods continued much as before, modified by popular books like Buchan's *Domestic Medicine*, which introduced the best of orthodox medicine of the city and had valuable sanitary propaganda.

The literate rural dwellers also did not abandon their self-treatment using their personal pharmacopoeias but the better roads and communications allowed more frequent conventional consultations with the city practitioners. Nevertheless large areas of Scotland had no trained medical man and even large islands like Arran or Mull had no practitioner as late as 1790. Hence health care must have been in the hands of local healers or ministers or the heritors. Though the gentry and ministers may not have treated themselves and each other as frequently as before, they still took on the treatment of the sick poor. The day-to-day life about 1755 of the Rev. George Ridpath, Minister of Stitchel (modern Stichill), five miles north of Kelso, shows that he looked after much of the ordinary illness in the community and consulted in his home or in the town each Monday morning.[20] For surgical problems, a surgeon-apothecary might come from Kelso, often staying the night with the minister. Thus the minister took on the role of healer and Ridpath's diaries show that he read many medical texts and made notes from them for his own use. The ministers also inoculated against smallpox and let blood regularly. The nobility also continued in practice and the Earl of Errol's brother was noted to hold a consultation weekly at Slains Castle in 1773. Lastly, the new printed periodicals of the 18th century began to carry medical recipes, and late in the century the first advertisements for patent medicines appeared.

Of the self-help methods most widely used, however, the most popular was the health holiday and particularly the use of mineral wells.[21] As noted earlier, the Reformation abolished faith in the divine healing by the sacred wells, but almost immediately another set of healing wells with chemicals in the water became popular. These waters, drunk in quantity over an extended period, certainly had marked effects on the body, inducing diarrhoea, vomiting and flow of urine.[22] The similarity of these effects to the evacuant therapy of the 18th century physicians is striking, and the early Scottish chemists hurried to analyse these wells with their new methods of analysis, seeking the healing ingredients.[23,24]

The development of a mineral well followed a fairly standard pattern. On the discovery of a well with water of a distinctive taste and different from the normal drinking water, a local reputation might grow up and this might lead to attempts by landowners or medical men to publicise the find.[25] If the well achieved any fame, then chemical analysis was carried out by a reputable academic and favourable comparisons made with other established spas. A laudatory pamphlet was issued and an industry then grew up round the spa catering for the visitors. If the resort was lucky, eminent persons might be attracted, which in turn brought others in and the social and intellectual life of the spa became important. David Hume, Joseph Black, Boswell and Burns used the Moffat spa for therapy and relaxation, and Hume, during his last illness, was sent to Bath. The water of the well might be bottled and sold, and 'Scarborough' water became popular and widely used.

One of the wells which achieved early fame in Scotland can be looked at more closely, namely the 'wine well' of Peterhead.[26] It became known in the 17th century as a result of an article in 1633 by a lecturer in medicine at King's College, Aberdeen and was at the height of its fame in the 18th century. The Old Pretender had landed there in 1715, since his arrival point ensured that he quickly met the aristocracy. Near the well, houses were built and sea bathing encouraged by the building of a natural bathing pool in the rocks. A virtue was made out of Peterhead's disadvantages, since the intensely cold sea bathing was alleged to have a strengthening effect on the constitution of nervous persons and even the fogs arising from the sea were considered to be medicinal. The links of Peterhead were also recommended for golf and bowls in the afternoon pastimes such as reading, talking, dancing, singing, cards and dicing were available. The fame of the resort grew and the town prospered. In 1759 the local Freemasons built a Lodge close to the well which contained a pump room, a tearoom and a ballroom, and two large inns were also built. In deference to the elegant company which the town welcomed in the season, the peat stacks and dung hills of the town were removed. The leaders of society were the local Dr Laing, minister of the Episcopal Church, the Reverend Dr Beattie, and the Queen of Scottish society, the Duchess of Gordon.

These wells faded in popularity late in the 18th century but others in Scotland rose in fame as their virtues were publicised by medical men, landowners and local hotel keepers. Attempts were made to draw patients from far and wide and to discourage Scottish patients from visiting the increasingly better known wells in England and the continent, but this effort ultimately was to be a failure. Nevertheless, in their time the Scottish wells, notably Moffat, Innerleithen (popularised by Scott in *St Ronan's Well*), Bridge of Earn, Strathpeffer and many others had much acclaim.

The literature which grew up round the spa cures is voluminous and makes dreary reading. In summary, there were four types of well. Firstly, the acidulous or mineral which liberated carbon dioxide as a fizzy gas, of which type none existed in Scotland. Secondly, the saline water (which produced diarrhoea and vomiting) as at Bridge of Earn and Pitkeathly; thirdly, the foul-smelling sulphur waters containing large amounts of hydrogen sulphide, as at Moffat and Peterhead. Lastly the chalybeate wells at Moffat and Peterhead contained iron.

Allied to the spa therapy was the use of bathing as therapy and a lasting belief in cold water as a stimulant arose – a view clearly coming from the stimulant system of therapy encouraged by some medical authorities. Of the sea bathing spas, Peterhead was particularly well known but another, the shabby resort at Brow Hill on the Solway Firth, is notorious since it was here that Robert Burns went during the last phase of his illness caused by a leaking heart valve. He waded daily up to his armpits in the sea and died a week after finishing this treatment.[27]

A lesser known health holiday, which involved retreating to a simple life in the country and drinking only the whey from goats' milk, also had a vogue. The resorts which provided this were at Callander and Luss and in 1740 it was recorded that in Glasgow in July, all the ministers were absent, being 'at the goat's whey.'[28]

In addition to these mineral wells and health holidays a modest and often clandestine belief in spiritual healing by wells persisted after the Reformation. The well of St Fergus at Kirkmichael in Banffshire was famous for the cure of skin diseases. It had to be visited after midnight, particularly on the first Sunday in May, and the power of the well apparently declined through the summer and was ineffective after September.[29] The well of St Maelrubha in Loch Maree was still used for treatment in the 18th century and even later. Patients were dipped or even dragged by ropes in the loch at midnight and votive offerings of strips of clothing and money were left in an oak tree on the island. Perhaps the best known of the healing waters was a pool in the river Earn at St Fillans. It became well known through another of Sir Walter Scott's works *Marmion*, and the pool and its power are also described in *The New Statistical Account of Scotland*. The patient suffering from mental illness was attached to a rope and thrown three times into the water to collect three stones from the bottom of the river on each immersion, making nine in all. The three stones were put on three cairns on the river bank. The patient was then taken to the chapel nearby, bound and gagged, and left overnight. In the morning, if the patient was found free of the bonds, a cure of the disease had occurred. It was estimated that at the height of its reputation two hundred people annually visited St Fillans for a cure.

Towards the end of the 18th century the popularity of these wells and pools waned. The local explanations for this loss of popularity and power were varied. It was said at St Fillans that cures had become rare after a sick bull was thrown into the pool in an attempt at a cure. The loss of potency of a well near Stirling was blamed on the local habit of mixing the water with whisky. But the real reason was the decline in the belief in magic and supernatural healing. The new explanations of disease and the new efforts to heal in the 18th century resulted from the Enlightenment: this theory and practice had no place for magic.

Quacks

The quacks and mountebanks of the 18th century are distinguishable from the orthodox medical men in much the same way as in the 17th century.[30] They were usually travelling practitioners, setting up in practice for short periods in the towns and then moving on. They advertised their skills by display in a way shunned by conventional 18th century practitioners and the remedies sold were cheap and hence available to the broad mass of the people. Though in Glasgow and Edinburgh the corporations of the physicians and surgeons sought to prohibit the practice of the quacks, they were still popular with the people, and the magistrates were not prepared to prevent them selling their wares or treating the sick. Thus the quacks continued to escape the control of the Colleges and outside the towns they were safe. A brief entry in the Session records of the Parish of Shotts suggests a successful and convivial visit by an itinerant to treat a patient on Poor Law relief:

> 1730 – To Mr. Green the Muntybag for couching John Roger's wife's eyes . . . £9 . . 6 . . 0
> – To a bottle of ale and a gill of brandie that was drank with the doctor £0 . . 4 . . 6[31]

The quacks' stalls were set up in the market places and as in earlier times a show of dancing or juggling might be given or a bawdy play acted to attract attention. After the crowd had gathered, the healer would extol his skills and sell his wares.

In the 18th century, the travelling healers often had some basic orthodox training. They also moved with the enlightened times and like the orthodox practitioners, modernised their methods, making a point of publishing and lecturing. One of the best known and interesting of these itinerants was John Taylor who had received an orthodox surgical education in London at St Thomas' Hospital but abandoned conventional practice to become a travelling oculist.[32] His activities in Edinburgh illustrate the methods of the travelling healers but also some of the problems in distinguishing them from the orthodox practitioners.

Prior to his arrival in town, he had bills and advertisements printed extolling his qualifications and listing the distinguished cures he had effected in the rich and famous. On his arrival he gave a public lecture. Thus, on his Edinburgh visit of 1744, he advertised that 'Dr. John Taylor, Oculist to His Majesty, will arrive at Mrs. Mackenzie's in Writers Court.' The audience for his lectures 'On the Eye' was limited to 300. By all accounts, the lectures were well attended not only by the curious but also by well-informed Edinburgh citizens, who were also welcome at the medical lectures in the university. The doctor helped the sense of occasion by lecturing dressed entirely in black and seated on an elevated dais. His lecture attracted some physicians and surgeons of the town: he then used this to his advantage by quickly readvertising that his lectures had been supported by Edinburgh medical men. The doctor stated that he was also prepared to treat the poor if they attended his lodgings at 8 o'clock and he even managed to raise a voluntary subscription to rent rooms for his surgical operations. His use of the newspapers was particularly deft, since the *Caledonian Mercury* printed all the material given to them by the doctor and included the statement that 'not one instance has yet appeared where he was failed of the success he had given hope of.' The Town Council were pleased with his efforts and admitted him as a burgess in the city. The Corporation of Surgeons then determined to act. They placed a statement in the *Caledonian Mercury* of 12th July 1744 saying that none of the professors had attended his lectures, though a few other members of the faculty had attended out of curiosity. Taylor's methods, they said, were 'most common and had been attended with very indifferent success', and many patients 'complain of being worse than before they came into his hands.' They contested Dr Taylor's claim about treating the poor:

> He had been oppressive to several in low circumstances by demanding exorbitant fees and intending having suits against them for small services or none at all, and notwithstanding his professing to serve the poor gratis he has by his advertisements induced several poor people to come from remote parts of the country and extorted money from them. He had also dismissed others of them because they could give him nothing.

Taylor replied by publishing a pamphlet *Syllabus or the exact description of 243 diseases to which the Eye and contiguous parts are subject*, and provocatively dedicated it to the Fellows and Presidents of the Royal College of Physicians. He then left for Glasgow, Aberdeen and Perth, and then returned to London. Five years later, in the spring of 1749, he returned once again to Edinburgh and the same routine was repeated.

A second travelling healer of interest was Dr James Graham (1745–94). Of Edinburgh origins and originally apprenticed to an apothecary, Graham never finished his training but roamed the world acquiring skills of an orthodox and unorthodox kind.[33] In America he picked up a superficial knowledge of electricity and magnetism from an acquaintance with Benjamin Franklin and later used gadgets of this kind as part of his trade. Indeed, Sir Walter Scott was taken by his father to see Graham in Edinburgh and a course of electricity was given in an attempt to help the old polio weakness of Scott's leg. Thus Graham, like Taylor, was less unorthodox than their detractors would suggest, and their conventional skills may have been considerable, in addition to the power of their charismatic personalities.

Graham travelled to Bath and then to London, where he built a lavishly decorated Temple of Health containing among other things a celestial electrified bed in which, for the substantial fee of £100, a childless couple could have fertility bestowed on them during a night's sleep. In London Graham was accompanied by his assistant Emma Lyon, later to be Lord Nelson's Lady Hamilton. Like other travelling healers of the time, he gave lectures on health for which a fee of two guineas was charged. Graham's fortunes in London declined, and in spite of lowering his fees he failed to regain his practice. He returned to Edinburgh to practise but his first lecture caused a scandal on account of its indecency. Though Graham suspected that the College was behind this outcry, it seems likely that the Magistrates acted on their own initiative and Graham was imprisoned in the Tolbooth. He never fully recovered from these reverses and though he was to become a well-known figure and health fanatic with some sensible ideas on hygiene and simple living, he died in modest circumstances near Edinburgh. Only one visit to Glasgow by Graham is recorded and it passed without incident though a well-known gossip stationed himself outside the doctor's residence to identify those who used his celestial bed.

Hospitals and help for the poor

As in the 17th century, the poor were perhaps fortunate to avoid the excesses inflicted on the rich by the trained medical men. For the poor there was the modest assistance given by the parish through the Poor Law, which sensibly decided in most cases to give money or food rather than medical help though occasionally, as in the 17th century, grants of money for visits to spas or for surgery are recorded. Otherwise the poor used their own traditional healing methods, local healing wells, local folk healers, amateur bleeders or the quacks. For the destitute sick there were the poorhouse hospitals. Very few of the medieval hospitals survived into the 17th century and even fewer of these small institutions for the old or feeble continued into the 18th century.

Thus institutional care for the sick started afresh and it started with the needs of the poor, if only because all others in society could have the necessary medical care in their own homes. For the destitute sick the parish authorities allocated part of the new poorhouses built in the early 18th century.[34] Thus Glasgow's Town's Hospital (1733) and Aberdeen's Poor's Hospital (1739) had beds for the sick poor as had the Paisley Poor House (1743) and the Dumfries Poor House (1753). These institutions had a sombre interior and provided a meagre diet.

In addition to these hospitals, in the 18th century a start was made on institutions primarily to house the non-pauper sick and which were set up by voluntary subscription. These were the new 'infirmaries'. The Royal Infirmary of Edinburgh (1729) was the first in Scotland,[35] but was quickly followed by the Aberdeen Royal

Infirmary (1742).[36] These new voluntary hospitals had a number of functions. They helped in teaching, they were a hostel for patients travelling from far, and they gave institutional care for the sick who were not destitute. Since most medical and surgical care in the 18th century was easily carried out in the home, the teaching and hostel function of these new voluntary hospitals was probably of importance. The managers in Scotland, unlike England, often included some of the medical men, and they drew up rotas for the physicians and surgeons of the town to attend the patients for periods of a few months to a year. From day to day, between visits by these doctors, the routine work was done by the apothecaries who lived on the premises and had a shop or by the medical students attending the hospital while training.[37] Later, the doctors in training took on the burden of these chores and a ladder of seniority and promotion appeared. The nursing services were poor and those employed were often unreliable or dishonest.

The annual report of the voluntary hospital was always an important event, since the managers were responsible to the subscribers for the efficient use of the funds. The clinical results of the treatment were of interest and in the first Report of the Royal Infirmary of Edinburgh a rough statistical review was given, a format used by the proud managers of other hospitals for centuries. The term 'cured' was flexibly employed and often meant 'restored to temporary health'.

Table 4:1

Condition of discharged patients: Edinburgh Royal Infirmary 1729–30

Cured	19
Improved	5
Incurable or dismissed for misbehaviour	5
Died	1
Total	30

Source: Annual reports of the Royal Infirmary of Edinburgh[38]

The Royal Infirmary showed great ingenuity in raising money. Apart from the money from regular subscribers, they charged those patients who could afford to pay, and they were also prepared to look after servants for a fee. Soldiers of the government army were admitted after the 1745 rebellion and had also to be paid for. Other funds were raised by weekly dances, entry money to the hot baths of the Infirmary and the renting out of vacant ward space to medical societies or other bodies. Apart from the hospital there was in some towns also a charitable dispensary and in others, salaried district surgeons had responsibilities for the sick poor.

The first Scottish dispensary appeared in 1776.[39] Andrew Duncan, professor of the institutes of medicine, set up a dispensary for the sick poor in Edinburgh.[40] This was supported by charity and its other object was to provide teaching for the students. Duncan was assisted by a number of colleagues and the service given to the poor by the dispensary even extended to home visits, which were carried out by Duncan's students. Other charitable dispensaries were founded elsewhere – Kelso in 1777, Dundee and Montrose in 1782, Paisley in 1786.

The institutional care of the insane was also slow to appear. Early Scotland had only patchy care for the insane, though the Town's Hospital in Glasgow from 1733 had 'six vaulted cells for mad people, the first of that kind in North Britain'. Robert Fergusson, the poet, died in a stone cell in the Edinburgh poorhouse in 1774. Otherwise the only place for the insane was the prison, or physical restraint in their own home. The first purpose-built mental hospital in Scotland was built in Montrose in 1781 after a spirited local campaign by Susan Carnegie had raised the money. The annual running costs were met by a church collection at the spring communion in Montrose Parish Church.

Thus the institutional provision of health care for the poor was patchy throughout Scotland. Glasgow and Dundee could manage without a voluntary hospital until the end of the century and neither had a dispensary. Only Edinburgh had both a large infirmary and dispensary, and the needs of teaching were as much a stimulus to the appearance of these institutions as were the needs of the patients. The Royal Infirmary in Edinburgh was a crucial innovation, since it was in medical teaching and research that Scotland was to lead the English-speaking world in the 18th century.

The Enlightenment

This rise of Scottish intellectual life is all the more remarkable because of the relative backwardness of Scotland at the beginning of the 18th century. In the Enlightenment Scotland had a particular eminence in philosophy, chemistry and medicine, also producing writers, painters and architects of genius. But in medicine, Scotland and Edinburgh had a particular authority. Out of this came not only successful research but a role in medical education which was to be unchallenged until the late 19th century. Also appearing were new ways of scientific communication in the appearance of the first journals devoted to medical matters, medical societies and a host of standard text books. This achievement in medicine by Scotland shows that cultural factors were amplifying natural ability in an extraordinary way. No less than four of the greatest names in European medicine were born and worked within a few miles and years of each other in the west of Scotland – Cullen, the Hunters and Smellie. Add to this that Tobias Smollett was a surgical apprentice in nearby Glasgow at about the same time, and the case for the investigation of the origins of the Scottish Enlightenment is easily made, and in particular, analysis of the eminence of Scottish medicine during this period.

At first sight, the cultural and political milieu of early 18th century Scotland does not appear to offer the conditions for intellectual growth. The Scottish universities were poor and backward. As late as 1696 a student had been hanged in Edinburgh for blasphemy. The Union of the Parliaments had removed rich and powerful patrons from Edinburgh and even the lesser gentry had returned to the country. There was also in progress a movement against the use of the broad Scots language and this interference in the natural method of communications might normally have been a threat to scientific innovation. This problem was described by David Hume in his famous synopsis of the paradox:

> Is it not strange that, at a time when we have lost our Princes, our Parliaments, our independent Government, even the Presence of our chief Nobility, are unhappy in our accent . . . is it not strange, I say, that, in these Circumstances, we shou'd really be the People most distinguish'd for Literature in Europe?[41]

Lastly, Scotland had largely missed the particularly successful period of European science and medicine in the 17th century and had awakened at a time of rather dreary European theorising and construction of sterile 'systems' to explain disease. Nevertheless, over a period of a few decades, Scotland changed from a relatively backward nation into a significant force in European cultural life.

Prelude

Before the 18th century, medical teaching in Scotland had been haphazard and was not regularly provided for intending physicians by the Scottish universities. Only the surgeons could attend rather half-hearted courses of instruction for the trainee surgeons and apothecaries during their apprenticeship in the town.

The training as a physician started with an M.A. degree taken at a home university followed by a move to the continent. In the early 18th century, Leyden was the favoured place as a result of the fame of Boerhaave who taught medicine as a practical skill, not a theoretical subject. Analysis of the origins of English-speaking Leyden students enrolled in the Boerhaave era from 1709 to 1738 shows the following mix of nationality in 746 foreign students, most of whom had preliminary education at their home university.

Table 4:2

Origins of English-speaking Leyden students studying under Boerhaave 1709–1738

Angli	352
Scoti	244
Hiberni	122
Britanni	7
Colonials	15
'Foreigners'	4
Not stated	2
Total	746

Source: Underwood 1977[42]

The nationalities used in the list show that both English and Scots often preferred their pre-Union title (though many entries in the matriculation album were Anglo-Britannus and Scoto-Britannus). The relatively large number of Scottish students is impressive and meant that a considerable number were leaving Scotland each year to study in Leyden. Their numbers are twice that of Ireland and only a third less than England. Many English students took an Oxford or Cambridge medical degree, but, dissatisfied with their entirely theoretical training there, dealt with this deficiency by practical instruction under Boerhaave.

Table 4:3 shows the pre-medical education and country of origin of those 298 English-speaking Leyden students – about one-third of all Boerhaave's students – who listed a previous university degree. Not all students with such a degree entered the information in the matriculation roll.

Table 4:3
Preliminary university education of Boerhaave's English-speaking students 1709–1738

		Country of origin			
First degree from		*Scoti*	*Angli*	*Hiberni*	*Colonials*
Edinburgh	39	33	5	1	0
Glasgow	29	13	6	10	0
Aberdeen:					
King's	10	10	0	0	0
Marischal	10	8	2	0	0
St Andrews	12	11	1	0	0
Cambridge	83	0	82	0	1
Oxford	56	2	49	3	2
Dublin	59	0	1	57	1

Source: Underwood 1977[43]

The figures are of great interest. The preliminary degree registered gives us some insight into the state of the Scottish universities in the early 18th century and shows that both Glasgow and Edinburgh attracted many students from outside of Scotland, almost certainly dissenters banned from an English or Dublin training by the Test Act. Of the two, Glasgow was the more cosmopolitan, attracting more English and Irish students than Edinburgh.

Thus figures are available to show that large numbers of Scottish students in the early 18th century were being trained in Leyden Europe's best medical school. Many stayed on the continent, or settled in England, but some returned to Scotland to practise. Those who settled in Scotland were probably uninterested in and impatient with the damaging and unproductive religious controversies which had split and hampered the country. They went back to create a new and stimulating intellectual environment and those settling in Edinburgh found that the anxious civic authorities were looking for ways to strengthen the town.

The great era

So successful were the early Scottish medical teachers that by the end of the 18th century Edinburgh and Glasgow were the dominant medical schools in Britain, and Edinburgh could claim to be pre-eminent in Europe from the middle of the century. This remarkable achievement in such a short time can be related to the interaction of a number of factors.[44]

The declining status in Scotland of the Church led many students to seek a career in medicine or law rather than in the Church. Added to this was a softening attitude of the Church towards the new thinking, particularly after the Moderates came to power. The legacy of Calvinism remained, however, and the Scottish students of the 18th century still regarded life as a serious journey during which intellectual effort was required, a view shared by the dissenting students who came from England and America. The philosophy of the highly successful Scottish 'common sense school' also had the assumption that innovations were to be of practical use, an approach which gave medicine an important position in the priorities of the Scottish Enlightenment. The sceptical philosophers of 18th century Scotland looked for comfort in this world rather than reward in the next.[45]

The Union of the parliaments was not of immediate benefit to Scotland, and private medical practice may have declined in Edinburgh after the loss of the rich and powerful men to London. But the later prosperity resulted in a new middle class of merchants and professionals in the 18th century and a need for more trained medical men.[46] With Boerhaave's death in 1738 Leyden lost its popularity with students and thus there was scope for medical teaching in Scotland and England. The decline of latin as a universal language also made the continental universities less attractive. The right conditions for the appearance of new Scottish medical schools thus appeared. The teachers for these new medical schools were immediately available, since Scotland had a cosmopolitan, talented cadre of medical practitioners, educated in Europe in the late 17th and early 18th centuries, ready to teach in the new medical schools.

Apart from the Scottish students, there were others who found a Scottish medical education attractive, since Scotland was the only country which welcomed them. From England, the nonconformists came north, excluded from Oxford and Cambridge. Numerous presbyterian students from Ireland, excluded from Trinity College in Dublin, came to Scotland. Later in the century those from England who would normally have travelled to the continent for further clinical training also came to Scotland, being prevented by the Napoleonic wars from travelling in Europe.

It was important that Scotland had not set up a medical school at St Andrews, as had been planned at the Reformation. A St Andrews medical school would have been a theoretical teaching establishment like Oxford, since no hospital existed nearby and it would undoubtedly have held back or prevented Edinburgh and Glasgow's development as medical schools. Had St Andrews flourished, Scotland's reputation, based on practical clinical teaching in Edinburgh and Glasgow hospitals, might never have appeared.

In Scotland's backward 17th century period no attempt had been made to follow the English example in setting up scientific institutions outside the universities. Bodies such as the Royal Society of London had been founded by scholars as a reaction to the conservatism of the English universities. In 18th century England, these societies competed with the universities and inhibited their growth. By contrast the Scottish societies were slow to appear and by following the rise of the universities did not compete with them.[47]

In Edinburgh (but not in Glasgow), the colleges of surgeons and physicians, for different reasons, did not oppose the rise of the university medical teaching. Medical teaching by the College of Physicians in Edinburgh had been specifically forbidden by their charter, and the Incorporation of Surgeons, as a craft guild linked to the Town Council, dutifully supported the plans for a medical faculty in the Town Council's university. This success in Edinburgh was also made possible by some far-sighted and skilful medical and municipal politicians. Once the medical school was set up, the early years were blessed with professors who worked amicably and in harmony with each other. The noisy disputes and litigation between the doctors in the 17th and 19th centuries were notably absent in the 18th.

Lastly, Scotland's educational system was a factor in producing the talent for the Enlightenment, though the extent of its contribution is far from clear. Certainly a large number of students reached university who would not have done so before and the relatively cheap and short university course was attractive. But analysis of the background of the leaders of the Scottish Enlightenment shows that they were mostly upper-middle-class scholars who might have received higher education in any case.[48] Whether or not they would have been able to travel to the continent for medical education is less clear, and it may be that the educational opportunities within Scotland for poorer children and students helped boost the growing medical school.

Thus the rise of Scottish medicine and medical education can be explained by this amplifying series of factors and Scotland, and Edinburgh in particular, could meet the need for doctors both in Britain and North America at a time when continental education was less attractive and when the status of the Oxford and Cambridge medical schools was declining.

Medical schools

The universities of Aberdeen, Glasgow, Edinburgh and St Andrews made almost simultaneous starts in the early 18th century in setting up teaching. The abolition of the regenting system (the teaching of many subjects by each teacher) started in Scotland in Edinburgh in 1708 and this allowed the rise of specialist posts. Aberdeen's King's College had kept up medical teaching in a small way by the post of 'mediciner' since medieval times and in 1700 a chair of medicine was set up. Patrick Chalmers was appointed to it, but his Jacobite sympathies led to his ejection from it. Though one of his successors, James Gordon, made a determined attempt at clinical teaching from 1734 onwards, expansion at Aberdeen was seriously inhibited by internal feuds between its two universities and the number of students did not rise to significant levels. In St Andrews a start was also made. The Chandos chair of medicine was set up in 1722 and though the first holder Thomas Simson was an enthusiastic teacher, on his death in 1764 his son succeeded him but failed to teach. With no hospital in the town, clinical teaching was also impossible.

Without exception, these early Scottish medical professors had studied at Leyden and they knew what was required to set up successful medical teaching. In Scotland, however, they were mostly unsuccessful: only in Edinburgh, and later in Glasgow, were they to succeed.

In Edinburgh medical education in part had already existed.[49] The training of surgeons had for centuries been met by apprenticeship in the town, and from time to time there had been periods of enthusiasm for communal teaching of these apprentices. The surgeons in Edinburgh had been granted the bodies of some executed criminals each year for dissection as an aid to teaching, and this had been carried out irregularly from medieval times. Another communal teaching project was the herb garden in Edinburgh constructed in 1656 for teaching the apprentices of the newly allied surgeons and apothecaries. This example was followed by others in Edinburgh and by 1704 six physic gardens had been established. Towards the end of the 17th century, there was discontent with the arrangements for the medical education and a number of attempts were made to arrange for teaching. The physicians settling in Edinburgh after their continental education saw a need for local training, and the surgeons found the apprenticeship scheme increasingly unsatisfactory. Various short-lived schemes were set up for teaching and though they did not last they all brought the ultimate solution nearer.

It is not clear if the first attempt in Edinburgh was a serious one. In 1685 the Town Council, temporarily in close alliance not with the surgeons but with the physicians, appointed three talented practitioners as professors of medicine. They were the Leyden-trained Robert Sibbald, James Halket and the unpredictable but gifted Archibald Pitcairne. In spite of these appointments, no organised teaching resulted and the appointments may have been intended as honorary ones from the start: certainly no salary had been proposed for them. The next move was the result of Pitcairne using the Incorporation of Surgeons to organise teaching, since his own College of Physicians had been prevented from teaching by the terms of its charter. Pitcairne had fallen out with the College of Physicians after a religious and political brawl and was also out of sympathy with the Town Council. In 1694 he induced one of the surgeons to claim a supply of bodies for dissection, to which request the Town Council agreed, having been reminded of the ancient corporate rights of the surgeons. The Incorporation of Surgeons, understandably aggrieved, quickly followed with a request of their own to reactivate their supply of bodies for dissection. The Council also agreed to this and added a sensible condition designed to improve teaching in the town. They ruled that a proper anatomical theatre was to be constructed by the surgeons and the surgeons agreed to do so. The last move in the prelude to the appearance of the medical school was that the Town Council agreed to provide a salaried position of professor of anatomy, whose teaching was to be carried out in the new anatomy theatre. Robert Eliot (or Elliot) was appointed to the post, the first of its kind in Britain. Though much of the prompting for these early moves had come from the physicians, the crucial developments which then followed were the result of a joint effort of the surgeons (notably John Monro, father of Monro *primus*) and the Town Council (notably in the person of George Drummond).[50] That the surgeons should be so powerful in Edinburgh is still slightly mysterious, since even in Scotland they had a lowly status and their training was largely by apprenticeship. But a university medical school was not totally irrelevant to their world, since some of the town's surgeons had been to Leyden, an unusual move for surgical training. It may be that the initiative by the Monros was an attempt to raise the status of surgery even higher in Scotland by providing the trainees with a full range of teachers in a university medical school.

The Town Council's interest in a medical school was more obvious. The acute loss of status after the Union of 1707 called for new civic enterprises and the presence of talented men in the town offered one way of restoring the fortunes of the town by creating a medical school. On the appointment of the professor of chemistry in 1713 for instance, the Town Council said that the post was set up because

> through want of professors of physick and chemistry in this kingdome, the youth . . . have been necessitat to travel abroad . . . to the great prejudice of the nation by the necessary charges . . .

This concern was often repeated in the announcement of new university posts thereafter.[51] Occasionally the Council added the hope that students might come from outside of Scotland to Edinburgh, in particular that the dissenters in England who could not be admitted to Oxford and Cambridge, would be attracted. But it was hopeless to train incoming students for the Scottish Church or to practise Scottish law. The only hope was to try to set up a medical school. In this Edinburgh was successful beyond any reasonable expectation.

The power of the Edinburgh Town Council to set up the medical school was unique in Scotland: only in Edinburgh was the university under the control of its local town council. The plan for a medical school was also helped by the absence of any major opposition in the town. Forty years previously the establishment of the College of Physicians in Edinburgh had been opposed by the university and Town Council, but they had been won over by the major concession that the College would not teach medicine. Thus the freedom of the university to set up a medical school had been established and the physicians were pre-empted from acting on their own initiative to set up medical teaching. The other major political force in the city which could have prevented the appearance of the university medical school was the Incorporation of Surgeons, reunited with the apothecaries in 1721. But they had links as a craft with the Town Council and some of the leading surgeons were behind the moves towards the medical school. Thus the surgeons did not oppose the university and Town Council in their plans for a medical school.

In the moves towards the medical school the Town Council's interests were represented by George Drummond (1687–1766) who in his frequent spells of public office in Edinburgh, notably as Provost, proved to be the town's greatest benefactor. Apart from promoting the medical faculty, he also planned the New Town of Edinburgh and it was said that

> from the year 1715 to the time of his death in 1766, nothing was done in regard to the College [i.e. the university] without his advice or direction. His care of the University not only extended to an accurate investigation how its funds were expended but he was of more essential service to procuring men of real talents to be appointed as Professors.[52]

It was said that, in the course of the fifty years during which he managed the city, he appointed all the professors.

The other person who played an important role in the early days of the medical school was John Monro (1670–1740), a surgeon educated as an apprentice but thereafter trained at Leyden and Padua. He was Deacon of the surgeons corporation from 1712–14 and a town councillor. Monro and Drummond, in a long and elaborate series of patient negotiations and appointments, developed the medical school into one which was to lead Europe. To pre-empt opposition to a medical school and win the approval of the numerous and highly sensitive factions of the medical men in Edinburgh took time and considerable political skill.

The first step came when a Mr David Cockburn requested the university in 1705 to grant him the ancient but previously unused degree of Doctor of Medicine (M.D.):[53] many think Monro pushed him forward as the first pawn's move. The university felt unable to grant the degree without help and requested the College of Physicians to examine the candidate instead and to report. The College agreed to do so, reported favourably, and Cockburn was made the first graduate in medicine of the university. Similar awards were made in the following years and the university began to be represented in the examination committee, helped by the appointment of James Crauford to a chair of physic and chemistry in 1713, an appointment planned by Principal Carstares, an admirer of Dutch education during his exile there. Cautiously the university took over the initiative and organised the M.D. examination with less and less help from the College. Monro then moved to strengthen the university teaching. He organised a vacancy in 1720 in the Town's chair of anatomy – both the joint holders mysteriously resigning – and he arranged for his son Alexander (Monro *primus*) to be placed in it. But, on the announcement of the new appointment, the chair now appeared as it had never done previously, as a joint Town Council and University chair: thus again the university teaching was strengthened. One unexpected event also helped. After a grave-robbing scandal in 1725, a mob attacked the anatomy rooms in Surgeons' Hall and Monro removed himself and his teaching to the safety of the university. Anatomy was now being taught within the university.

In 1726 the Town Council, at the prompting of the College of Physicians, declared that a school of medicine should be set up in the town teaching 'medicine in all its branches'. Thus the important agreement was reached that a group of teachers rather than one anatomy professor was required. The argument used was again that the Edinburgh students would have no need to travel and that students might be attracted in to Edinburgh. Alternatively it may be that the Council was concerned at the appearance of other teachers in Edinburgh and hurried to set up a group with official status.

Thus the medical faculty was formed in February 1726. A petition from four teachers of medicine in the city proposing a medical faculty in the university with themselves as professors was accepted by the Town Council. John Monro was patron to this group: even the wording of the petition may have been his. Alexander Monro was relieved, having thought that he had to do all the teaching as professor of anatomy and 'for though he would not disobey his father, yet he thought the task designed to be imposed too great for him to bear'. The first appointments were of John Rutherford and Andrew Sinclair to be professors of the theory of medicine and Andrew Plummer and John Innes as professors of medicine and chemistry. These four and Alexander Monro now formed a formal medical faculty within the university. John Monro's plan was complete. Success did not come immediately and the teaching of some of the subjects was unsatisfactory. But the faculty existed and success came later.

Throughout the century the Monros continued their dominance. Alexander Monro *primus* (1697–1767) son of John Monro taught until 1756, when his son Alexander Monro *secundus* (1733–1817) took over, handing over the chair to Alexander Monro *tertius* (1773–1859) in 1804. Only with this fourth Monro did the nepotism fail.

An idea of the rapid growth of the Edinburgh medical school can be gained by the figures for the enrolment in the anatomy class, as shown in Table 4:4

Table 4:4
Number of students enrolled in the Edinburgh anatomy class 1720–1800

1720		57
1730		83
1740		130
1750		158
1760–70	(Annual average)	194
1770–80	,, ,,	287
1780–90	,, ,,	342
1790–1800	,, ,,	over 400

Source: Struthers[54]

Those who took the class intended to be physicians or were surgical or apothecaries' apprentices from the town. The figures should be treated with caution in concluding anything about the output of trained practitioners, since not only did some students attend the class twice but lay people were welcomed to the lecture course. However the figures are close to the number of student tickets sold for attendance at the Royal Infirmary. 104 tickets were sold in 1742 and in 1751 the number had risen to 150, and one can conclude that these were the number of serious students of medicine in these years.

The earliest students were from Scotland, but success meant that many others were attracted, particularly as the lecture courses were relatively cheap and no religious tests were applied to applicants. The non-residential university was also attractive to the young men who disliked the residential restrictions elsewhere. Nor were there any language difficulties and Monro *primus* boldly lectured in English, one of the first Edinburgh professors to do so.

Information on the origins of the students is not available except for the minority who chose to graduate M.D. Of those who did so between the years 1726–1799, the country of origin is shown in Table 4:5

Table 4:5

Country of origin of Edinburgh M.D. graduates 1726–1799

Scots	237
North America and West Indies	195
English	254
Irish	280
European	26
Others	143

Source: Sloan[55]

These numbers confirm the attractiveness of Edinburgh and the great range of students appearing for medical education. To the Scots it meant that intending physicians no longer had to travel to the continent and that the surgical apprentices had splendid local teaching in subjects of interest to them. The students could be young apprentices, or those just finished an M.A. degree or were older practitioners who returned to add formal teaching to practical skills. The Irish students appeared since they were banned from Dublin or English education and came instead to Scotland. English students looked north since Edinburgh was anxious to take the nonconformist students denied entry to Oxford and Cambridge. The students of North America, many of them Quakers, came from Virginia, South Carolina and Pennsylvania.[56]

The attraction of Edinburgh to the American students was, perhaps, not only the prospect of a fine medical education:

> Just as the literati of Scotland had viewed themselves as provincials when they encountered the urbane culture of London's drawing rooms, men concerned with the life of the mind in Philadelphia, Boston and New York probably had a similar reaction. Thus they admired the Scots for their unique success in creating a culture that was both national and cosmopolitan; they yearned for a comparable development in America.[57]

Benjamin Rush, who visited London after study in Edinburgh and made the acquaintance of Samuel Johnson must have been hurt when ridiculed by the lexicographer, 'I am willing to love all mankind except an American,' said Johnson of the meeting. The only time that the American students were less than welcome in Edinburgh was at the time of the War of Independence when the Scots reacted to the events with solidarity with England. The American visitors shut themselves in their rooms when new American victories were announced to avoid the reproaches of the Scots.

The Edinburgh professors were paid a small basic salary or nothing at all, and charged each student a fee for the course of lectures. In the 1796 session the income from these sources for some of the professors in the university is shown in Table 4:6 and it emphasises that the anatomy class was still the most lucrative.

This system of payment by results was vigorously upheld by the Scottish *literati*. Of the class fee system, Adam Smith gave a typical defence:

> I have satisfied myself that the present state of degradation and contempt into which the greater part of these [European and English universities] have fallen arises principally from the large salaries which in some universities are given to professors and which render them altogether independent of their diligence and success in their profession.[58]

In addition, the Scottish professors also had an income from giving board and lodging in their homes to students, a practice universal among the teachers, physicians and surgeons, and one which must have greatly benefited the students and pleased the parents of these young men. Joseph Black, while a student in Edinburgh, stayed in the house of the professor of philosophy. It could be costly and rich parents might be charged up to £40 for a year's board and lodging. The professors also earned handsome publishers' fees for their textbooks. Table 4:6 also shows that the number of students taking each subject of the medical school varied considerably. Since no formal curriculum existed the numerous apprentices in surgery and pharmacy, and the intending physicians and interested lay persons who joined these classes, chose a mixture of courses to suit their needs.

Table 4:6

Teaching income of some Edinburgh university professors 1796

Chair	*Salary*	*Class Fee*	*Persons in Class*
	£	gn	
Logic	52	2	87
Moral philosophy	102	3	95
Institutes of medicine	0	3	97
Anatomy	50	3	326
Midwifery	0	3	126
Materia medica	0	3	66
Chemistry	0	3	253

Source: Chitnis[59].

Thus an unusual situation had developed which had been in existence from the early days of the medical school. Though the medical teachers were within a university, there was no curriculum and each teacher was paid only by the students he attracted: in spite of this the degree of M.D. could be awarded to anyone after finishing a medical course of their own choosing. While elsewhere in Britain the surgical apprenticeship or physicians training was rigorously laid down and the students had no control over what was taught, the *Lernfreiheit* in Edinburgh was not only flexible but was ultimately controlled by the students through their financial approval of individual teachers.[60] This anarchy in the teaching proved to be highly successful and many of the stars of the Edinburgh medical school had taken unorthodox courses of study, of whom the most notable was Cullen. But it must have been less successful in other cases and the university's willingness to grant the optional M.D. to virtually any student at the end of minimal training or to those established in medical practice who wrote back to Edinburgh for it was to cause trouble later.

This curious structure of the medical school ensured that the students played a vigorous part in the new medical school and the presence of many older men and their cosmopolitan origins made the student body responsive and articulate. The students organised themselves into a number of societies which also drew in many members of staff. The most notable of these was the serious-minded Royal Medical Society (founded 1734) which met on Saturday nights, having circulated the paper to be discussed ahead of the meeting.[61] The students were active in their own interests and successfully joined the complex negotiations which successfully attracted Cullen from Glasgow. Later they urged that room should also be made for Black to return to Edinburgh.

Such was the cohesion of the medical school and the mutual interest of the teachers in keeping up their income that the century apparently passed without serious disruption of the structure of the medical school: even the '45 rebellion caused hardly a ruffle in work.[62]

In the rise of the Edinburgh medical school, the building of the Royal Infirmary was a crucial factor, and as suggested earlier it was built as part of the plan for teaching medicine in Edinburgh. The poorhouse hospitals of Scotland were largely refuges for the old and feeble, and were unsuitable for teaching. Of the university towns St Andrews did not have the potential for a large hospital, and the poorhouse hospital built in Glasgow remained in the hands of the town doctors, who declined to accept university teaching. Aberdeen had a suitable voluntary hospital opened in 1742, but the university failed to exploit it. Only in Edinburgh was the ideal realised and again only because of the planning skills of a small number of persons. In the origins of this new hospital, John Monro and George Drummond can be seen at work again. It was they who ensured that the new hospital was part of the new medical school.

The first moves towards a hospital in Edinburgh came with the appearance of an anonymous pamphlet in 1721, probably written by the Monros, calling for a hospital.[63] The motives, as far as can be judged from the pamphlet, were charitable, economic and educational:

> As men and Christians we have the strongest inducements and even obligations to this sort of charity . . . That humanity and compassion naturally prompt us to relieve our fellow creatures when in such deplorable circumstances as many are reduced to, naked, starving and in utmost distress from pain and trouble of the body and anguish of the soul: that as relief of these is a duty, so it is no less advantage to the nation, for as many as are recovered in an Infirmary are so many working hands gained to the country: that students of physic and surgery might hereby have rather a better and easier opportunity of experience than they have had by studying abroad, where such hospitals are, at great charge to themselves, and a yearly loss to the nation.

This first effort failed, but a second attempt was successful, largely because it was sponsored by the Royal College of Physicians. Together with George Drummond, then in one of his spells as Lord Provost, they raised £2,000, including help from a special collection throughout Scotland's parish churches. A small hospital with six beds was opened.[64] The first patient to be admitted on 6th August 1729 to the new Infirmary was a girl with anaemia from Caithness.

The hospital was not big enough from the start and, spurred by a threat from the surgeons to run their own hospital, a new financial appeal, again supported by donations from throughout Scotland and elsewhere in the world, raised enough to open the new Royal Infirmary in 1741. No less than £379 was donated by the Quakers of the north of England. The grand scale of the plan for 228 beds exceeded Edinburgh's local needs and clearly allowed for the needs of teaching, as well as the treatment of the sick gathered from a distance. Scotland's much travelled doctors would have seen the enormous Hôtel Dieu hospital in Paris, but the model for Edinburgh came from the small hospital at Leyden. Even so the eventual size of the Edinburgh Royal Infirmary was huge and it seems likely that it was planned to use the hospital as a hostel for patients from all over Scotland, who would have difficulty finding accommodation in Edinburgh.[65]

The physicians and surgeons of the town took it in rotation to treat the patients and to teach the students of medicine. Clinical teaching became more firmly established in 1748 when John Rutherford was appointed to give formal clinical lectures based on individual patients. The Edinburgh medical school was thus developed along the lines that Boerhaave had pioneered: his textbooks were used by the clinical professors.

Glasgow failed to equal the early eminence or growth of the Edinburgh medical school, yet the circumstances in Glasgow were similar, indeed apparently more favourable than those in Edinburgh.[66] The University of Glasgow had a constitution which allowed for the teaching of medicine: the strong single Faculty of Physicians and Surgeons might seem to have been an advantage. Talented men like Cullen and Black emerged to teach in Glasgow and the area had also produced the Hunters and Smellie. Moreover Glasgow prospered in the 18th century and, though its population was initially smaller than Edinburgh, it increased rapidly. In 1703 the power of Glasgow to grant the degree of M.D. was tested in exactly the way in which Edinburgh had been started on its way towards a medical school.[67] In that year Samuel Benion, a nonconformist minister from Shropshire and an M.A. of Glasgow, applied for the M.D. degree and was granted it after an examination.

The reasons for the failure of the Glasgow medical school to thrive in the same way as Edinburgh are of interest and illuminate the skill of the Edinburgh pioneers. The obstacles to similar developments at Glasgow were in the university itself, the lack of a hospital and the opposition of the Faculty of Physicians and Surgeons in Glasgow.

In the early part of the 18th century, Glasgow University was thriving as a training ground for the large numbers of new ministers required for the restored Church, but it was in the hands of strict presbyterians who took their instructions from the General Assembly of the Church of Scotland and clearly hoped for a return to the old days of Calvinism. The new thinking on the continent and England did not interest them, which along with the new secular medical practice and research, were regarded as dangerous. The Assembly looked in vain for even one text of philosophy suitable for the universities but found only unsuitable material. They concluded that:

> For Cartesius, Rohault and others of his gang beside what may be said against their doctrine, they labour under this inconveniency that they give not any sufficient account of the . . . old philosophy which must not be ejected.[68]

Only slowly and with difficulty was this direct interference of the Church thrown off by the universities; a Parliamentary Commission of 1727 finally accomplished this. Edinburgh University had from the start been run by the Town Council and hence was not liable to this direction by the Church. Nor was it so concerned with training men for the ministry.

Glasgow however did make a start of the teaching of medicine in appointing John Johnstoun to the chair of medicine in 1714 – the same chair abolished by the Church in 1646. Their other appointment in the same year may have been a mistake. Thomas Brisbane was elected in 1720 to the combined chair of botany and anatomy, but it then appeared that he considered that his duties were mainly to teach botany and it also emerged that he had considerable distaste for anatomical dissection – the essential subject for the early medical schools. The students appealed to the Principal to intervene and arrange for anatomical teaching, but in a crucial decision he declined to confront Brisbane. In Glasgow there was another problem. There was opposition to the development of university medical teaching by the Faculty of Physicians and Surgeons who felt that they alone should supervise the training of surgeons and the licensing of physicians in Glasgow. They could also claim that they provided the necessary teaching, though it was irregular and lacked continuity. The medical professors appointed to Glasgow University were also practitioners in the town and usually good Faculty members: their first loyalty was to the Faculty.

The next problem was that there was no sizeable hospital in Glasgow to support clinical teaching. Though the Town's Hospital was largely a poorhouse, it did have some beds for the sick and had a small operating/lecture theatre, but it was run by the town's doctors and they made few moves towards teaching.

It is little surprise, therefore, that Cullen, Black and others after successfully teaching small numbers of students in Glasgow were attracted from there to the new opportunities in Edinburgh, taking with them their loyal students. Cullen went in 1756 and Black in 1766. Both found private medical practice irksome and diverting, and Cullen complained of the time spent on long visits to patients in the country. On the other hand teaching could pay well and success in Edinburgh could reward them without interfering with scholarship.

In Edinburgh a new scientific community with associated societies and publications grew up round the nucleus of the medical faculty whilst in Glasgow this was delayed. It was, however, recorded that William Hunter once proposed to Cullen that they and Black should return to Glasgow and set up a medical faculty which would rival Edinburgh. It is not known if this was a serious suggestion, but if so, it is interesting to speculate on the fame of a school headed by such a triumvirate.

Influence abroad

The great output of the Scottish medical schools in the 18th century and later made the Scottish doctors prominent in medical practice throughout the world, notably in the armed forces and in the design and operation of new medical schools of Britain, Europe, the Empire and beyond. No other medical school competed with the Scottish output and their broad training in medicine and surgery also made them qualified to lead. Looking at the influence on America alone,[69] it is calculated that in the 100 years of the Edinburgh medical school after 1750, there were 650 students from North America graduated M.D. plus an unknown number who merely took the classes: about 60 Americans graduated in Glasgow in the last half of the 18th century.[70] Thus the American link was the most striking one and it arose from the emigration from Scotland and North America which had occurred earlier and continued. In the 17th and 18th centuries, many Scots and Scots-Irish left their native land for a better life or were banished after the rebellions, and became prominent in America, tending to settle in the less developed Middle Atlantic and Southern States where they were joined by others involved in the new trade acoss the Atlantic.

The first Scottish practitioner traced to America was John Johnston, an apothecary from Edinburgh, born in 1661 who settled in New York. The first physician noted was Cadwallader Colden from Duns, who settled first in Philadelphia in 1708. To these early physicians fell a number of tasks in the community – the practice of medicine and the development of the educational system, and often also the politics of the colonies. Moreover, they continued to look to Scotland for renewal of their intellectual life and in the mid-1700s this link was supervised by Benjamin Franklin who gave the Americans letters of introduction to Edinburgh.[71] This link is seen most clearly in the rise of the small schools and colleges like New Jersey College (later to be Princeton University) which in 1768 persuaded a presbyterian minister from Edinburgh, John Witherspoon, to be its President. The man who recruited him was Benjamin Rush, then studying medicine in Edinburgh, and both he and Witherspoon were to sign the Declaration of Independence. Curiously enough, another Edinburgh medical graduate, John Fothergill, on whose advice Franklin relied in medical matters, exerted himself in London towards a peaceful solution of the American problem. To the young Americans, Scotland was attractive, not only as the land of their origins, but because of the Scottish political and religious toleration then appearing and in Edinburgh the Quakers also made them feel at home. The Edinburgh teaching was unrivalled and the only criticisms by the students was that the success of Edinburgh resulted in crowding at the clinical teaching sessions and their resulting inability to teach anatomy in the 'Paris' manner, namely allowing the students to do dissection. Many, therefore, took extra time to visit and study in London – 'walking the wards' – and taking extra private anatomy classes with the Hunters or the other respected private teachers George Fordyce and William Hewson, both of whom were trained in Scotland.

The first medical school in America was the Medical Department of the College of Philadelphia, and it was designed and staffed entirely by Edinburgh graduates. William Shippen and John Morgan, who had been in Edinburgh in 1761 and 1763 respectively, set it up in 1765 and were joined by Rush and Adam Kuhn, who had studied in Edinburgh in 1767. Even the design of the hospital used for clinical teaching, the Pennsylvania Hospital, was based on the Edinburgh Royal Infirmary. The second medical school in America was King's College New York, now Columbia University and opened in 1767. The moving spirit in this venture was an Edinburgh graduate, Samuel Bard, and four of the six founder professors were from Edinburgh. In the American War of Independence, the Edinburgh graduates took the highest ranks in the medical services, as did Edinburgh medical men in the British forces. One Scots surgeon even fought against the British Army in two different wars and for two different causes. Hugh Mercer of Aberdeen was in the Prince's army in the '45 and fled to America after Culloden. Under Washington, he was made a Brigadier-General and died at the battle of Princeton.

Adam Mabane, a Scottish surgeon's mate on the staff of General Amherst was first to settle in Canada and the first Canadian to return for training in Scotland did not do so until 1793 when John MacCulloch travelled to Edinburgh from Sarnia.[72] The first Canadian medical school was the Montreal Medical Institution and the founders had all studied at Edinburgh: even the French l'Ecole de Médecine et de Chirurgie was set up in 1843 by five Edinburgh graduates. McGill University had started teaching medicine in 1832. Its founder and financial patron had been James McGill, a merchant from Glasgow.

The Scottish medical men reached all parts of the world.[73] One of the first of Scottish practitioners to respond to Tsar Peter's 1702 appeal for craftsmen and professional men to help the reconstruction of Russia was a Scottish surgeon, Robert Erskine.[74] Later the Russian health services were reorganised in the 18th century by Alexander Crichton. William Stokes was later to do the same in Ireland. South Africa, New Zealand, South America and Australia all had pioneers from Scotland, as had India and South America. The broad self-chosen Scottish medical curriculum encouraged scholars with interests well beyond narrow professionalism, ranging from Roget (of *Thesaurus* fame) to Mungo Park the explorer, and the eccentric 'Balloon' Tytler, the Edinburgh surgeon who pasted together the scrappy first editions of the *Encyclopaedia Britannica*. In botany the early students of medicine or arts travelling to or returning to America put to use their training and gave their names to a number of species – Colden (coldenia), Alexander Garden (gardenia), J R Poinset (poinsettia), Caspar Wistar (wisteria), and John Mitchell (mitchella repens). Numerous other students achieved fame in other fields having studied only briefly in Edinburgh as part of a general education – notably Oliver Goldsmith.

The Edinburgh medical school seems also to have been attractive to radical political thinkers and the American fathers warned their student sons that there were many dangerous notions around in Edinburgh 'which would normally be a bar to public confidence'. The list of political activists among the medical students is impressive – Rush, the signatory to the American Declaration of Independence, Thomas Emmet, an Irish Nationalist eventually imprisoned in Fort George near Inverness and whose younger brother Robert was hanged in 1803, Joseph Bassas de Roger, a Spanish refugee and perhaps the most dangerous of all, Jean Paul Marat, who may have taken an orthodox period of study at Edinburgh under the assumed name of John White.[75] Many of the Edinburgh students later supported the French Revolution, and this forced Thomas Beddoes to resign from his Oxford Chair. William Maxwell, Robert Burns' friend and doctor had even been in the escort taking Louis XVI to the guillotine.[76]

Influence within Britain

The Scottish universities were increasingly providing an education which was not only advanced and based on sceptical philosophy and scientific methods, but also cut across the traditional divisions within the medical men's ranks. In the Scottish medical schools the students were choosing classes which trained them in both surgery and medicine and the university was prepared to grant the degree of M.D. to these strange hybrid healers while in England the physicians continued to have an increasingly outdated Oxford or Cambridge university training with surgeons continuing to be trained as apprentices. In one area this new type of Scottish graduate was particularly successful. The Scottish medical training was of value to the army, navy and the East India Company, all of which were increasing in size and faced considerable health problems in their foreign ventures. The medical services of these organisations became largely staffed by Scotsmen, and in particular those from Edinburgh. This success of the Scottish doctors in the armed forces was not only the result of their broadly based education and their ability to cope with the new complexity of warfare and exploration. Their success as physicians and surgeons to the armies and navies arose from the unexpected outlet that it gave for their investigative skills and the scientific attitudes gained from the lectures of their famous professors. Paradoxically while the professors had little scope for experimentation or trials of public health measures, in the armed forces the situation was different. The problems of disease were increasing and the value of preserving the trained men in an increasingly sophisticated army and navy was being realised. Thus the navy went to sea for longer periods and the mortality from scurvy on these voyages was alarming to the authorities: the armies were larger and the death rates even in camp or barracks were increasing. To meet these problems, the authoritarian nature of the armed forces gave the opportunity to medical men for prolonged observation of human patients and gave them opportunities for treatment and prevention. Ironically, while the Scottish medical teachers achieved little themselves in the treatment of disease and could not even begin the necessary work of public health, their pupils in the army and navy managed to innovate in both areas.[77] Thus Lind's discovery of the curative and preventive value of lime and lemon in scurvy was as the result of careful scientific trials and must be the only significant therapeutic innovation of the 18th century which was not derived from folk medicine or the quacks, and was the application of pure reason, albeit to a man-made problem. The second major advance by the Scottish military men was the introduction of sanitary and other preventive methods by Pringle, Blane and Trotter. These changes revolutionised the health of the forces.

James Lind (1716–1794) was a native of Edinburgh and had studied medicine there.[78] His careful observations on the navy's worst disease were made when physician to the Naval Hospital at Haslar. He urged the use of lemon juice in preventing scurvy, advice that the dilatory Admiralty eventually took. He also published work on the necessity of sanitary arrangements and hygiene. In this, he was largely following the pioneering work of Pringle in the army. Sir John Pringle (1707–1782) was an Edinburgh student in 1727 and practised in Edinburgh.[79] At the age of 35 he became an army physician and eventually Physician-General to the army under Cumberland, in which capacity he returned to Scotland against the forces of Prince Charles. The death rate in the army for reasons not related to fighting was increasing and his introduction of elementary sanitation and hygiene made great reductions in this loss. These methods were described in his classic work on sanitation and prevention of disease *Observations on the Diseases of the Army* (1752). He was also responsible for successfully proposing the concept that the wounded on each side in war should be protected from attack, a principle later enshrined in the Geneva Convention.

In addition to the medical men of the armed forces, there were increasing numbers of Scottish graduates practising in England, and frequently clusters of trained medical men re-created in England the Edinburgh environment by founding scientific societies and debating clubs. Of these the best known and influential was the Birmingham Lunar Society and which included Scottish-trained men like William

Withering, Erasmus Darwin, James Watt, James Keir and Matthew Boulton and into whose company were drawn Joseph Priestley, Baskerville the printer and Josiah Wedgwood. Lastly, there were medical students who turned to science and technology like William Roebuck, who was a successful chemist in Manchester, but returned to construct the first blast furnace in Scotland, and Thomas Beddoes who, after his resignation from the chair of chemistry at Oxford, set up the Pneumatic Institute in Bristol which employed Humphry Davy.

Publishing

There were many other products of this great period of self-confidence and radicalism in Edinburgh and a stream of books, many of which were published in Edinburgh, was one feature of the 18th century. The medical teachers had great success with their treatises and Cullen's book on medical practice became a standard text.[80] As well as the successful medical books by these teachers and the texts by their pupils like Lind, Trotter and Pringle, two others can be noted which had vast influence and significance beyond their immediate readership. The first was a complication of drugs, the Edinburgh *Pharmacopoeia*. The second was a popular treatise on health care, Buchan's *Domestic Medicine*.

The Edinburgh *Pharmacopoeia* was first published in 1699 and in the next 110 years went through ten editions in latin and two editions in English.[81] Though not the first of its kind, it became one of the most authoritative. The full title was the *Pharmacopoeia of the Royal College of Physicians of Edinburgh* and later in 1864 it joined the London and Dublin *Pharmacopoeias* to become the *British Pharmacopoeia*. As described previously the early editions of this Edinburgh work merely recorded and encouraged the absurd polypharmacy of the 17th century, but by 1756, at a time when the Edinburgh Medical School had reached the peak of its reputation and the physicians' status was secure, the *Pharmacopoeia* was cleared of many of the more ludicrous remedies and the fame of the book rose with this break with the past. Strong criticism of the old prescriptions had come from the new leaders of the medical faculty in Edinburgh and their embarrassment with the text led to the cull. Professor Alston also had some acid comments to make. Of the use of burnt live toad, he asked that

> these innocent animals be killed before they are burnt . . . for I assure you the powder will be none the worse for it. Is not burnt mouse as good as burnt toad?[82]

In the 1756 edition, the number of animal extracts had also been reduced from 47 to 27, and many of the more outrageous remedies removed. By 1774 this process was almost complete, though the millepede powder remained till 1800. The number of drugs of some value steadily increased, though the compilers had many problems of judging efficacy. Thus digitalis, one of the most effective drugs known, had appeared in the first edition, was dropped from the fourth in 1774, but reappeared permanently in 1783, doubtless gaining a reputation for toxicity through the difficulty in preparing extracts of constant potency. The *Pharmacopoeia* had great influence and was preferred by many to other similar compendia. The 1772 edition was pirated by a London publisher and there were latin editions printed in ten different European cities, together with Dutch and German translations. The *Pharmacopoeia* of the Massachusetts Medical Society, published in 1808, acknowledged that it was adapted from the Edinburgh book, with 'little variation from that excellent work', and the Massachusetts *Pharmacopoeia* in turn went on to be adopted almost entirely as the first *United States Pharmacopoeia*.

The second publication of lasting fame arising from the Edinburgh medical school at the time of the Enlightenment was William Buchan's *Domestic Medicine* of 1769.[83] The intention of the author was in 'laying medicine more open to mankind'. In this Buchan was opposed by his colleagues since, as we have seen from the *Pharmacopoeia*, much of the emphasis of early 18th century medical practice was based on obscurantism and baffling over-elaboration of prescribing in an attempt to secure medical practice as a profession. Buchan's philosophy took the opposite direction since he attempted to explain simply to the general public the theory and treatment of disease. Indeed, his attitude was quite anti-professional: 'Sensible nurses often know disease better than those bred to physic.' The book appeared in numerous editions for almost a hundred years, only disappearing in Britain in 1846. It was translated into seven languages and enjoyed an even longer life in America, where it lasted until 1913 having outsold its 18th century rival, John Wesley's *Primitive Physic*. Buchan was probably helped greatly in preparing its first edition by his publisher William Smellie, the compiler of the early *Encyclopaedia Britannica*, another product of the Scottish Enlightenment. Buchan, disappointed at failing to obtain a chair in Edinburgh, moved to London. He achieved immortality by his work and was buried in Westminster Abbey.

Buchan met the new mood of the Enlightenment and the desire for knowledge of a practical nature. He fell foul of the colleges in doing so, since they had a vested interest in convincing the general public of the advantages of their orthodoxy and preferred the secrecy of latin prescription to Buchan's openness. In one other aspect, the book was revolutionary. It was characterised by emphasis on sanitary principles and the prevention of disease and in this it drew heavily on the teachings of Pringle in his text *Observations on the Diseases of the Army*. Buchan took Pringle's recommendation to the armed forces of clean clothing, elementary sanitation, ventilation and the prevention of overcrowding and applied it to civilian life. Buchan emphasised that, in dealing with sick patients, a change of clothes and bed clothing was desirable, and that the doctor should make a habit of washing his hands. The section on child health is particularly sensible and far-sighted 'almost one half of the human species perish in infancy by neglect,' he stated, and his recommendations included simple hygiene and education of the mothers. Buchan also showed concern for occupational disease and in particular drew attention to the plight of the Scottish miners.

The third edition of his book in 1774 also called for public health measures:

> We are sorry indeed to observe that the power of the magistrate is very seldom exerted in this country for the preservation of health. The importance of a proper medical police is either not understood or very little regarded.

Despite this early concern, there was little Scottish or English concern for public health for a century, but in Germany the cameralist tradition was continued when Johann Frank published his proposals for a medical police who would act to prevent or deal with problems of public health. Even Adam Smith did not discuss the need for a healthy work force. Only when epidemics returned in Britain was anything done. However, Buchan's book may have been read by those who were to be the sanitary reformers of the 19th century.[84]

Thus the Enlightenment gave Edinburgh a tradition of publishing that was to last into the 20th century. Edinburgh was also to be the home later of a pharmaceutical and instrument-making industry of whose products the microscopes were particularly successful.[85]

Scientific Societies

In the 17th century, scientific communities in Europe had developed from learned academies, rather than from universities, but because of the delay in the start of the Scottish revival, Scotland's scientific community started in the university and spread out.[86] This was fortunate since the new societies helped rather than hindered the university and ensured a close scientific group. The first purely clinical society for the doctors was the Medical Society in Edinburgh in 1731. It immediately expressed a concern for the number of medical texts available and encouraged the publication of research in 'a page or two', thus producing 'more authors and fewer books'. Their product was the first successful medical periodical in Britain – *Medical Essays and Observations*.[87] The students' Royal Medical Society followed in 1734 and of the general scientific societies, the Philosophical Society of 1737, (later the Royal Society of Edinburgh), and the Edinburgh Select Society (1754) were enormously successful in a town fond of debate and formal and informal conviviality. All these societies amplified the output and achievement of the university and medical school. In Glasgow the growth of similar organisations was slow, but they appeared at the end of the century.

Medical men

The reputation of the early period of the Edinburgh medical school had resulted from excellent teaching by Leyden-trained Scottish surgeons and physicians. In the later 18th century this Scottish reputation for teaching was added to by the conduct of highly original research in Edinburgh and Glasgow. This second wave of medical teachers and scientists was largely trained in Scotland. Of new Fellows of the Edinburgh College of Physicians in 1680–1710, 80% had been trained abroad: in the period 1750–1770, it was only 15%.

By the middle of the century Edinburgh was at the height of its fame and the city was dominated by the professional men and the *literati*. In the absence of a Court, Privy Council or Parliament, there was instead an aristocracy of intellectuals thrown together in a small town and nightly forced out of their insanitary houses into a convivial tavern life. The broad friendship of this group, their mutual affection and the breadth of their authority is illustrated by events during the last illness of David Hume, the great philosopher, whose scepticism encouraged much of the other endeavours of the Scottish Enlightenment. In this illness, Hume was looked after by William Cullen: Sir John Pringle in London was also consulted and was involved with the treatment.[88] A journey to the spa at Bath was decided upon, though Hume was characteristically unconvinced that any good might result. On the painful journey south, the group met John Home, the playwright, and Adam Smith hurrying north because of the news of the serious state of Hume's health. At Bath, Hume was examined by John Hunter. Hume died shortly after his return to Edinburgh and in his last days was attended by Joseph Black. Before his death, James Boswell repeatedly visited the house in the expectation that the philosopher would accept the existence of God at the last. The reputation of the Edinburgh medical school in the mid-18th century rests largely on the teaching and research of Joseph Black (1728–99) and William Cullen (1710–90). The high regard in which Cullen was held is perhaps difficult to justify immediately. Certainly he was highly thought of as a teacher. His textbook of medicine was used until the 19th century, and his concern for his pupils and their affection for him is clear in the considerable correspondence between them. But Cullen is not asssociated with any major research discovery nor did he promote any lasting insight into disease or therapy. The part that he played was a more subtle one.[89] His first contribution was to continue the reform of the Edinburgh *Pharmacopoeia*. His second contribution was his ability to encourage talented colleagues and promote their work. It was Cullen who brought William Hunter into partnership with him in Hamilton and encouraged him to go to London for further training. It was Cullen who encouraged and supervised Joseph Black's crucial early research in Glasgow and helped him later in Edinburgh. Cullen's other claim was an unusual one. He successfully resisted the application to clinical work of the philosophical attitudes of the stars of the Enlightenment around him, notably the inductive methods of the Scottish philosophers, applied so successfully to chemistry by Black. Cullen realised correctly that insights into disease mechanisms and therapy were unlikely until the pedestrian job of classification and systematisation was accomplished. In the event, this was not even started until a century later and Cullen's own attempt using methods similar to those of Linnaeus in botany, are now forgotten.

Perhaps Joseph Black also sensed that in clinical medicine little progress was possible, and his incisive mind found a challenge in chemistry instead.[90] His first great discovery arose indirectly out of a project on lime-water started in Glasgow using the methods taught to him by Cullen. On moving to finish his medical studies in Edinburgh, Black continued to consult Cullen about the work but finding that the same project was also being investigated by his professors, Robert Whytt and Charles Alston, Black changed to another problem to avoid the slightly acrimonious debate between his teachers. With only a short time left to complete his thesis for graduation, he chose to look instead at magnesia alba (magnesium carbonate) and showed that its loss of weight after heating was the result of the loss of 'fixed air'. This discovery of carbon dioxide can be said to have initiated the modern era of chemistry.[91] The work was written up hurriedly in time for graduation and was modestly placed second to a description of the control of gastric acidity, added to pad out the otherwise slim work which Black feared had no clinical relevance. Black soon returned to Glasgow to take Cullen's place. There he demonstrated the phenomenon of latent heat, a finding brilliantly exploited later by James Watt, then employed in Glasgow, in the construction of his revolutionary steam engine.

Medical science

But while chemistry was flourishing, the understanding of the mechanisms of the body and investigation of disease was making little progress, at least in civilian practice. Though the philosophers of the Enlightenment urged the use of the practical observation and quantitative experiment and the method had enormous success in the physical sciences, no start was made with comparable measurement in biological science. Physicians like Cullen measured the patients pulse rate, but never thought to use the new thermometers which had been exploited so successfully by Black in demonstrating the release of latent heat. It is also remarkable that Black and Cullen with their combined talents in botany, chemistry and medicine could not realise that the human body created carbon dioxide and that plants consumed it.

Moreover, while medical men continued to deplore empiricism they continued to obtain most of the useful therapies from unorthodox sources. Digitalis, inoculation and vaccination came from folk medicine, cinchona bark came from native medicine in Peru and even quack methods of dissolving bladder stones were closely studied, as were the successes of the mineral wells. In desperation some 'rational' systems of disease were devised, seeming to miss out the essential stage of observation and classification, and a tribe of would-be Newtons obstructed progress with their search for a single cause of disease, for a final doctrinaire answer to all questions of health.[92]

No such system was better known, or did more damage, than that of John Brown, a pupil of Cullen.[93] Brown was born into a poor family in 1735 (or 1736) in the village of Lintlaws. He had considerable intellectual power and as a student he was helped by the Edinburgh professoriate, who waived their teaching fees in helping Brown to train successfully in medicine. During this time he earned money by rendering into Latin his fellow students' theses for the M.D. degree. He was befriended by Cullen who took him into his home as a secretary and tutor.

Brown was successful as a physician and about 1780 announced his own system of physiology and disease, using a newer form of the hydraulic model of the body based on Haller's finding of natural 'excitability' in organs independent of their nerve supply. This was used in Cullen's own teaching, but Brown made it the basis of his medical treatment, while Cullen based his clinical practice on pragmatic observation, rather than theory. In the Brunonian system all disease stemmed from over- or under-activity of the body – asthenia or sthenia – of the system; hence medical therapy had to be directed towards stimulating the body or quietening it. Among Brown's remedies for these states were laudanum (opium) for stimulation and alcohol for sedation. Brown himself took opium regularly for gout, and perhaps became addicted. His remarkable powers of persuasion and oratory resulted in an unusually committed support and he had vocal and loyal followers of his doctrine among the students in Edinburgh. Brown and his supporters provoked a clash with the teachings of Cullen and confrontation with the gentle Cullen followed: in Edinburgh, duels between the students supporting the rival factions had to be forbidden. Brown's reputation faded quickly in Edinburgh, and after his failure to gain a chair, he moved to practise in London, but failed there also. He died in 1788.

In Europe and America the humble origins of Brown and his iconoclasm harmonised well with the revolutionary atmosphere, and enthusiastic supporters appeared there also. In Mexico translations of his work appeared before those of the works of Newton. In the University of Göttingen, troops were called in to pacify his noisy supporters after two days of rioting in 1802 between students. Support for Brown in Germany persisted until the 19th century. His system of treatment, which eventually collapsed following better knowledge of the workings of the body, did however form an alternative to the exhausting medical treatments of the 18th century by purging, vomiting and diuresis. Brown's opposition to these methods gives him a modest place in medical history.

The problems of success

The remarkable role of late 18th century Scottish medical education within Britain is made clear by the fact that of the university-trained British graduate medical men in the period 1751–1800, no less than 87% were trained in Scotland, a situation resulting not only from the reputation of the medical schools in Scotland but also from the eclipse of teaching at Oxford and Cambridge and the decline in continental education.[94] This explosive rise in the output of Scottish graduates inevitably led to their domination of medical practice and teaching throughout much of Britain, the Colonies, the armed forces and even in Russia and elsewhere. However this huge output of doctors did cause problems. The first problem was providing adequate instruction in anatomy: the second was that those settling in England met opposition to their training and their M.D. degree.

To provide teaching for these large numbers of students in Scotland became increasingly difficult. Though the lectures which were the cornerstone of the teaching gave no problems, and which might be repeated during the day if the classes grew too large, it was in anatomy and clinical instruction that the problem arose. Anatomy could be taught by lectures, but the students expected at least demonstrations on dissected corpses, and personal practical dissection if possible. Bodies for dissection were extremely difficult to obtain in Edinburgh and though the law was vague and magistrates were lenient with body-snatchers, there was the anger of he Edinburgh mob to consider. Thus the anatomists often had difficulty getting material even for demonstrations. Clinical instruction of such large numbers was also difficult and the Edinburgh teaching could not be very personal. As a result it became common later in the 18th century for the Scottish students to spend time in the London hospitals and even at the private anatomy schools there.

The Scottish Medical Degrees

In spite of the success of the Scottish medical schools, there was a problem which their graduates had to face on moving to England. Some English authorities declined to recognise the Scottish qualifications. This barrier was not as high as it might seem, since it was possible to practise in England outside of London without any inquiry into the legitimacy of any degree or medical training claimed. But if the practitioner wished to join the army, navy or the East India Company, or even be a surgeon to a slave trade ship, or join the College of Physicians in London, the problem of the 'Scotch' degrees appeared. The problems were of two kinds. Firstly, the diplomas given by the Faculty and College in Glasgow and Edinburgh to their surgeons and apothecaries after training by apprenticeship in the town were not recognised for the armed services or the East India Company. Secondly, those who trained as physicians in the medical schools of Scotland could not join the London Royal College of Physicians, and hence had difficulties in establishing themselves in London as physicians.

The surgeons fight

The problems over the recognition of surgeons' diplomas in England began immediately after the Union in 1707 with a poignant event.[95] The tiny Scots navy – three ships in all – was joined to the English navy. One ship had a surgeon, John Campbell, and though the Scottish officers were issued with new British warrants, Campbell was not and was required instead to submit himself to the examination of the London Company of Barber-Surgeons. The struggle from then on to abolish this profitable metropolitan monopoly was a long one, and it needed skill and perseverance on the part of the Edinburgh College of Surgeons. They faced a considerable array of independent Boards running the army, navy and the East India Company who continued to rule that the London Company of Surgeons should be the only licensing authority for their medical staff. This monopoly suited all involved – it meant revenue for the London surgeons and ensured reliable minimum standards for the employers. Moreover, the increasing stream of Scottish doctors into England and London was resented and the submission of the Scots to this discipline was doubtless thought to be well deserved. The Scottish graduates were not prevented from taking these posts – which they did in large numbers – but they had to take the London examination in addition to their Scottish training.

The first success for the College of Surgeons of Edinburgh – who fought these battles without help from either the Glasgow surgeons or from the Edinburgh physicians – came in regard to the least reputable of the outlets for surgeons, the posts on the slave trade ships. Concern for the appalling conditions on these ships had appeared and when draft legislation finally appeared in 1788 it was proposed that a surgeon be appointed to each slave ship. The Bill made the London Company of Surgeons the only licensing body but the Edinburgh surgeons prevailed on Henry Dundas, who, in the absence of any democratic parliamentary mechanism, was Scotland's powerful manager. He altered the Bill and when the Act appeared in 1789 it conceded that a diploma from the Edinburgh surgeons was acceptable as a qualification. Next to give in to the Edinburgh College was the army when, hard-pressed for surgeons for the Napoleonic Wars, it conceded the right for Edinburgh to license surgeons' mates. The Admiralty followed in 1797 by recognising the Edinburgh diploma for surgeons' mates. By 1799 Dundas was President of the Board of Control for India and again the Edinburgh surgeons successfully appealed to him to recognise their diplomas for service with the East India Company. The tasks remaining were to gain recognition for the licentiates as full surgeons to the army and navy. In 1808 the time was ripe: Dundas was Secretary for War and First Lord of the Admiralty. Before he could be used by the College, however, a scandal overtook their patron and recognition for the army posts had to be postponed, but the rehabilitation of Dundas in 1813 allowed it to go through. The last, and most difficult task was to make the navy yield, and the case was successfully made by Dundas's son in 1825.

London physicians

In civilian practice, a similar problem with the Scottish degrees existed. While there was no serious dispute that the surgeons who had studied in Scotland were well qualified when seeking the military posts, the London opposition to Scottish trained physicians attempting to work in that city went deeper, and was based on concern about their Scottish training and its alleged faults.[96]

London had been invaded by Scots after the Union. Their ambition was resented, particularly at times of Jacobite activity, and among them were numerous talented medical men – the Hunters, the Douglases, Armstrong, Hamilton, Arbuthnot, Pringle, Clephane and many others. In London the demarcation between physicians and surgeons was still maintained, largely through the power of the conservative Royal London College of Physicians. In London, surgeons, apothecaries and men-midwives were regarded as a lower stratum of practitioner and their activities were still under the control of the College. Moreover, the rules of admission to College membership were plain: the applicants had to be graduates of Oxford and Cambridge. The problem of the Scotch degrees had appeared in a small way at the time of the Union of the Crowns in 1603. James VI and I took a strange assortment of healers with him to London but included in this group was his orthodox physician, Dr Craig, whose admission to the London College was requested by the King.[97] This was questioned by the College on the grounds that Gray was not English. 'Wee purpose', said the King crisply, to naturalise him 'out of hand'. The King went on to lecture the College on the unity of the United Kingdom. In the 18th century, however, the pressure came from the numerous Scottish practitioners settling in London who could not meet the entry qualifications. To accommodate the new and mobile Scottish and foreign graduates, the College devised a second and inferior type of membership – the licentiate, and up to three were admitted each year from 1761–5.

The inferior status of the licentiates was increasingly resented and relations between them and the College became bitter. A particular complaint was that the licentiates were not allowed to enter the College buildings. By 1765 however, the licentiates were becoming more numerous and politically stronger. The fellows only outnumbered the licentiates by 74 to 63 and in 1767 the aggrieved licentiates, having failed with legal action to gain satisfaction, organised themselves for direct action.[98] With William Hunter in their number they resolved to storm the College, and this they did, breaking windows and manhandling the servants of the College. Having broken down the hall door, the licentiates poured in and sat among the College fellows then in session. This event caused a stir and London was entertained when the events were used in Foote's satirical play *The Devil upon Two Sticks*.[99] At least one of those Scottish graduates was not amused at the way he was portrayed, since the humourless John Fothergill tried to have the play banned.[100]

To the fellows of the London College, there was some justification in their resistance to the admission of the licentiates, particularly the Scottish ones. Firstly, many of the Scots were still teenagers, having gone early to university and then completed a medical course, which was flexible and self-chosen, in about three to five years, whereas the English graduates required eight or even twelve years at Oxford and Cambridge. Secondly, the Scots graduates were widely trained in surgery, medicine and midwifery and were practising as general practitioners. There were even full-time men-midwives like William Smellie, and this was anathema to the College. It was also known that the Scots were shaky in Latin and some knew no Greek. To the College, admission of such people would mean reducing the status of the members to the level of tradesmen. Lastly, there was concern over the M.D. degee held by some Scottish-trained medical men, and in this the College had more genuine cause for concern.

The problem of the 'Scotch medical degrees' – as it was called – had arisen in an innocent way. Before the rise of the Scottish medical schools, the universities in Scotland had the right to award the degree of M.D. and occasionally did so to those returning from a continental medical education. This was a source of a modest income to the professors, and St Andrews granted many such degrees in the 17th century, though no medical teaching was provided. Part of the St Andrews M.D. fee went to the upkeep of the library. When Edinburgh and Glasgow started medical teaching in the 18th century, the M.D. was optional at the end of the course but many, particularly the surgeons, declined to take the degree as it involved additional expense. However after some years in practice, many found that the M.D. degree was more attractive and if they had achieved a reputation as a physician, the degree helped them to charge greater fees. Many established medical men in Scotland therefore requested the degree of M.D. from a university later in life. The regulations for the degree varied from university to university and the minimum required was a fee (about £10), and one or two testimonials to the doctors skill from other practitioners. The doctors did not have to apply to their own university and could choose another, possibly because the fee or the paperwork involved there was less or a graduation thesis was not required. In particular, the Aberdeen or St Andrews degree was easy and was granted by post, and the number of distinguished 18th century practitioners who took their M.D. this way was considerable. Cullen, though he studied medicine at Edinburgh, was awarded a Glasgow M.D.; Pitcairne, in middle age, took an Aberdeen M.D., and Jenner obtained a Scottish medical degree by post, as did William Smellie at age 45. Peter Middleton, a professor of pathology and physiology at King's College, New York, from 1770, wrote back to St Andrews for an M.D., and study of the early fellows of the College of Physicians in Edinburgh shows that a 'postal' St Andrews M.D. was almost the commonest degree held.

Though this system was understandable in a small country with a compact profession many of whom were known to each other and when the university degree was optional, the later expansion in medical education left the awarding of the M.D. degrees in this way open to abuse. The earliest unusual use of the Scottish M.D. was by dissenting ministers in England, who in rural places took on the care of the sick, as did their Anglican counterparts. While the Anglicans were protected by a Bishop's licence to practise, the nonconformist ministers were unprotected and were occasionally threatened with penalties for the illegal practice of medicine. To these men a Scottish degree offered a legal solution and the first two Glasgow M.D.s went to such ministers. From 1712 onwards Glasgow University made obtaining the degree more difficult by requiring a thesis and when another dissenting minister from Chapel en le Frith enquired in 1729 he found that the Glasgow requirements were too difficult. He then tried Edinburgh and was refused, but on applying to Aberdeen and enclosing the necessary testimonials from three doctors who knew him, the protective M.D. was awarded.[101]

Though the majority of persons applying for the postal degree, or even for the degree awarded after an examination, were experienced and useful healers of some kind, there were thought to be exceptions, and to the College of Physicians in London the 'Scotch' M.D. held by these ministers and other strangely variegated practitioners was an object of suspicion. Those who grudged the Scots their success in London and opposed their entry to the London College made the most of any abuse of the Scottish degrees. The worst case of a spurious M.D. was that of Samuel Leeds, who managed to obtain an Edinburgh M.D. in spite of being an illiterate London brushmaker. He then applied for a post at the London Hospital, though the Scottish community warned the hospital of his pretensions in good time. These incidents debased the standing of the other Scottish medical graduates and 'Scotch degrees' became the butt of satirists. William Hunter wrote to Cullen on 'how contemptuously the College of Physicians here [London] treat our Scotch degrees indiscriminately'.[102] Cullen also thought that there were brokers in London who sold Scotch medical degrees and the quack, Dr Green, was thought to have a degree from St Andrews awarded without visit or examination. Cullen, fearing for the reputation of the Scottish medical education, took action on behalf of Edinburgh University and proposed a minimum two year period of study before the degree could be granted. He put the proposal to the Chancellor of the University, the Duke of Buccleuch, who in turn asked the advice of his old tutor, Adam Smith. Smith took a characteristic stand against a university monopoly and defended the loose M.D. regulations. He held that medical merit would always be rewarded and that there was no need to change the arrangements. Moreover, he had in mind the need to protect the private teachers, notably the Hunters in London, whose enterprise he admired. In practice, he wrote

> the persons who apply for degrees in the irregular manner complained of are the greater part of them surgeons or apothecaries who are in the custom of practising as physicians; but who being only surgeons and apothecaries are not fee'd as physicians. It is not so much to extend their practice as to increase their fees that they are desirous of being made doctors . . . Adieu, my dear Doctor . . . I am afraid that I shall get my lug in my lufe [ear in my hand, ie taken severely to task] as we say, for what I have written.[102]

Though Glasgow had introduced tougher rules in 1755 as did Edinburgh later, the universities of St Andrews and Aberdeen continued to award the degree in spite of having no local teaching. Thus the complaints against the system continued.[103]

In London the fight by the licentiates to become full members of the College of Physicians continued and in 1784 the College made concessions to the licentiates, allowing them the use of the College building and giving the President power to admit two licentiates each year to the fellowship. However in 1793, after four Scots and four foreign graduates had been admitted, the nervous College put an end to this portal of entry and thereafter admitted only one licentiate. They continued this exclusiveness into the 19th century and survived the scandal and investigation of the medical care of the navy on Walcheren Island, during which it emerged that only the physicians of the London College could be appointed as physicians to the navy. The College survived another crisis in 1833, when a Bill granting equal rights to Scottish graduates appeared in Parliament, but was withdrawn. Until 1858, the London College never gave in to equal rights for the Scottish graduates, but in that year the Medical Act abolished any geographical limitation of medical practice.

5
The industrial revolution 19th century (1)

Nineteenth century health and health care in Scotland were dominated by the social changes produced by the industrial revolution. In the Highlands a hardly less serious problem arose when the agricultural and economic system became unable to support the growing population there. These problems compelled central government reluctantly to drop the policies of *laissez faire* and to intervene directly in the life of the nation, notably in the new Poor Laws and public health legislation. In the land of Adam Smith this intervention was resisted by informed opinion and the voluntary principle upheld as long as possible.

The health problems arose from the rapid growth of the Lowland towns and a large scale migration of people from the Highlands to the industrial central belt. Edinburgh grew fairly gracefully, but Glasgow's unfettered capitalism led to a social crisis and the return of major epidemics. Of these the most theatrical was cholera. The drama of the appearance of cholera forced communal action and the rise of the public health movement. With the slow acceptance of the need for legislation and taxation, both local and national, to procure the common good, the self-inflicted damage of the industrial revolution was slowly overcome.

Medical therapy at the beginning of the 19th century was almost unchanged from the previous century and there was even a strong revival of the use of blood-letting and evacuant therapies, particularly to deal with the increasing problem of infectious diseases. However the discovery of the successful prevention of smallpox by vaccination was the first of a number of undoubted therapeutic advances in the 19th century, and while medical therapy advanced slowly, progress was more notable in surgery and in this Scotland made crucial contributions. The new methods of anaesthetics and antiseptics of the mid-nineteenth century onwards enabled not only the small number of known surgical procedures to be more humanely and effectively used, but also made possible a wide new range of surgical treatments. Though Scotland made significant contributions to these discoveries, these signalled the end of the great era of Scottish medical teaching and research and the quality of medical education declined. Thereafter, the continental medical schools led the way, while Scotland lagged behind, inhibited by antagonism to physiological research and opposition to state support of research.

The 19th century saw the first appearance of state medical services as a result of the new Poor Laws. The working class at the early part of the century had a low opinion of medical help, but as healing methods improved, those in regular work and with reasonable wages sought ways to pay for medical attention, and the small friendly societies, insurance schemes and works clubs all steadily expanded and increasingly employed their own doctors. Also aiding the working class were a mass of voluntary bodies concerned with health, notably the increasing number of voluntary hospitals and dispensaries.

In considering the main events of the 19th century, it is clear that in all aspects of health care – public health, medical education and medical practice – the first half of the century was a time of uncertainty and tension within Scotland, and that these problems were more acute than in England. The deterioration of health as a result of the industrial revolution, the decline in the quality of Scottish medical education and the problems of reform of medical qualifications all called for measures by central government, yet informed Scottish opinion was against this increase in the power of the state and the separate Scottish legal system and the distance from Westminster also contrived to delay the necessary measures in Scotland until mid-way through the century. Thus, a description of health and health care in 19th century Scotland is divided into a description of the problems which dominated the first half of the century and an account of the solutions which appeared in the second half.

The medical schools and doctors

By the start of the 19th century, the fame and output of the Scottish medical schools was still increasing. In 1750 the number of students studying medicine at Edinburgh University had been about 158 (counting students at all stages): by 1800 the number had increased to about 650. The numbers reached a peak in 1815 of 820 to meet the needs of the war, fell in the middle of the century, and then rapidly rose to no less than 2,003 in 1890. Glasgow had only about 20 students in 1750 but by 1800 the number had almost reached 100.[1] In 1815 a peak was reached of 232, followed by a fall in numbers towards the middle of the century, as in Edinburgh, and then a rise to a total of 800 by 1890, by which time Aberdeen and St Andrews had substantial medical schools also. In Edinburgh and Glasgow the total number of medical students was even greater since many others attended the successful extramural schools and private teachers. Until the first of the new London medical schools started teaching in 1821, Scotland had a virtual monopoly of university medical education and in the first half of the century almost 95% of doctors in Britain with a medical degree had been educated in Scotland.[2] The medical services of the armed forces continued to be dominated by the Scottish trained medical men as were the government services of the Empire, such as the Indian Medical Service and the Colonial Medical Service. It is not surprising therefore that the early pioneers of scientific tropical medicine in the later 19th century were Scots, like Sir Andrew Balfour, Sir David Bruce, Sir William Leishman and Sir Patrick Manson, the 'father of tropical medicine' and discoverer of insect vectors of disease.[3] The Scottish schools could hardly help but produce the 19th century leaders of the medical profession in Britain and the Empire.[4] This included the men who established the reputation of Guy's Hospital – Thomas Hodgkin, Thomas Addison and Richard Bright, and Charles Hastings founder of the British Medical Association. Dublin's Abraham Colles, Dominic Corrigan and William Stokes studied in Edinburgh. The founders of the new medical schools in England – Birmingham, Middlesex, University College and even the reformed Oxford School – and other medical schools elsewhere throughout the world like Bombay, Calcutta, Otago, Sydney, Lima, Dalhousie and Kingston, Ontario were from Edinburgh. The Russian armed forces medical services were still run by Scottish doctors, and the tradition of reforming the health services of the British armed forces continued with the reforms of Sir James McGrigor. The explorers Archibald Campbell in Tibet and John Rae in Canada were medical students at Edinburgh and the school also gave some medical training to Charles Darwin, W.G. Grace, Charles Tupper (Prime Minister of Canada) and Samuel Smiles, editor of the *Leeds Times* and author of the Victorian classic *Self Help*. Edinburgh medical graduates dominated early New Zealand politics.[5] Edinburgh also trained the education pioneer James Kay-Shuttleworth, the philanthropist Thomas Barnardo, also Arthur Conan Doyle[6] and the daring Chinese correspondent of *The Times*, George Morrison. In Hong Kong James Cantlie, the founder of the Hong Kong medical college, sheltered and encouraged the left-wing Chinese leader, Sun Yat Sen,[7] and Edinburgh's Henry Marshall, in command of the Royal Army Medical Corps, made vigorous protests at the methods of British colonialism in Ceylon,[8] thus continuing a Scottish tradition of radicalism in the Empire. Sir John Kirk in Zanzibar helped the abolition of the slave trade.

The extramural medical schools

The output of the Scottish university medical schools was added to by the numerous extramural teachers and medical schools which grew up round them in Edinburgh and Glasgow.[9] In Edinburgh, this growth had not been encouraged, but the free enterprise teaching system naturally produced lecturers who thrived in teaching those subjects in which the university was deficient. The university sought to create a monopoly of teaching by using the increasing popularity of the M.D. degree at the end of the course to insist that only their teaching was valid. But not for the first time, the Town Council stepped in and, using its ancient powers over the administration of the university, decreed that the extramural teaching be recognised. Though this was a necessary step in the early 19th century and saved Edinburgh's reputation, it later prevented the rise of large university departments. But the success of the extramural teaching in Edinburgh was not only the result of university students seeking better or extra tuition, since the College of Surgeons' own highly regarded licence could be obtained after courses from these talented extramural teachers or at the university. The early extramural teachers were to be found around old Surgeons Square, and later they formed groups of teachers and distinct schools, notably the Brown Square School started by Syme, the Argyle Street School and the short-lived Queens College.

In Glasgow extramural teaching had developed earlier and since the university medical school had been less well organised there was no bar to the extramural classes as counting towards a degree.[10] Of these, the best known was the Anderson's College medical school opened in 1796 as a result of a grandiose plan for a new university in the will of Dr John Anderson, formerly professor of natural philosophy in the University of Glasgow and patron of James Watt.[11] He was keen to settle old scores with his former colleagues whom he held, with some justification, to be preventing the reform of the university. Earlier he had gone so far as to call for a Royal Commission to investigate the affairs of Glasgow University. The plan in his will was grandiose, but it was commented that

> never was there an instance of wider disparity between the magnificence of the intentions and the narrowness of the means.

The plan for Anderson's University also ranted against the staff of Glasgow University, naming them as 'drones, drunkards, triflers'.

Anderson in fact left only enough money for one professor of anatomy, but from this shaky start, this medical school grew to offer an economical alternative to the university classes and also gave an outlet for talented young teachers. It grew steadily and eventually had more students than the university in the period 1840–60, a time when the extramural schools were also rescuing Edinburgh teaching. In David Livingstone and Lyon Playfair it had two famous alumni. In Glasgow, other extramural medical schools were founded – the College Street School (1796), the Portland Street School (1827), the Royal Infirmary School – often called St Mungo's College – (1876) and the Queen Margaret College (1890).[12]

Education

The quality of the Scottish medical schools suggested by their numerical dominance is less convincing when looked at more closely. Moreover the internal problems of the universities, demonstrated by the success of the extramural schools, were increasing. The intellectual sparkle, which had been the feature of the 18th century, waned as the 19th century progressed, but a number of factors combined to keep the Scottish schools still popular and pre-eminent within Britain in spite of their fading performance.

Firstly, the decline of Latin as the universal language created a language barrier to studying medicine in Holland or in France or Germany, and the Napoleonic wars closed the continent to students in the early 19th century. Secondly, within Britain, Scotland had initially little competition. The London hospitals and private teachers there had failed to organise medical education, arising from a failure to join in a co-operative effort. Though many eminent private teachers were active in London, no corporate bodies started teaching medicine until the 1820's. England's other problem was the decline in Oxford and Cambridge medical teaching as a result of their attachment to a long, purely theoretical training in medicine. The pattern of medical education in early 19th century Britain is seen in Table 5.1 and shows the preponderance in Britain of Scottish medical graduates in the first half of the 19th century.

Table 5:1

Place of training of graduate British medical practitioners, 1600–1850

	Oxford and Cambridge	*Europe*	*Scotland*	*Total*
1600–1650	599	36	0	635
1650–1700	933	197	36	1,168
1700–1750	617	385	406	1,408
1750–1800	246	194	2,594	3,034
1800–1850	273	29	7,989	8,291

Source: Newman[13]

These figures should be treated with caution, since they refer only to graduates and hence not only omit those who chose not to graduate, but also those trained largely by apprenticeship. Thus in listing only the graduates, the very large number of surgeons and apothecaries trained by apprenticeship are omitted, diminishing the figure of those trained in England. Nevertheless the number trained in this way was rapidly diminishing in the early 19th century. Scottish university education, though troubled, met the growing need for medical men in an increasingly affluent society and the needs of the armed forces and Indian Medical Service at a time when the continental education was less attractive and teaching at Oxford and Cambridge had declined.

The problems

In trying to cope with the number of medical students, Scotland still had the two problems which had first appeared in the 18th century.

The first was in trying to give adequate teaching to these large numbers of students: clinical teaching was unsatisfactory and the anatomists still had a shortage of human subjects for dissection. The huge number of medical students and the essential need of the anatomy teachers to maintain the attractiveness of their classes by practical demonstrations of anatomy led firstly to the acquisition of anatomical collections – Bell's museum was bought for Edinburgh in 1825, and Glasgow had welcomed the Hunterian collection in 1807. But these were not a complete substitute for fresh human material in the teaching of anatomy, and the demands led to an ever-increasing search for human bodies. This could only be met by the usual method of the removal of bodies from graveyards, and while this was more easily accomplished in the anonymity of the growing 19th century towns, the magistrates could no longer be relied on to be lenient. In the early 19th century the medical students were responsible for most of the night-time missions and, while the teachers and colleges made hypocritical pronouncements of displeasure they not only shut their eyes to the methods used to procure bodies but in Glasgow at least, encouraged students to obtain corpses by excusing successful students from fees for the anatomy class. The students and teachers also rationalised their actions as being in the nature of a post-mortem thus, they suggested, aiding knowledge of disease. The anatomists also claimed that the continental medical schools, who did not have problems with the supply of bodies, were becoming highly regarded and to sustain the reputation of the Scottish schools a supply of bodies obtained by any means was essential. As the practice increased, and since the law was vague and only a handful of ancient patrolmen guarded the streets of the Scottish towns, the citizens had to guard the graves of their own recently buried dead. Permanent watch houses were built at the graveyards and heavy mortsafes or vaults were constructed to protect the coffin at least until the body was of no use to the anatomists. These expensive measures could not be used by the poor, who had no alternative but to set a vigil over the grave.

The inevitable scandal grew nearer when in 1814 a Glasgow anatomist was prosecuted for receiving exhumed bodies, but escaped on a technicality. It was in Edinburgh in 1828 that the crisis occurred. In Edinburgh and London, but not Glasgow or Aberdeen, the work of the anatomy students had begun to be aided by professional grave robbers to supply the considerable needs of the anatomical teachers. The teaching of anatomy in Edinburgh was carried out by a number of lecturers, and Monro *tertius*, professor of anatomy and an uninspired teacher was losing students to the extramural teachers. Robert Knox (1791–1862), the best of these, had after a brilliant early career succeeded to the anatomy teaching post in the Surgeons' Hall with no less than 504 students enrolling for his 1828 session. Knox, a forceful and punctilious teacher, lectured three times in the day to meet this demand and had also promised the students that fresh anatomical specimens would be available. Scarcity of bodies was pushing up the price demanded and this supply of corpses offered rich returns to the Edinburgh underworld. It is likely that Knox dealt with these suppliers in exactly the same way as did his competitors in Edinburgh and his instructions to his anatomy room porters and the students who did the nightly rota for receiving bodies were similar to those of other anatomy teachers, though Knox paid well for bodies. His misfortune was to be patronised by the plausible pair – Burke and Hare.[14] Of the ninety-six bodies supplied to Knox in the year 1828, about one sixth were supplied by these operators. But Burke and Hare had no time for the uncertainties of grave robbing and had murdered sixteen of these subjects delivered to Dr Knox. Eventually one of those murdered was recognised: Hare confessed and gave evidence against Burke, who was hanged. Knox maintained a dignified silence, and was acquitted of blame by an inquiry. To mark the occasion, his students presented him with a gold cup, an event deplored by the *Scotsman* newspaper. But vilified by the public and abandoned by colleagues who had used similar methods, he resigned from his post in 1829. The necessary legislation in the Anatomy Act was quickly drafted and passed in 1832, allowing any unclaimed bodies for anatomical dissection. The legislation was effective, and in Glasgow alone there was soon double the number of bodies required for teaching. It was the first legislation to affect routine teaching and practice in Scotland.

The other problem facing both Glasgow and Edinburgh was that the medical schools were becoming increasingly old-fashioned both in their staff and in their teaching. While the Scottish medical teaching tradition had been based on anatomy and was directly paid for by the students attracted to the teacher, continental medical teaching was threatening Edinburgh's reputation by a new system of salaried university posts. This successfully allowed the holders to be free of heavy teaching commitments and allowed them time to carry out research into the new sciences of pathology and physiology. However in Scotland, and in Edinburgh in particular, there was resistance to these developments. The old habit and custom of students paying the professors the fees for a course and the examination had served the medical school well in the 18th century. The professors of the early 19th century stubbornly taught their old subject or subjects, and declined to split them into reasonable subsections. They also declined to appoint assistants, since their fees would be split. There was no lack of good applicants for the Scottish chairs, since the income was considerable and the summer vacation was long.

Thus in the early 19th century the payment of the professors by the class fee system was preventing the necessary development of the sciences in the universities. In chemistry for instance the need was for practical chemists to aid industrial expansion. Teaching bench work was unrewarding to the teacher, who needed considerable personal expenditure to supply equipment, yet could expect fees from only a small number of students. It was much more rewarding to continue teaching large numbers of students in the lecture theatre. In Edinburgh Thomas Hope (1766–1844) professor of medicine and chemistry from 1799–1844 was one of the most successful teachers ever, attracting 500 students in 1820. With this success, he had no need to support practical chemistry seriously, nor did he write or conduct research. His one new enterprise was however highly successful – his lectures on chemistry for the ladies of Edinburgh attracted 300 women in 1826 and drew in £700. Study of the chair of anatomy and surgery at this time also illustrates these problems. Alexander Monro *tertius* (1773–1859) refused to split his own subjects into the two parts, thus holding back the teaching of surgery and the development of the medical school. Worse still, his own teaching was indifferent and, deserted by the students in favour of the extramural teachers and with his own income declining, he was in no position to appoint assistants in anatomy in the university. Thus many talented Edinburgh surgeons and anatomists either taught extramurally or like Sir Charles Bell and Sir William Fergusson had left for London or elsewhere to find scope for their talents. Moreover in Monro *tertius* it was clear that old Edinburgh nepotism was no longer working, since he was emptying the anatomy class rooms, and it was alleged that he was reading out his grandfather's notes – including the phrase 'when I was at Leyden'. He even managed to give the young Charles Darwin a temporary distaste for anatomy. Even though the Town Council made the appointments to the chairs, nepotism was still possible and though the appointments were for life, in the professors declining years they often appointed a son or other relative as a substitute. When thus established it was seldom possible not to appoint the incumbent when the chair fell vacant.

One way of dealing with this problem was for the university to look for funds to support the appointment of new professors, and the universities accepted government money to set up 'regius' chairs. This move only resulted in further difficulties, since the old established professors safeguarded their income from examinations by refusing to take the new professors into the administration of the university thus excluding them from a share in the examination fees. Another complaint was that the regius chairs were appointed from London and could be given to doctors unknown to Scotland. The greatest success in the regius chairs was the appointment of Lister to Glasgow – though the method of appointment was criticised and he had a frosty reception. The worst appointment was an earlier one, that of Charles Badham to the Glasgow chair of medicine in 1827. The Glasgow correspondent of *The Lancet* remarked that

> the gentleman seems to be wholly unknown to the medical and literary rulers of this western emporium . . . but after several days of investigation it was ascertained that he was the author of a small duodecimo on Bronchitis.[16]

This hostility seems to have been justified, since in 1841 Badham retired to the south of France and arranged for most of his Glasgow salary to be sent out to him for life.

In both Edinburgh and Glasgow the problems multiplied. The once fruitful relationship between the Edinburgh Town Council and the university turned sour.[18] Following a complaint by the Edinburgh obstetricians to the Town Council over the lack of status of their subject, the Council used their power to command the university to introduce this useful subject into the medical school teaching in 1825, an idea that was ahead of its time. The university, ignoring or forgetting the Town Council's ancient constitutional powers, turned down their advice. The Council, to demonstrate its power descended on the university in full municipal dress as a Visitation, the first for 120 years, and read out an order on the subject. This was eventually obeyed, but the resentful university thereafter determined to seek a new constitution freeing them from the Town Council. They also took legal action against the Council but lost: they appealed to the higher courts, but again the Town Council's constitutional power was upheld. At the end of the case it was commented that the legal papers had 'exceeded every other case for bulk.' During the legal battle, the Edinburgh Town Council defended their position by saying that while the problems at Edinburgh University might be considerable, they were nothing to compare with those in Glasgow University 'where academic freedom existed.' Certainly the Edinburgh Town Council had a remarkable record since the foundation of the medical school of good appointments to its chairs and wise policy decisions.

In Glasgow, the problems were indeed as numerous though in the early 19th century the Glasgow medical school began to rival Edinburgh and the number of students rose sharply, since not only had the university some talented anatomists like Granville Pattison and Allan Burns but also men like Thomas Thomson professor of chemistry from 1818–52 and William Hooker, professor of botany from 1820–41. The Glasgow extramural schools were also strong, and all the chemistry teachers were teaching practical chemistry. Thomson in particular was a reformer. He understood that the changes in science occurring in Europe meant a new era of laboratory research and he attempted to move the university faculty to keep up with the events on the continent.[18] In this he was inhibited by holding a regius chair and hence was excluded from the administration of the university and from receiving revenue from examinations. But he managed by threats and complaints to get the university faculty, i.e. the Principal plus the 13 holders of the older chairs, to build the best chemical laboratory in Britain, perhaps even in Europe, though he continued his protests against 'the old monkish part of the establishment' and his lowly status in the regius chair. However the other problems he faced were insurmountable and his attempts to modernise the whole medical school were a failure. The main obstacles were the two inactive professors in the ancient chairs of anatomy and medicine. The first professor was in his seventies, and the second was the absentee Badham: neither taught and their lectures were given by substitutes.

Thus in both Glasgow and Edinburgh the quality of medical teaching was declining.[19] They were not alone in their difficulties since although St Andrews had been sharply criticised for granting the M.D. degree by post it actually increased the numbers of degrees granted in this way. Between 1836 and 1862 no less than 1,885 such degrees were awarded, and the fee had risen from £14 to £36 in 1822.[20] This steady source of income was vigorously defended on the grounds that all those receiving the degree were established practitioners, that the degree was not a licence to practise and that it helped those taught by the talented extramural teachers in Glasgow and Edinburgh. In Aberdeen, the two universities remained split and effective medical teaching was impossible.

Thus all four Scottish universities were in trouble for different reasons. A Royal Commission on the Universities in Scotland was set up to enquire into and remedy 'certain irregularities, disputes and deficiencies . . . in the Universities of Scotland'. It worked anxiously for four years to find solutions for the internal constitutional problems in each institution, and eventually made proposals in 1831. Parliament's preoccupation with other more urgent reforms delayed the necessary legislation until 1858. The new constitutions for the universities gave Edinburgh its desired freedom from the Town Council, united the universities in Aberdeen and disciplined St Andrews by limiting its awards of the M.D. degree to ten each year and only to practitioners over the age of forty. In all three medical schools the regius chairs were raised in status to the level of the older ones.[21]

Continental challenge

At the time that Thomson was struggling in Glasgow, chemistry was improving rapidly on the continent, and Scottish opinion, still reluctant to invite government support, nevertheless envied the results of state support in France and Germany. In particular the French government's highly successful £40,000 competition for a new method of making soda was admired in Britain. A clear demonstration of the continental supremacy was that the American students no longer came to Scotland and were to be found instead in France and then in Germany.

The Scottish universities were not in any way ready to meet this challenge. Edinburgh rightly felt that the German medical men who had so uncritically supported the doctrines of John Brown could therefore have little to offer. Had not Adam Smith also demonstrated that a salaried system of teaching, as on the continent, could not be productive?[22] Thus when Europe was opened up again to travel after the Napoleonic Wars, Scotland and Edinburgh were unprepared for the new ideas from France and Germany and only grudgingly admitted the lead from these countries.

The continental challenge to the failing Scottish system was made clear by a curious event in Edinburgh which showed the impending loss of authority in education and research to Germany. The doctrine of phrenology was first propounded by Spurzheim and Gall in Germany about 1800. It held that the parts of the brain had separate functions and if these functions were well developed, the brain and the area of skull over the part was correspondingly enlarged. Spurzheim was a serious scholar and accomplished anatomist, but Edinburgh's response to this challenge to its medical supremacy was to attack phrenology and Spurzheim, notably by a hostile polemic in the *Edinburgh Review*. Spurzheim himself hurried to Edinburgh to face his critics and dissect the brain in their presence.[23] The leaders of Edinburgh medicine could not be convinced, but Spurzheim's skill at dissection won some converts, notably the young Dr George Combe who became an ardent disciple and supporter of phrenology. In Combe's memoirs he says that his admiration for Spurzheim arose from the brilliance of the dissection of the brain by Spurzheim and commented adversely on the low standard of anatomical dissection in Edinburgh of the day.

By the middle of the 19th century, the leadership in European medicine was conceded to have passed first to France and then to Germany. This French success was the result of the enthusiastic post-revolution development of a sound knowledge of disease by systematic post-mortem dissection, and the later German medical reputation came from their experimental research into physiology – the normal mechanisms of the body – and their work in practical chemistry.

That the Scottish medical schools and the new and old English ones failed to follow the European lead is clear : neither pathology nor physiology became well established until later in the 19th century.

The reasons for the delay are numerous. In this declining phase of the Scottish medical schools, the old ways were held to be sacred. Moreover, the method necessary for advancing pathology was post-mortem dissection, which was considered by the Scottish general public to be similar to grave-robbing, and because of these attitudes the benefactors and managers of the voluntary hospitals often discouraged post-mortem examination. The new physiology required animal experiments and this was opposed by the general public and also by those supporting the hospitals through charitable funds. One of the few Scottish contributions made to the understanding of physiology was Sir Charles Bell's anatomical discovery of the two nerve paths going into and out of the spinal cord, a discovery which he shared with the French physiologist Magendie – a favourite target of the British antivivisectionists. Since Bell was reluctant to carry out animal experiments, this great discovery was exploited on the continent and formed the basis of the new understanding of the nervous system which emerged from Germany.[24] In Britain, Bell instead became known for supporting a return of conventional religious wisdom into understanding the mechanisms of the body and his Bridgewater treatise *The Hand: its Mechanism and Vital Endowments as Evincing Design* catches the spirit of this unproductive trend in medical development, one which had been absent in 18th century Scottish thought.[25] The theory of evolution also had a cool reception in Scotland, and the professor of anatomy in Edinburgh, John Goodsir, Monro *tertius*' successor, opposed it in his declining years in Edinburgh.

The second reason for the emergence of strong medical schools and research in Germany was the involvement of the German state in the universities by the creation of salaried posts. While in Scotland each subject usually had one professor only, by the mid-19th century each German professor and his salaried assistants shared the teaching. In Scotland, the staff to student ratio was 1:30, but in Germany it was 1:11.[26] This gave the staff in Germany more time for research which was not of the old anatomical kind, but into physiology, in which the European medical schools began to excel. Complementing this in Germany was the growth of medical specialities like study of the ear, eye and brain, whereas Britain remained wedded to generalism, and only slowly hospitals for diseases of the eye began to appear. Even in hospital and clinic building the German state had a role, while in Scotland the interest of a philanthropist had to be aroused to endow a hospital. However, individualism and self-help were still sacred principles in Scotland and England, and it was held that only in dire social or national emergencies should government intervene: medical science was not one of these.

University degree difficulties

In addition to the problems of declining vitality in the Scottish universities, their numerous medical graduates had problems practising in two places – England and, surprisingly, Glasgow. The Scottish graduates of the early 1800's not unnaturally felt themselves qualified to practise both medicine and surgery in Scotland and England, but two institutions sought to challenge this. In Scotland the corporations of surgeons in Glasgow and Edinburgh had, through their ancient charters, the right to regulate the local practice of surgery which from ancient times had been taught by apprenticeship in the town. In Edinburgh the College of Surgeons was very successful and its licence was highly regarded, and it did not oppose the trend towards a university training for the surgeon. In Glasgow, however, the Faculty of Physicians and Surgeons did not have a national reputation and its members and hence its income came largely from local sources. To protect its vital interests, the Faculty was determined to maintain its ancient rights. The University of Glasgow was equally determined to allow its graduates to practise anywhere, and particularly in Glasgow.

The Faculty decided to act when a growing number of graduates in the expanding and rich city of Glasgow began to practise medicine and surgery without attempting to join the Faculty and in 1815 it went to law with a case against four selected practitioners in the city.[27] The selection had been carefully made, since each doctor had a degree from a different Scottish university. In the case of the graduates of Edinburgh and Glasgow, the court upheld the legal power of the Faculty's claim under their ancient charter of James VI and ruled that the graduates were practising illegally in not being members of the Faculty. The University of Glasgow appealed against the decision, but the appeal was unsuccessful and the university then set up the new degree of C.M. (Chirurgerie Magister) in 1816 as an alternative to the M.D., the new degree having an emphasis on surgery. This was not necessarily a deliberate provocation of the Faculty. There were other practical reasons for instituting the degree, in particular the Passenger Acts of the 1800's requiring that all ships carrying more than fifty passengers should have a ship's surgeon. These surgeons were required to have a surgical licence from the colleges of surgeons of Edinburgh, London or Dublin (but not Glasgow). The University of Glasgow's new degree met the regulations and for the first time a university degree was accepted in Britain as a surgical qualification. In spite of protests from all the British doctors corporations, the degree became established and was popular, and holders of it appeared in Glasgow setting up in practice without the blessing of the Faculty. In 1826 the Faculty took legal proceedings against three selected holders of the new surgical degree who were not members of the Faculty. The surgeons appealed to the University for help, and the medical professors decided with reluctance to fight the case since the University had no corporate funds and any expense had to be borne out of the professors' incomes. Again the University lost the case, but appealed to the Lords, in spite of protests by some of the professors at the rising costs of the fight. In the Lords, long legal arguments on the original charters of the University and Faculty were made. The University held that its Papal Bull allowed it to teach any subject and to qualify graduates to practise anywhere. They conceded that in medieval times surgery had fallen in status but contended that in the universities of Italy, whose constitutions Glasgow had copied, surgery had always been held in great esteem and was taught as an academic subject. The Faculty's case was simple and was based on its charter from James VI. It was contended that the charter gave the Faculty the legal right to regulate surgical practice in the whole of the West of Scotland and that in any case surgery was a practical skill to be taught by practitioners, not by a literary body such as a university. After many delays, the Faculty's case was again upheld, and its exclusive privilege to license the practice of surgery in Glasgow was maintained. The case alienated the two sides for decades and the reputation of both suffered. In the course of the struggle, the University prevented the Faculty gaining 'Royal' status, thus postponing this elevation until 1909.

The legal battle had been bitter and expensive, and the fees for the University totalled £2,217. The only sources of money to pay the legal bill were the professors' income and the library fund. Both were used. Worse still, no one had won. The unsatisfactory nature of medical qualifications throughout Britain were only remedied by the reforms of the Medical Act in 1858. Even before this the qualifications of the University and the Faculty were both legally recognised. The Faculty's battle with the University had also so pre-occupied it that it failed to look outwards. The Edinburgh College of Surgeons, on the other hand, had exploited the opening opportunities in the Empire and in the army and navy for its licentiates and was already feeling its way towards a postgraduate role. The University of Glasgow was weakened and diverted at a crucial time in its history.

The debate in Glasgow also illustrates the confusion in the medical qualifications of the early 1800s. There were the university courses and degrees, the qualifications and classes produced by the extramural medical schools, the surgical apprenticeships and the postal degrees. Quacks and imposters also existed, but the cost of legal action by the colleges prohibited regular monitoring and prosecution in their areas. Moreover the fines of about £4 were easily paid and the quacks often welcomed the publicity of a prosecution.

Apothecaries Act

The movement for proper regularisation of qualifications took on momentum in the 1830's, just when the Faculty and the University in Glasgow were locked in their mutually destructive struggle. To obtain national agreement among the doctors on medical degrees and training was no easy task since there were still considerable status differences within their ranks, particularly in London. There the physicians regarded the surgeons as craftsmen, and the surgeons viewed the apothecaries as jumped-up grocers. These distinctions were not so apparent in Scotland, since the surgeon-apothecary was well established as a general practitioner, and hence apothecaries did not exist in Scotland. Their role was taken over by the new dispensing chemists. Ironically, it was from the apothecaries that the first move for reform came with the passage of the Apothecaries Act in 1815.[28] The Act was deliberately weak and limited in its intention and applied only to England, but was so badly framed that there was an unexpected outcome which threatened the London medical establishment and caused consternation in Scotland, thus accelerating the moves towards reform. The reason for the Apothecaries Act was the rise of the apothecary as the general practitioner in the growing small towns of late 18th century England. 'Pure' physicians and surgeons tended to remain in the large towns and in rural areas the apprentice-trained apothecaries and the more broadly trained Scottish surgeon-apothecaries had taken over as general practitioners.

In spite of their success in becoming recognised as practitioners, the English apothecaries had a number of grievances. Firstly, they were looked down on by the physicians and surgeons. Secondly, the apothecaries were prohibited by law from charging a fee for attending the patient and hence could only make a living by surcharging heavily on the drugs they dispensed. The third problem of the apothecaries was that as the population expanded they became overstretched, and chemists were taking over some of the apothecaries' work. The apothecaries in England set up a pressure group and in an early show of professional solidarity, they pestered Parliament for legislation to allow them to be recognised as medical practitioners. All other medical bodies seem to have been uninterested in these moves, except the College of Physicians in London. It decided that there was a possibility that the Bill might be passed and give the apothecaries the right to treat patients. The College decided to attempt to weaken the Bill rather than oppose it, and ensure that the apothecary remained, as they put it, the 'physician's cooke'. The College's amendments were incorporated and appeared to give them satisfactory power over the apothecaries and they were content to let the Bill go forward. The Bill was passed quickly and without fuss at the end of a busy Parliament in 1815. The main proposals of the apparently innocuous Act were that all the apothecaries, and hence all drug dispensers, should serve a five-year apprenticeship, and the Society of Apothecaries could inspect all shops and test the drugs sold. It was not long before the full powers given unintentionally under the Act were realised: all practitioners who prescribed drugs came under the Act. Even the apothecaries had not realised the extensive privileges given to them.

The Scottish universities and colleges had not been consulted and had ignored the legislation: they were also poorly represented in Parliament. After some battles in the courts, the widest possible interpretation of the Act was upheld, and all general practitioners in England, including a very large number of surgeon-apothecaries from Scotland who made up their own drugs, were ruled as coming under the Apothecaries Act and were required to satisfy the London regulations. Complaints within England became loud and injured in tone:

> It does not seem quite so reasonable that because the apothecaries have ceased to be grocers, they should be forthwith invested with the entire regulation of the practice of medicine in England.[29]

But it was in Scotland that the complaints and protests were even more justifiable. The Scottish universities and colleges had been accustomed to sending well qualified surgeon-apothecaries or M.D. graduates to work in England, and they now found that the new and oppressive regulations prevented their graduates from settling in England unless they complied with the apothecaries' regulations, which meant another long, formal apprenticeship in London.[30] The Report of the Royal Commission of Inquiry into the Universities of Scotland in 1831 concluded that

> the statute really confers upon the Apothecaries the monopoly of licensing all the general practitioners in England and Wales. The result of the operation of this statute is to exclude the whole of the graduates of the Scottish universities from practising in England unless they have served the requisite apprenticeship in London. The direct effect of the enactment is to vest the monopoly of practice in a class of persons of very inferior education.[31]

In 1833 a Scottish physician was indicted and convicted for practising as an apothecary without the London qualification. The Society of Apothecaries sent threatening letters to Scottish licentiates in England insisting that they acquire the Society's certificate. Only the enormous amount of administrative work required by the Apothecaries' Society prevented litigation against all those breaking the new Act, and there were many petitions from the Scottish graduates in England. The respected *Edinburgh Medical and Surgical Journal*, almost exhausted in its constant battle with the apothecaries and the London College of Physicians, became paranoid and concluded that there was a plot to support the apothecaries in England by the London College arising from

> from a deep, fixed, and determined hatred to the Scottish Universities, and every one who avails himself of their means of instruction.[32]

The unexpected power gained by the apothecaries gave the crucial push towards reform and regulation of the medical profession. There had been vigorous previous attempts. The College of Physicians of London had proposed a simple plan in 1804 which extended their power to the whole of England, a proposal which was ridiculed by the members of other professional groups. The next attempt in 1810 had more success and was the result of a strenuous and single-minded effort by one man, Dr Edward Harrison, an Edinburgh graduate in practice in Lincolnshire.[33] His scheme proposed a register of qualified practitioners, and minimum standards of training for physicians, surgeons and apothecaries. He took his plan to London and won the support of the Presidents of the Royal Society and the Royal College of Physicians. This group met regularly and attempted to enlist the help of other medical bodies in Scotland and Ireland. These corporations were largely unhelpful, but Dr Harrison pursued his campaign and interested the Treasury and William Pitt in his reforms. The main opposition, however, came from the College of Physicians in London who saw a threat to their status. The College of Surgeons of Edinburgh were uninterested, though the Glasgow Faculty encouraged his efforts. After a six-year struggle, Harrison gave up in 1811.

The first event in the final stage was an enquiry into medical education which reported to the House of Commons in 1812. The pressure for reform was led by Thomas Wakley using his editorship of *The Lancet* for a crusading movement towards medical registration. By this time the Scottish universities and Edinburgh doctors' corporations were eager for medical reform which would remove all geographical restrictions on practice by their graduates and licentiates, though the Faculty of Physicians and Surgeons in Glasgow was guilty of just such actions in their fight to preserve the monopoly of licensing surgeons to practise in Glasgow. The concern for 'equality of education and opportunity' in Scotland arose from two problems. Firstly the Apothecaries Act had badly shaken the Scottish medical world, and called for repeal in some way. Secondly the College of Physicians in London still refused to admit Scottish graduates.[34] Their regulations did not absolutely forbid such an election, but as the *Edinburgh Medical and Surgical Journal* observed

> on nearer approach, such a series of fosses and palisades, of barbicans, drawbridges and portcullises, and of all the nicer machinery of patent bolts and locks, which the astuteness of the legal mechanist and architect, stimulated by the fears and jealousies of the inmates, have devised to guard the entrance . . .[35]

The opposition by the London College to the Scottish degrees continued to be based on the claim that the training was too short and variable, that the Scottish graduates were trained in trades such as surgery and midwifery, and even then lacked the practical skills resulting from an apprenticeship. Hence they could not take their place in polite society as physicians. While Edinburgh could claim that their education was sufficient, the London authorities could still point out that Aberdeen and St Andrews still gave the degree of M.D. by post. Edinburgh medical men were also occasionally enraged by patronising accounts from England of the usefulness of a Scottish education. A member of the London College of Physicians wrote of Edinburgh:

> Such schools, in the present extended scale of colonization, and martial temper of the empire, have become absolutely requisite. Were the school of Edinburgh on the footing of the English universities, few would be the labourers going out to harvest. For what highly accomplished physician would depart and sit down to be frozen in Newfoundland, Hudson's Bay, or the Orkneys, or broiled for a pittance in the West Indies, or starved in a little dirty Scotch, Irish or Welsh borough, or waste his health, his vigour, and his talents, amongst the outcasts and convicts of New Holland . . . ?[36]

There had been a number of determined efforts by Scottish graduates to gain admission and a legal battle by Dr C. Stanger from 1796 almost succeeded. Other distinguished Scots in London like Sir Gilbert Blane ignored the College and even refused their Fellowship. But London medicine was changing, and changing in the direction of the type of medical education in Scotland. The enrolment at Oxford and Cambridge had fallen and practical teaching in London was increasing rapidly. Moreover, members of the College of Physicians were clandestinely doing some general practice.

In these new circumstances, all the teaching bodies agreed that medical reform was necessary, and the insistence of the new employing authorities like the Poor Law Boards, the prisons and the voluntary hospitals in appointing only 'properly qualified' practitioners emphasised the chaotic state of medical education. The Parliamentary process was to be long and arduous. Eventually the sixteenth version of the Bill was passed. The interim Bills give interesting variations on what was to be finally the scheme setting up a General Medical

Council and a 'multiportal' entry to the practice of medicine, and the interests of the universities or the colleges or the medical schools from time to time gaining the upper hand.

The sixteenth Bill was passed to become the Medical Act of 1858. It made allowance for a General Council of Medical Education and Registration to be set up, responsible to the Privy Council. Its duties were the establishment and maintenance of a Register and examination of any qualifications claiming to produce a medical practitioner. Branch councils were set up in Scotland and Ireland. The earlier plan to abolish the powers of colleges of physicians and surgeons to license was not pursued and their power to award medical qualifications equal to the universities was maintained. The established medical organisations were allowed to nominate the majority of members to the General Medical Council.

In much of the negotiations prior to the Medical Bill, the Scottish universities were prominent as a result of their position as the biggest producers of medical graduates in Britain. Having suffered from parliamentary neglect, not only under the Apothecaries and Anatomy Acts, but also from the badly framed Scottish public health legislation, they managed to defend successfully their position under the Medical Act. A hard lesson had been learnt in ignoring the new power of the state, and the dangers of inattention to the affairs of the distant parliament were now clear.

Doctors

The practitioners in Scotland in the early 19th century were disputatious and proud and were flourishing through the increasing use of their services by the new merchant class, who could afford the fees previously only paid by the upper classes. Many town practitioners could hope to be rich if their reputations were established. While the 18th century had been largely free of brawls and litigation between doctors, this broke out again with vigour in the 19th century, and in Edinburgh this was particularly notable. In that town there was by then not only the possibility of great success in private practice, but the chance of fame by teaching, which was well rewarded by the fees paid directly to the teacher by the individual students. Success in teaching also meant that the teacher was known to his pupils and they might spread his name as a practitioner. The famous feuds in Edinburgh thus centred round the battle for patients and students.

The University and the voluntary hospital – the Royal Infirmary – became involved since it was now established that a doctor's reputation could be made by success in the hospitals. The first famous Edinburgh confrontation appeared at the turn of the century. An anonymous pamphlet appeared entitled *Guide to Gentlemen Studying Medicine in the University of Edinburgh* (1792). It was reasonably factual and informative but went on to denigrate all the teachers and professors – except James Hamilton, the obstetrician.[37] James Gregory, the professor of the practice of medicine and a great polemic writer himself, responded by attacking Hamilton in the street and thrashed him with his stick.[38] On being fined £100 for this attack, he said that he would pay double for another opportunity. Later Hamilton himself was slandered by Dr Andrew Duncan senior and successfully won £50 in the courts. The surgeon Robert Liston criticised the Royal Infirmary and was excluded from it in 1822, and later the equally famous Edinburgh surgeon James Syme openly invited patients dissatisfied with other surgeons to come to Edinburgh. On another occasion he tore up the works of Sir J.Y. Simpson in front of a class of students. Professor John Lizars criticised Syme's surgical methods and accused him of not being honest about his results. Syme replied that he regarded Lizars – whose star had faded in Edinburgh – as 'being beyond the pale of professional respect and courtesy'. Lizars dragged Syme into court, but lost. All these charges and counter-charges were followed closely by the gossipy medical journals of the day and *The Lancet* was notably well informed on the Scottish feuds.[39] The most miserable piece of denigration was also one of the last in a half-century of private and public controversy and litigation, when J.Y. Simpson, at the height of his fame, attacked Lister's antiseptic methods anonymously in *The Lancet*.

Medical practice

In the early 19th century, medical practice in Britain and Scotland was still in a primitive state. The Edinburgh physicians in particular had turned their backs on the attempts made by Cullen and others to introduce simple treatments and their emphasis on the *vis naturae medicatrix*. The dominant medical practitioner in Edinburgh, James Gregory, was clearly determined it was said, 'to seize nature by the throat' and he and his colleages purged, vomited, bled, and poulticed their patients deliberately to the point of exhaustion. This lead was copied elsewhere, and in America in 1799, the three physicians attending the last illness of George Washington (two or whom were Edinburgh University graduates) ordered blood-letting, tartar emetics, calomel salivation and blistering of the skin for Washington's fatal respiratory obstruction. On the same day elsewhere in America, Benjamin Rush won a law suit against a satirist of these methods, of which he was a notable advocate. The treatment of many diseases was by these methods, and therefore the medical management of many conditions had a rather similar look. Thus puerperal fever and retained placenta were managed by blood-letting and evacuant therapy, as was scarlet fever, measles, cholera and many other diseases. Local blood-letting using leeches was used in whooping cough, and any localised infection.[40]

It is little wonder that the physicians of the early 19th century were regarded with suspicion by the general population and it is not surprising that they now had to face not only new cults within the orthodox medical world, notably homeopathy, mesmerism and phrenology, but also a new secular self-help movement. This developed from the mineral spa therapy, then declining in popularity, and was the hydropathic movement started in Germany by a layman, Vincent Priessnitz. This new water cure was not based on water containing chemicals but on the use of pure water for drinking and bathing, and a simple life style encouraged at the spa. The doctors were initially hostile to this therapy.[40] The *Edinburgh Medical and Surgical Journal* summarised Priessnitz's training thus:

> He received such an education as suited the son of a Silesian farmer, and was destined to the same useful occupation.

But the doctors wisely decided to support the new water cure, and many Scottish practitioners founded or administered the new wave of hydropathics built later in Scotland and which were more successful in attracting patients than had been the Scottish mineral spas of the later 18th century.

There was however one innovation in the early 19th century which gave the medical men a powerful preventative weapon. The discovery by Jenner of the prevention of smallpox by cowpox vaccination had been the result of careful study of folk lore. While the benefits of the earlier method of inoculation against the disease were controversial, Jenner's discovery was rapidly shown to be effective. Practitioners throughout the country quickly obtained a supply of fluid from Jenner and in Scotland the first to obtain some material for use was Thomas Anderson, a surgeon in Leith.[42] By 1800, vaccination was widely practised and accepted. The first English vaccine institution was opened in London in December 1799, and in 1800 the Edinburgh Dispensary started vaccinating: in February 1801 it opened a separate Vaccine Institution. In the first two years, 1,204 children of the poor in Edinburgh were vaccinated. In addition, the Dispensary did valuable work in investigating methods of preserving and packing the virus for despatch to the Highlands. These new methods also allowed them to send the vaccine to America and the West Indies, since the numerous Edinburgh graduates contacted Edinburgh for supplies. The Institute also appealed to the parish ministers in Scotland to carry out vaccination and simple instruction in the method were sent to them along with a supply of lymph. In Glasgow similar provisions were made and in May 1801 the Faculty of Physicians and Surgeons in Glasgow started vaccinating free at their hall in St Enoch's Square. In the first five years, 10,000 persons in Glasgow were vaccinated. There seems to have been a split in the Glasgow medical profession at that time, and a rival and successful 'Cow-pox Institution' was opened in St Andrew's Square. Aberdeen opened a Vaccine Institute in 1803.

About 1809, doubts about vaccination arose, led by publications from Thomas Brown of Musselburgh which were quickly taken up by informed and uniformed opinion.[43] The controversy raged for some time until it was realised that the immunity wore off with time and that a second vaccination might be required, a proposition denied until the last even by the enthusiastic supporters of vaccination. By 1854, the Poor Law required its doctors to vaccinate free and in 1868 the Royal College of Physicians of Edinburgh could insist that all intending fellows produce a certificate of having studied vaccination. There is little doubt that the introduction of vaccination prevented many deaths from smallpox but it was followed by a rise in measles deaths in the early 19th century thus leading to moralising on interfering with God's will, and the appearance of the depressing Doctrine of Replacement – that since weak infants would be struck down by measles, it was hardly worth preventing smallpox. There was some truth in this cynicism, since the deaths from smallpox probably took away those least well fed, and these same children, because of their low immunity, were also liable to death from measles. Vaccination against smallpox was not made compulsory in Scotland until 1864, ten years after England, another example of the Scottish 'legislative gap' of the times. Many towns omitted to carry out regular vaccination and were saved from epidemics only by the immunity in neighbouring areas; notable defaulting towns were Kingussie, Hamilton, Hawick and Beith.[44] It was perhaps the success of vaccination and the physicians concern that they had little effective therapy to offer (an impotence cruelly demonstrated during the cholera epidemics) that led the Scottish physicians, particularly those in Edinburgh, to be active in concern for the prevention of disease, and some, notably W.P. Alison, headed the political demands for reform of public health and the Poor Law as did Andrew Buchanan and Robert Perry in Glasgow.

Though the physicians had little to offer, surgical practice was improving. Syme and Liston in Edinburgh and John Burns in Glasgow were leaders in Britain. The reasons for this Scottish success are not clear, but the great tradition of anatomical teaching doubtless played a part, and the higher status of surgery within Scotland must also have been important. The main changes in surgery were that operations for bladder stones and hernia had become part of the skills of the trained surgeon. In the Edinburgh surgical school a range of other heroic surgical procedures were also carried out in spite of the lack of anaesthesia and antisepsis: removal of diseased bone and tumours in the breast and even the tongue and jaw were reported. The painful early moments of these operations were carried out at great speed to reduce the ordeal for the patient, though the ligature of the blood vessels and closure of the tissues thereafter was done more slowly. In Edinburgh in 1829, James Syme carried out his most extensive operation on a conscious patient.[45] The patient had a cancer of the bone of the left cheek, and Syme excised the whole of this maxillary bone which involved ligature of a number of large arteries and a considerable amount of cutting with a saw. The patient survived. The great expansion of surgical practice only occurred when anaesthesia and antiseptic methods appeared later and the earlier unpleasant surgical experiments could become humane routine procedures.

For the first time in Scotland, an idea of the fees charged by the doctors in private practice is obtained. At the start of the 19th century, a number of organisations published scales of recommended fees, which suggested that they were attempting to reach a wider range of potential patients or seeking to prevent the undercutting of fees by the doctors themselves. The fees listed were only for consultation and home visits since there were no hospital or clinic admissions for the fee-paying patients: all illness was looked after in the patient's own home, or by consultation at the practitioner's rooms. The scales recommended by the various organsiations show that the fees were much the same throughout Scotland and the *Rules adopted by the Medical Society of the North* and published in Inverness in 1818 may be taken as typical.[46] The introduction states that there had been difficulty experienced by the public in estimating the reasonableness of fees charged by doctors. The Society had therefore unanimously agreed to publish a list of fees. In the introduction the pamphlet states that the fees varied according to the social class of the patient, and since

> medical fees have invariably been regulated by apparent wealth, hence the division of the community into classes.

The Medical Society adds the sensible explanation that

> these regulations are by no means intended to confine the liberality of the higher classes or to preclude the humanity of the practitioner to the lower.

There were four social classes and in Table 5:2 examples are taken from two of the groups – the highest and lowest. This scale of fees was put out under the names of both physicians and surgeons. It shows that in that town the physicians were prepared to lower their fee from the traditional guinea in order to increase their practice. It is seen that even the routine fees of the early 19th century practitioners were high. Other observations on this scale of fees are that consultation by letter was still used and that blood-letting was still common. Attendance after death and preparation of the body was a profitable surgical service. It is interesting to note that apprenticeships in surgery could be obtained in Inverness or nearby.

Table 5:2

Scale of medical fees charged in Inverness 1818

	Higher Class	*Fourth Class*
Single visits during the day	£0. 10. 6.	£0. 2. 6.
Visits during ordinary hours of rest	£1. 1. 0.	£0. 5. 0.
Single visits to country not exceeding 4 miles	£2. 2. 0.	£0. 10. 6.
exceeding 4 miles charge/mile (excluding hire of chaise or horse)	£0. 5. 0.	£0. 2. 6.
Professional advice at the practitioner's house	£1. 1. 0.	£0. 2. 6.
Consultation by letter	£1. 1. 0.	
Surgical Operations		
Major – Amputations, lithotomy, hernia, mastectomy	£21. 0. 0.	£2. 2. 0.
Minor – Hare lip, hydrocele	£5. 5. 0.	£1. 1. 0.
Orthopaedic – Reduction of fractures	£4. 4. 0.	£0. 10. 6.
Dressing ulcers, per week	£2. 2. 0.	£0. 7. 6.
Vaccination	£1. 1. 0.	£0. 5. 0.
Extraction of Teeth	£1. 1. 0.	£0. 2. 6.
Blood Letting	£0. 10. 6.	£0. 2. 6.
Delivery of Child	£10. 10. 0.	£1. 1. 0.
Wrapping in cere-cloth	£30 – 10 gns	
Apprentice Fees (3 yrs)	£20 – 30 gns	

Source: Medical Society of the North.[47]

Highland doctors

Inverness was an affluent county town: medical practice in the rest of the Highlands in the early 19th century was quite different. It was known that there were few doctors in the Highlands and with the growth of new medical knowledge, reliance on the minister, land-owner and other amateur doctors was becoming less acceptable. A survey was carried out by the Royal College of Physicians of Edinburgh in 1852 in an attempt to determine the numbers and work load of practitioners.[48] Letters were sent to the ministers and doctors of 155 parishes in the Highlands and Islands and the figures showed that while 62 parishes were adequately supplied, 52 were only partially supplied, and 41 were rarely, if ever, visited by a doctor. The population of these 41 poorly supplied parishes, which were largely in Ross, Sutherland and the Islands, totalled 34,361. From these parishes, the ministers wrote about the lack of medical attention and considered that human life was often lost through lack of attention. The Island of Mull obtained its first doctor in 1850 and during Garnett's visit in 1798 he noted that the nearest doctor was in Inveraray.[49] The College also found that in a number of places, Shetland in particular, the ministers and the landowners still gave medical help, and that in some districts the parish midwife was the only person who could treat disease. The replies of the doctors gave interesting data on the conditions of practice in these times. Most of the doctors had been in practice for up to twenty or thirty years in the Highlands, and they reported that their ordinary daily travel was between three and fourteen miles: journeys of a hundred miles to reach a patient were occasionally undertaken. Horses or ponies were the normal method of transport: the doctor usually owned two such animals and used them on alternate days. Sixteen doctors out of the total of 53 who replied had a horse and trap and seventeen used a boat every day. The fee for travel was 1/9d a mile. All reported that a large proportion of their patients paid nothing at all for medical help, and the College's report concludes with this testimony:

> Many of them appear to be activated by true philanthropy, doing their best, in the most unfavourable possible circumstances, to manifest the benevolent spirit of their profession . . . much regret is expressed that they are, for the most part, very poorly remunerated.[50]

The view of the College was that the conditions were deplorable and their proposals to improve matters were radical and ingenious. Firstly, they felt the government and landowners should help to pay the salaries of medical practitioners in some of the poorer areas. Secondly, that some of the medical officers of the army and navy who were then not in work but on half-pay, should be directed to serve in these neglected parishes. The College also suggested the purchase of a few small steamships to take the doctors from place to place. Lastly, the College suggested that the landowners give medical practitioners a small farm on their land, thus giving financial security.

In spite of the College's progressive ideas, little was done and indeed they could exert no political influence. It could be argued that at the start of the 19th century the Highlands suffered little from having few orthodox practitioners, since medical and surgical skills were seldom of clear effectiveness, and local healers were resourceful. Moreover, the problem in the Highlands in the early part of the century was the food supply and not the availability of medical men. But as the century progressed, the lack of qualified practitioners trained in the newer methods of surgery, anaesthesia and midwifery put the Highlands at a considerable disadvantage. While the Highland Poor Law medical services were a useful advance it was not until the Dewar Report of 1912, that any way was found to attract good doctors in adequate numbers to the area.[51]

Self-help and folk medicine

In the early 19th century the last traces of the practice of medicine by the Scottish nobility can be found, since some diaries and journals still have collections of medical recipes. In the country the ministers continued their medical work and in the Borders in the early 1800's the Rev. Nicol of Traquair vaccinated before each communion service, and the Rev. Ballantyne let blood on each Sunday before church. The increasingly well-organised and confident medical profession slowly took over from these other sources of help, though in rural places there remained a distrust of the medical men, and the Scottish Poor Law authorities seriously considered in mid-century placing some of their early medical services in the hands of the ministers and educated farmers.

Early 19th century folk medicine in rural Scotland is fairly well described and the methods were a continuation and improvement on the earlier ones.[52] The herbs used were spinach, parsley and garlic, but the doctors methods of induced vomiting and diarrhoea were not used nor was blood-letting common. However, induction of the flow of urine by drugs such as broom, juniper and foxglove was used. Seaweed was applied to joints affected by rheumatism, and warts treated by applying spittle. Eye diseases were treated with extracts from the common eyebright or the eyes were touched by folk healers credited with powers of healing. Coltsfoot was used widely in asthma and spreading erysipelas was treated by flour put on the part affected or by poultices of the rose plant with fresh butter or wild geranium. Interestingly, the ancient method recorded centuries earlier by Martin Martin for the treatment of jaundice by burning with a red hot poker was still in use, as was the surgical removal of the uvula. The disease of phthisis – which included tuberculosis – was common in the Highlands and was dreaded. It was considered to be infectious, and a good diet was emphasised with treatment by extracts from the black spleenwort or a jelly from deer horns. The other approach was by manipulation and massage. Each area had women skilled in this chest massage, for which the fee charged might be a half pound of butter per session. Milk, particularly very creamy milk, was also thought to be useful in phthisis. Healing charms were sometimes used in the treatment of phthisis and the massage therapy was often accompanied by mutterings of snatches of verse, details of which the masseuses were reluctant to give. Other incantations were still in use for disease and written charms for the toothache were worn round the neck. Magical methods were even more overt in the treatment of other diseases. For epilepsy a black cock without a white feather was buried in the place where the patient had their first fit. An alternative was to take parings of the nails of the patient's fingers and toes, wrap them up with a sixpence in a piece of paper on which was written the name of the Father, the Son, and the Holy Ghost, and this package then tied under the wing of a blackcock and all buried in a hole dug at the spot where the first fit occurred. Another remedy for the sufferer was to drink water at dawn out of the skull of a suicide victim or one who died a violent death. The treatment of whooping cough also involved a number of rituals. The patient might be passed under the belly of an ass, drinking milk from it and a charm muttered at the same time. Travelling healers hired out their donkeys at 6d a time for this cure.

Unqualified practitioners were also common. Those thought to have healing powers in the Highlands in the early 19th century were, as always, the seventh son, particularly if a daughter had been born before and after the series of sons, and even the water blessed by such healers was considered to be effective in disease. Another interesting but mysterious group of healers were the bone-setters who used manipulation in chronic disease, but also treated fractures and dislocations.

In the towns doubtless folk healing methods were also used but herbs would be less available. An alternative source of help was the travelling healer and his wares. As in the preceding two centuries, these travelling quacks differed from the trained practitioners. While orthodox medical practice now recognised various diseases, but had rather an inflexible evacuant therapy for them all, the travelling quacks still favoured the older ideas of nosology though their remedies were also cure-alls for a multitude of ailments. While conventional medical treatment continued to be unavailable or to be ineffective, expensive and exhausting for the patient, the mass of the people preferred the simple alternative treatments of folk-medicine or the travelling healers.

The clash between these traditional remedies and orthodox medicine is described by Dr Gourlay in Lentrathen in Forfarshire.[53] During an epidemic of fever (probably typhus) in 1819 he commented that

> the existing prejudices among the lower classes prove the greatest obstacle to the efficient practice of the country surgeon; I found it no easy matter to persuade them to the necessity of losing blood for the cure of the fever, the old people declaring that in their time no such thing was ever allowed or thought of. At my first visit, I found it necessary to bleed as a matter of course, and the flow of blood continued until syncope supervened which, in most, happened upon losing 32 ounces. To some I ordered an emetic of tartrate of antimony but only to those who had a desire to throw up. A dose of calomel and antimonial powder was administered at bedtime as would procure three evacuations from the bowel.

It is doubtful if Dr Gourlay was doing much good: it must be asked if he was causing harm.

Voluntary hospitals

In this period, the other towns of Scotland slowly followed the early Edinburgh and Aberdeen example in setting up a hospital for the sick poor by means of public subscription.[54] By the early part of the 19th century such hospitals had been built in Dundee (1798), Glasgow (1794), Dumfries (1776), Paisley (1805) and Inverness (1804). Perth (1838) and Montrose (1839) followed later. Dr Gray's Hospital at Elgin (1807) was unusual in being founded and endowed by one person, and Dr Gray could insist that 'no expense be incurred under pretence of meeting to consult for the benefit of the hospital'. These new hospitals meant that most towns of consequence had a hospital aided by voluntary subscription, and it was often the biggest local charity. The hospitals continued to be inventive in raising money and in Aberdeen, Glasgow and Edinburgh considerable money was now raised from student 'tickets' to attend the hospital. The huge success of Edinburgh teaching meant that in the early 19th century, one sixth of the income of Edinburgh Royal Infirmary came from student fees. This overcrowding led to a hospital regulation requiring the students to remove their hats when attending the surgical operations 'both to allow others to see, and as a mark of respect for the operator.'

Admission of patients to the voluntary hospitals was limited to those recommended by the subscribers who provided a 'line' and the needy might trudge the city to obtain such a line. The very poor might not be admitted, as the poorhouse could deal with them. All patients had to leave the hospital within a fixed period, usually forty days, and funeral expenses were to be guaranteed by the person giving the line. Apprentices and servants were not to be admitted, as they could be looked after in their master's home or were treated for a fee. Some illnesses were not thought suitable for admission and this list varied from hospital to hospital. Usually pregnant women were not admitted, nor were those with chronic, incurable or infectious diseases like itch, venereal disease, cancer or smallpox.

These voluntary hospitals had become of increasing importance to the local medical men, since while the 18th century managers had been content to allow all or most of the local practitioners to attend the hospital in rota, this system had usually proved difficult and unsatisfactory to run. In most voluntary hospitals the local doctors had been forced to accept that only some of their number be appointed as the doctors to the hospital. The growing status of the hospital and the contacts with the influential managers (and hence with potential private patients) meant that these posts were eagerly sought. They were the first moves in the eventual dissociation of hospital consultants from the general practitioner. The method of making these appointments varied from town to town, but in Edinburgh and Glasgow there was one feature which ensured that a high standard of appointment resulted. In England the voluntary hospitals had not been erected with the needs of teaching medicine in mind, and hence the managers were always lay persons. English appointments of doctors were frequently made as a result of influence and lobbying and with no attempt being made to assess clinical skills. In Scotland, however, the use of the hospitals for teaching had resulted in the early inclusion of medical men as managers and hence medical appointments were more based on clinical abilities.[55] Even within Scotland there was a major difference between the administration of the Edinburgh Royal Infirmary and the Glasgow Royal Infirmary. While in Edinburgh the shrewd founders had placed university representatives among the managers, thus ensuring that the university professors could teach and practise in the hospital, in Glasgow the University was poorly represented on the Board of the Royal Infirmary, and the powerful Faculty of Physicians and Surgeons who ran the hospital excluded the university staff from teaching or practising in the hospital until the middle of the century. For the first time the voluntary hospitals were prepared to pay their medical staff, and after 1807 Glasgow's Royal Infirmary granted £50 per annum to its physicians and £20 to the surgeons. The apothecaries were also replaced by resident doctors about this time and a resident superintendent was first appointed to the Edinburgh Royal Infirmary in 1837. The organisation of the Edinburgh Royal Infirmary in the 18th century has been described earlier: the day-to-day administration of Dundee Royal Infirmary in the early 19th century can be studied here.[56]

The hospital was maintained by subscriptions and each subscriber could recommend patients for admission. These patients were to appear on Thursdays at 11 o'clock for examination, but those coming from a distance, or fever cases or accident cases could be admitted without a line. Only a minority were treated free and it was usual to charge 3/6 per week to the recommending subscriber, who was also liable for burial expenses or 10/6 per week if his patient could not leave the hospital when treatment finished. Later the finances of the hospital improved and after 1828 no charges were made for the patients. The hospital drew its finances from a large number of sources and charged for any soldiers treated in the hospital and also for out-patient use of the hot and cold baths and the 'electric machine'. Apart from subscriptions, donations and income from investments, it obtained a share of the fines paid to the Dundee police, donations from the mills and the proceeds of charity events. The annual meeting of the governors of the hospital was a great Dundee event with a civic procession headed by a band. This was followed by a church service, sermon and collection, which in 1811 raised £68.13.2½d. This event must have been too successful, since in 1818 it was discontinued because of 'the evils which these occasions produce by occasioning idleness and dissipation'.

The domestic arrangements in the Dundee Infirmary in the early 18th century were simple. The town surgeons took it in turns to attend the hospital, at first changing every two weeks, and later every year. They visited the hospital regularly and between visits a resident apothecary administered treatment, held the drugs, and ran the hospital. For many years the chief nurse was the apothecary's wife and these two were the only night-time attendants. Otherwise, the other nurses were untrained, unreliable and frequently disciplined for rudeness or drunkenness. The diet in Dundee Royal was wholesome: the 'full diet' gave porridge, night and morning, with bread and 'good broth' or 'flesh meat' at dinner. Ale or beer was served with all three meals. Smoking in the wards was forbidden and the sheets were changed once a fortnight.

In the early part of the 19th century the voluntary hospitals began to experience the effects of the deterioration of health in the growing towns. All the hospitals admitted cases of 'fever' – usually typhus – or relapsing fever and in 1816 even the new hospital beds built at the Glasgow Royal Infirmary were filled with fever cases, and by 1818 the number of fever cases seeking admission was 'overwhelming' in spite of a surcharge of £3 to the subscriber for each case sent in. In the same year Edinburgh and Aberdeen Royal Infirmaries had similar problems and both had to take over other buildings as temporary fever hospitals. This was not a measure to isolate the cases, since between the crises fever cases were taken into the main hospital and informed opinion held that this was a safe policy, provided the ratio of fever to ordinary patients did not exceed 1:6. But the recurrence and worsening of the fever problem led to increasing overcrowding and difficulty within the hospital, with rising death rates and a marked increase in the infection of surgical wounds. Even the chapel in the Edinburgh Royal Infirmary was taken over as a ward in the 1848 epidemic. In Glasgow there were complaints when it became clear that most of the fever patients were Irish and even in Edinburgh measures to prevent this Irish drain on the charitable purse were considered.

The rising problem in the community also severely strained the early medical services developed under the old Poor Law. In the towns the parish or the poorhouse often employed a medical man to look after the indoor and outdoor poor. In Glasgow this organisation centred on the poorhouse – the Town's Hospital – and until 1816 one surgeon (which at that time meant a general practitioner) only was required. In that year three more were appointed and Glasgow was divided into four medical districts. In 1817 a fifth surgeon was added and in 1818 a sixth was required.[57] To these men fell the task of dealing with the rising problem of epidemic fever (typhus) and cholera later. They took on the task of isolation of cases, the fumigation of the houses and administration of the cholera hospitals.

Thus the medical services of the early 19th century were under strain. At first, the problem resulted from the economic depression after the Napoleonic Wars: later it was the result of the industrial revolution. This urban crisis and the no less important problem in the Highlands can now be considered.

Industrial revolution

The marked expansion of the industry of the Scottish lowland belt in the 19th century was based on the tobacco trade, the expansion of the cotton industry and, later, the growth of the iron and steel industry. As a result the towns grew in size and Glasgow had a 20–30% increase in population in each decade of the early part of the century. To accommodate this increase, high density housing appeared and rooms were repeatedly sub-divided. In Glasgow and Greenock in particular, overcrowding and squalor unequalled in Britain appeared. Malnutrition was widespread and the old Poor Law proved difficult to administer in the new situation of rapidly growing towns and a migrant work-force. Conditions were therefore suitable for the return of serious epidemic and non-epidemic disease, notably typhus, relapsing fever and cholera.

While this deterioration in health is obvious from descriptions of the conditions of the times, it is not possible to give complete statistical support to these literary accounts. Regular notification of cause of death in Scotland was not enforced until a time when the height of the crisis was past. But careful early 19th century work in Glasgow by early pioneers of social statistics, notably Watt and Cleland, allows a glimpse of the health of that town before the great urban crisis.[58] A crude death rate of 25 per 1,000 in the 1820's increased to 30–35 per 1,000 in the troubled years of the 30's and 40's, but reached 56 per 1,000 in 1847, falling thereafter as public health measures became effective. The high death rates were from a number of causes. Measles became a major killer, though smallpox had been largely controlled. Scarlet fever and diphtheria which had not been a problem at the start of the century became serious later, but above all, it was cholera that claimed the attention of doctors, sanitarians and politicians. The incidence of other diseases can only be guessed at. There were claims that typhus had almost been eliminated from Edinburgh by the start of the 19th century but then became serious: certainly the statistics given in the annual reports of the voluntary hospitals confirm this. Later in the century, obstetricians claimed that they had not noticed the problem of rickets in their patients until the 1850's.

The towns became notable, not only for disease, but also for crime, alcoholism, prostitution and infanticide. In Glasgow in 1819 there had been only 89 arrests for criminal offences, but by 1854 there were 3,176: pawn shops abounded and in Glasgow in 1841, one house in ten sold alcohol. In the 1850's 450 brothels existed in Glasgow which spread venereal disease widely in the community.[59] Abortion was a routine way of limiting family size and patent abortifacients became openly advertised. Infanticide may have been common and these deaths often occurred when a child was in the care of a local baby-minder whose methods were not questioned or investigated. Much commoner was simple neglect of a baby or failure to feed a sick infant, and even the voluntary hospitals did not consider it worth while taking in children under two years of age or even older ones who had failed to thrive.

The poor were exploited and put at risk by food suppliers whose infected meat and fish were sold off cheaply and without inspection. Milk was regularly adulterated with water, and could also spread tuberculosis from infected cows and scarlet fever from its handlers. The water supply also was dangerous and in Glasgow in 1804, there were twenty-nine public wells and several private companies providing the water. The growth of the town meant an increasing industry for collecting food from the country for sale in the towns and the need to mix food, particularly milk, from numerous sources prior to distribution amplified the effects of a single infected source.

For private industry to provide the water supply and the mechanism of food distribution conflicted with the public interest.

In addition to the health hazards of these living conditions, work conditions also became dangerous. Whereas in a rural society, the agricultural working day was limited by the hours of daylight and children could not be exploited because of their lack of physical strength, the opposite was true in the new factories. The working day could be extended by artificial lighting and the children put to work for prolonged periods. Legislation gave only modest protection, but the Factory Act of 1833 put a ban on employing children under nine and later the Ten Hours Act of 1847 restricted the working day. New diseases appeared as a result of the new industries – lead poisoning, manganese poisoning from the bleaching industry and the dust diseases of the lungs of miners and grinders. Unguarded machinery was an increasing source of accidental injury. There were occasional compassionate employers like Robert Owen at New Lanark and James Smith of Deanston, both of whose factories were safe, well ventilated and heated, and had arrangements for education and welfare of their workers. But the majority of employers took advantage of the absence of legislation to extort the maximum work from their labour force, young and old. Faced with the choice between these factories or no work at all and in the absence of trade unions, the work force was powerless to counter their exploitation. They were also at the mercy of fluctuations in trade and, in the troughs of the trade cycle, unemployment increased and health deteriorated in a way reminiscent of a medieval mortality crisis. Health care for the mass of the people was poor or absent. Even as late as 1871, the causes of 24% of Glasgow deaths were not certified, since a doctor had never attended the patient and no cause of death could be given.

Conditions inside the hospitals mirrored those outside. Just as the cities were overcrowded and dangerous from infection, the hospitals had, as a result of overcrowding and heavy bacterial contamination, an epidemic of wound infection and other disease, which made admission and treatment dangerous. The poor therefore often fled from the hospitals or refused surgery when offered.

Early 19th century society was poorly organised to meet the problems. Local government was undemocratic and had virtually no staff or money to carry out the necessary reforms. The Poor Law in the towns was breaking down, unable to cope with the new situation. National government was remote and unrepresentative and it also lacked an administrative civil service: the Treasury funds were used mainly for war and expansion of the Empire. Moreover, the separate Scottish legal system was a nuisance to Westminster and even when Parliament acted in England the corresponding reform in Scotland was delayed and badly framed. The middle class were reluctant to part with money, either as national taxation or as local rates, to procure the common good. Anything that interfered with industry or trade was deeply suspect and in Scotland the principle of non-interference was sacred. Only slowly and painfully were the necessary reforms made and each improvement in sanitation, water supply, public health and food supply could only come after public outcry, followed by investigation by reformers and then local or national legislation. Each step was opposed by conservative forces or special interests and each battle had to be fought separately in each town of Scotland.

Perhaps the greatest factor ensuring reform and improvement was the appearance of cholera.[60] Its rapid spread and malignancy gave an uncomfortable demonstration of the ineffectiveness of medical treatment and its occasional spread to the middle class areas of the towns and the interruption of trade and social life aided the demands for legislation on public health. The method of spread of infectious disease was still unknown in the early 19th century but it was undeniable that these diseases predominantly affected the population in the overcrowded and insanitary working class areas. Thus it was considered that an infectious 'miasma' arose in these parts of the town or it was tempting for moralists to suggest that intemperance and lack of religious faith had led to this divine punishment on the poor. But slowly, those favouring other mechanisms won the argument.

The first major cholera epidemic in Britain was in 1832, and it affected Scotland particularly badly. Having spread from the Far East, this epidemic appeared first in Sunderland in December 1831. Local businessmen tried to dispute the diagnosis and discourage reports of its presence. By January 1832, it reached Haddington and Edinburgh and was in Glasgow via Kirkintilloch by February. By the autumn, it had reached Dumfries and elsewhere throughout Scotland. The measures against cholera were pathetically similar to those against the plague, the only difference being that the plague regulations had been tougher. In dealing with cholera, business interests and the arguments about its causation prevented full quarantine regulations. Strict measures against cholera only appeared in some places: the minister of Arbirlot put a *cordon sanitaire* round his village and there were no deaths.[61] 'Our trust was in God and prevention,' he said. The 1832 epidemic was the worst of all the visitations by cholera and the death rate in those attacked reached 50%. It attacked some areas but by-passed whole towns capriciously and each epidemic had bizarre resemblances to previous ones. In Leith in 1848, the first case notified was in the same house as in the earlier epidemic of 1832 and in Pollokshaws, Glasgow, the first case died in the same bed and room as in the earlier epidemic. Cholera scared people, and there was even a suggestion that fear itself predisposed to infection with cholera. Other features of cholera failed to help the 'contagionists' view that it was infectious, and the spread by infected water rather than personal contact was baffling. Thus in the Town's Hospital in Glasgow where the poor were accommodated two in each bed, the partner rarely caught the disease from an afflicted bedmate. The nurses and other staff seemed immune from the disease also, or less badly affected. Of the four cases among nurses in Glasgow, none were fatal.

Nevertheless, unlike the usual 'fever' – i.e. typhus – cholera did spread into the middle class districts. The first case in Rothesay was 'a respectable lady in comfortable circumstances' and the second case was 'old Dr. Fyfe', though it was explained that he was 'intemperate and irregular in his habits.'

Public opinion demanded that something be done, but the action taken was designed more to give an impression of firm leadership, calming the fears of the people rather than provide effective prevention. Moreover, as the expert advice given to parliament was split even on the issue of the infectivity of cholera, stringent measures could be avoided by government. The 'contagionists' held that cholera could pass from person to person directly or via clothing or goods. The supporters of the 'miasma' theory held that infection appeared as a result of harmful effluent from rotting or stagnant material. These theories had quite different practical and political consequences. If contagion was the method of spread, then full quarantine regulations were necessary. If the miasma theory was correct, then public health measures and sanitary reform alone were required.

The government, having been given uncertain advice, were reluctant to bring business to a halt and managed to avoid harsh measures. They set up a central Board of Health and encouraged the appearance of local boards. The policy of management of the epidemic was simply to attempt containment by isolation of those affected and only weak recommendations on quarantine were made. The choice of persons for the national and local boards was designed to give reassurance to the citizens that everything possible was being done. Prominent citizens and reputable doctors were chosen rather than anyone with experience of the management of cholera in other countries. The voluntary quarantine policy proved disastrous in the west of Scotland, since the commercial users of the Forth and Clyde canal failed to cease trading and almost certainly spread the disease from the east to Kirkintilloch and thence to Glasgow, in spite of a last minute attempt to stop travel between these two towns.

Once in Glasgow, the disease was dealt with as it had been managed shortly before in Edinburgh. Circulars were issued giving hints to the middle class on early treatment and exhorting the poor to strict temperance. A large fever hospital was set up at Mile End in Glasgow together with five temporary cholera hospitals. A primitive ambulance was gifted to the Board of Health and regulations were made for disinfecting the houses of sufferers. The dead were to be buried quickly in new, isolated, burial grounds. The dung hills of the town were removed. The doctors agreed on a treatment for the disease – a mixture of mustard and common salt to induce vomiting, bleeding from a vein and friction applied by nurses to legs and arms, followed by morphine in toddy with the patient kept warm and given stimulants of whisky, cayenne, and ginger. The value of bleeding in fevers was becoming controversial, and some Glasgow practitioners had rightly decided that in advanced cholera, the removal of the usual one or two pints of blood was harmful. The traditionalists continued to blood-let, even warming up moribund patients in a bath to obtain enough blood from the arm veins. Ironically, a new treatment of cholera by intravenous injections of saline was experimented with in Scotland during this epidemic, with Thomas Latta, a surgeon in Leith, arguing correctly that lack of fluid was the problem. He tried this treatment in four cases, three of which recovered promptly. His report on his method was noted by the London Board of Health, but was only one of many other remedies sent to them. The Edinburgh doctors considered his methods but were also unenthusiastic, and with the passing of the epidemic, this major advance in treatment was laid aside.

The Board of Health in London monitored the progress of the epidemic in Scotland and sent inspectors from London to advise and report. The inspectors had a difficult time in Scotland. They met opposition not only from those with business interests, but also and less obviously, from the poor. The poor regarded the activities of the ruling class during the cholera epidemic with considerable cynicism. To them the deaths from cholera were only part of a continuous mortality from other infectious diseases and the new hospitals, inspectors and regulations were regarded by the poor with suspicion. In particular, the early burial of the dead was contrary to established customs. The separate burial grounds and the post-mortems carried out by the doctors on cases dying in hospital also aroused hostility among the poor. Hence the Board of Health inspectors were made unwelcome and occasionally assaulted or stoned. The special cholera ambulance in Edinburgh was also attacked and in Glasgow a mob of about 1,500 people in the Gorbals chanted 'medical murderer' at a surgeon visiting a cholera victim.

The worst incident in Britain came in Glasgow when one of these fears of the poor was shown to be justified. In 1832 six out of seven recent cholera graves in the new Paisley graveyard were found to have been opened and bodies removed, certainly for the anatomists use. A mob set out for Glasgow and smashed the windows of all the doctors houses, except of one who was thought to have denied that cholera was in the town. A troop of the 4th Dragoons had to be called in to control the situation. As the epidemic passed, regulations were relaxed, the streets became used again and church services resumed. It was hoped that each epidemic would be the last, and as a future Medical Officer of Health wrote of these epidemics:

> The play was over and the old props were not even stored away: they were burned.

But each epidemic was not the last: cholera returned in 1848 and in 1853 and typhus was ever present, becoming epidemic following any year with bad trade figures. It was a greater killer than cholera. Cholera was undoubtedly the greatest force for reform in 19th century Europe and those countries and areas which it did not reach often lagged behind in sanitary reform. The drama of the spread of cholera, the high mortality in those affected, the occasional middle-class cases and the threat to commerce, all called for action. Cholera also put an end finally to the concept of the divine causation of disease. In 1832 the draft English Cholera Prevention Bill did not have any reference to the vengeance of God, but the corresponding Scottish Bill did reluctantly have references to the infliction of disease by God. For the last time in public affairs, during the 1853 cholera epidemic the officials of Edinburgh asked Palmerston to proclaim a national day of fasting and humiliation in the hope of divine intervention in the progress of the disease. Palmerston gave them a sharp answer, suggesting the construction of some drains and toilets instead. The problems of cholera decreed that health came before commerce. The measures eventually brought in included the restriction of trade and business, and reform of public health. These measures will be considered later.

The Highlands

Though the problems of the towns forced the best known of the 19th century health legislation, the troubles in the Highlands of Scotland were, in an unobtrusive way, the earliest stimulus to the intervention of the state.[62] In the Government's action to deal with the conditions on the emigrant ships sailing from the Highlands and its later action to deal with the famines in the north can be seen an early, though reluctant, admission of national responsibility for the common good. Two factors forced intervention in the Highlands. First, a unique situation had developed there in which people deeply attached to their homeland were removed from their farms and forced to live at the coast, there sustained in greatly increasing numbers by a precarious food supply and the risky kelp industry, both of which collapsed. Secondly, the Highlands had a class structure resembling the Scotland of 100 years previously, namely a handful of rich and often absentee proprietors with a large number of people living close to destitution. Whereas in the Lowlands there was now a well-off middle class who would answer voluntary appeals to deal with poverty and who shared between them the funding of the old and new Poor Laws, in the Highlands there were only the landowners, some of whom had financial problems themselves, and many of whom felt no obligation to assist in dealing with the immense problems of the area.

The Highlands had changed after the defeat of the rebellion of 1745. Of particular significance was the ending of the clan kinship and thereafter the new attitudes of the chiefs. The new chiefs were concerned to increase the income from their considerable land holding and the advice offered to them was that the ancient system of small mixed farms should end and that sheep be reared instead. The problem of what to do with the large number of displaced small farmers was to be solved, in theory at least, by moving them to the coast where they would be given small lots of land (crofts), and put to work in new industry. On the east coast, factory work was planned and fishing was to be encouraged. On the west coast, the kelp industry – the collection of seaweed for alkali production – was a labour intensive solution to the proposed clearances. Though this ideal was achieved in a few places, most of the Highland clearances of the people to make way for sheep were accomplished without alternative plans for work. In some places, the reluctant farmers and their families were removed by force and controversy over the methods used and the damage done remains to this day.

The suffering of those who decided to emigrate rather than settle in the coastal crofts is not disputed. The earlier emigrant ships of the 18th century were reasonably well equipped and not overcrowded. Conditions deteriorated. The rush of emigrants, the result of the Highland clearances of the late 18th century, later led to vicious profiteering by the shipowners and a dismal trail of disease and death. Many of the ships left from Highland coastal towns without going through any formalities at any port and hence the number of people leaving and the conditions on many of these ships are unknown.[63] However, even the facts about the ships which did register before leaving show that abuses existed. In 1791 a 270 ton ship left Skye for the Carolinas with 400 emigrants on board, each provided with berths 18 inches broad between decks 2 feet apart. Two ships – *Sarah* and *Dove* – left Fort William in 1801 for Canada and of 700 on board, 100 died, probably of typhus. There was a remarkably prompt government response in 1803 to deal with these abuses, and it was the first national intervention of its kind. On closer inspection, the motives behind this legislation were less admirable, since the government action came after the prompting of the Scottish landowners through their Highland Society. Their memorandum on emigration was sent to Parliament through the Scottish 'managers'

Charles Hope and Henry Dundas, and it showed that the landlords appeared primarily concerned at the loss of rents from the new crofts on the coast and the loss of a labouring population rather than with the problems of the emigrant ships. The memorandum pointed out that, in the years 1773 to 1803, the emigrants had also taken away £100,000 in cash 'lost to this nation for ever'. The memorandum went on to estimate that the number of people thinking of leaving that year was about 20,000. The government sent Thomas Telford north to report and to survey communications. His report showed the reasons for the emigration fever and he recommended some control of the emigrant ships and a scheme of public works in the Highlands. The legislation which resulted was the Passenger Vessels Act (1803), the first of many similar acts controlling the emigrant ships, and it laid down severe restrictions for operating these ships, including provision for a surgeon in any vessel carrying more than fifty persons.[64] To the delight of the Highland proprietors, this Act had its desired effect. The cost of a passage to North America trebled and emigration sharply declined. The coastal Highland population steadily increased and the tiny crofts were further subdivided for the new members of the families. This increase was only made possible by two special factors. Firstly, the kelp industry was successful in providing employment, particularly on the west coast and secondly, the population were prepared to survive on a basic diet of potato and fish – mostly herring. During the early years of the 19th century the kelp industry was still successful and, though the crofters' labour was greatly exploited, it was at least some form of work. The factors responsible for the success of the kelp industry were also the reasons for its sharp collapse. The Napoleonic Wars had increased the need for home-produced alkali and the kelp industry prospered as a result of this local demand. But with the peace of 1815, imports of cheap alternatives became possible. In 1827 the price of kelp collapsed and the industry failed, in spite of pleas by the landowners for intervention by the government. The tenacious Highlanders clung on in increasing poverty to their tiny patch of land, which provided them with potatoes as their only means of survival, a dependence which led to disaster.[65]

There had been earlier warnings of the crisis to come. The potato crop had been poor as a result of storms in 1772 and 1783 and the crop had failed partially in 1816 and 1836, but the communities had always survived the winter till the next year. But in 1846, a new disease struck the crop with speed and widespread destruction. The potato blight, the fungus *phytophthora infestans* which had earlier destroyed the Irish crop and killed large numbers of people by starvation, reached Scotland in 1846. Starting in Skye, it destroyed almost the entire Highland crop thereafter, leaving not only no food, but no seed potatoes for the next year. Any food reserves not destroyed had been eaten by the autumn and the people in some areas were starving. Diseases like typhus and scurvy appeared, and the spread of cholera was only checked by the distance between the communities and their use of pure spring water.[66] An appeal to the government was made and though it had not acted in Ireland, faced with a similar imminent disaster in the Highlands, the government acted quickly and decisively, though with many private reservations about the wisdom of doing so.[67] The Treasury sent Sir Edward Coffin to the Highlands to study the problem and to advise. Coffin did not share the conservative attitudes of his superiors at the Treasury. He confirmed that a disaster was likely and that local and national help was required to feed the hungry people. Locally, he urged the landowners to release funds and take advantage of government-assisted public works, which gave schemes to pay their tenants, hence providing money to purchase food. A small number of the proprietors responded, notably MacLeod of Dunvegan, who ensured that all his 8,000 people were fed and he nearly ruined himself in doing so, as did Matheson of Lewis. The worst response was from the absentee Gordon of Cluny, owner of the islands of Barra, South Uist and Benbecula, whom Coffin unsuccessfully tried to bully and then had to threaten. Coffin proposed to intervene directly and he wrote to Gordon saying he would leave Parliament to decide

> whether or not you should be legally responsible for the pecuniary consequences of this just and necessary intervention.[68]

Gordon reluctantly provided food for his tenants, but it may be that deaths from starvation occurred in Barra. Even this was not a free handout of food, but a loan, and the crofters were still paying back the cost years later. While Coffin was mobilising the local effort, a national rescue was on the way. Two ships with supplies of government meal were sent and arrived in December 1846 and food depots were set up in Tobermory and Portree. Coffin tried to restrict the food distribution only to places where the proprietors could not manage the relief themselves, but eventually the food was sold to all in need. Coffin had to contend with the nervous Treasury and particularly the powerful Sir Charles Trevelyan, the Assistant Secretary, who told him that nothing was to be done to interfere with local commerce and the market forces. This gave Coffin a problem, since the local entrepreneurs, including the landowners, were profiteering during the famine and the local price of meal had risen to double the normal level. Coffin's solution was to use the more reasonable prices charged in Glasgow, but even this started rising sharply in the winter as a result of a general scarcity in Britain. Coffin appealed to Trevelyan for a lower price but received back only instructions of strict Treasury orthodoxy – 'we cannot force down the prices of provisions without disorganising society.'

Fortunately, the government's emergency relief operation was quickly supported and taken over by other voluntary efforts. One usual source of aid was absent however. In the towns, the Poor Law would have stepped in, but in the Highlands of 1847, this mechanism did not exist. The Church in Scotland had split in 1843 and the Free Church had separated itself from the Church of Scotland. In the Highlands the vast majority of the crofters had joined the Free Church, thus putting themselves beyond the Poor Law organised by those remaining in the Church of Scotland – often only the minister and a handful of landowners and farmers. Not surprisingly, therefore, the first body to augment the government's rescue operation was the Free Church, who quickly obtained £15,000 of meal and transported it by boat to the areas in need. In addition, an interdenominational Central Board of Management of the Fund for the Relief of Destitute Inhabitants of the Highlands appeared in Edinburgh and Glasgow and continued the relief during the three years of the famine, 1847–50, raising no less than £250,000 during this time. The grateful Treasury offered the Board assistance with information on needs in the north and then bowed out, not without this parting homily from Trevelyan:

> Next to allowing the people to die of hunger, the greatest evil that could happen would be their being habituated to depend upon public charity.[69]

Evaluation of the success of the operation is difficult. Certified numbers and causes of death are not available for the Highlands in this period nor are there any figures on the number of deaths available from burial records. The suffering of the Highlands can only be judged from contemporary accounts made during these harrowing times and the record is confused by polemic and partisan publications.[70] However, it is clear that though a few deaths from starvation may have occurred, the rescue operation, particularly the early part, was a success. After the 1846 famine, the Highlanders concluded that the only solution was to leave and this was often aided by schemes of the landowners for an assisted passage.

Emigration was now encouraged. It was judged therefore that the early Passenger Acts were too strict and the regulations were eased. This new wave of emigration was encouraged by the landowners and, if anything else was needed to spur them on, it was the new amended Poor Law. This led to a compulsory local poor rate in each parish to aid all the poor of any denomination and since no middle class existed in the Highlands, the landowners took the full burden of this levy. Anxious prospective purchasers of Highland estates enquired first about the poor rate and often found it was three times the town level.

Though the emigrant ships in this new wave of departures were not grossly overcrowded, the journeys to Canada and elsewhere could be hazardous, as a result of shortage of food and the danger of typhus breaking out on the journey. During cholera epidemics the disease might also get on board ship with disastrous consequences, and even the average death rate on the British emigrant ships in 1847 was almost 10%. The governments of America and Canada often protested at the dumping of ill, dying and destitute Highlanders on their shores, often with no plans for their employment having been made. In Canada, special quarantine and general hospitals were set up on the east coast, notably on Grosse Island, to deal with these suffering emigrants, and almost 1 in 3 emigrants admitted to these refuges died.[71]

The Poor Law

Reform of the Poor Law was a central issue in 19th century Scottish politics and was to have important effects on medical practice later.[72] The 'old' Scots Poor Law dated from statutes of 1574 and 1579 and in several respects differed from that in England. The Scottish Poor Law has not won the admiration of all social historians because it was alleged to be mean and run by amateur administrators. The Poor Law was supported by money raised by collections in church, together with the fines imposed by the Church on moral offenders, and occasional contributions or assessments on the landowners. In Scotland, no relief for the fit unemployed was given, except for short spells. It also seems likely that the parishes in Scotland may have deliberately chosen to spend their money on schools rather than on the Poor Law and the success of Scottish education may have been at the expense of poor relief. Very few of the Scottish parishes resorted to a compulsory tax to raise the money for the support of the poor, though this was common in England. In the towns of 19th century Scotland, however, the rapid increase in population stretched the old Poor Law to the limit and there were even court cases in which the poor attempted to establish a legal right to aid and even to medical help.[73] The old Poor Law was unsuitable in the new towns for another reason. While in rural parishes the Poor Law had enabled the minister to give money in accordance with the needs of particular persons, the new poor of the towns were unknown to the parish ministers and the number of paupers created a severe financial strain on the urban parishes. Requests by the poor for relief were frequently answered by the suggestion that the applicants should return to the parish of their birth, advice which was particularly inappropriate for Highlanders driven from their homeland. However, there were occasional alternative sources of poor relief in the towns from charitable organisations, e.g. in Glasgow from the Trades House or private charities.

The old Scottish Poor Law had its staunch supporters and with great effort money was raised by charity to meet the deficiences of the Poor Law in the early 19th century. The first urban crisis came in 1813 with the end of the Napoleonic Wars and the resulting post-war trade depression. Beggars reappeared in Edinburgh and, after penal methods failed to disperse them, soup kitchens were provided and money was raised by the Committee for the Relief of the Working Class. The problems in Glasgow were similar and £10,000 was raised for the destitute. In 1832 similar difficulties recurred as a result of the cholera epidemic. In 1837 the cotton spinners strike also called for action and a committee in Glasgow raised £8,200 for relief by soup kitchens and hand-outs of food and fuel. It was hoped that each crisis would be the last and those who organised the relief continually hoped to be able to turn their attention to good works at home and abroad. But the problems of the Victorian towns multiplied and its citizens had to conclude that the health and welfare problems of Scotland were as bad as those of the heathen and that a change in the Poor Law was required. This was accomplished in 1845.

But this was only part of a series of major legislative measures affecting health, health care and medical education in Scotland in mid-century, the problems of each having been described above. The background to the remarkable entry of the state into Scottish affairs in the period 1845–1867 can now be studied and the reasons for the well-known delay in the appearance of Scottish legislation can be analysed.

6

The entry of the state 19th century (2)

The middle of the 19th century saw not only remarkable changes and improvement in medical and surgical care, but a flurry of legislation affecting health care, public health and medical education. The Poor Law was reformed in Scotland in 1845, and in a remarkable period in mid-century came the Universities (Scotland) Act of 1858, the Medical Act of the same year, the Public Health (Scotland) Act 1867 and the Lunacy Act (Scotland) 1857 as well as minor statutes and Police Acts. There was also legislation on the notification of death (1854) and to make vaccination compulsory (1864). Almost all these necessary reforms for Scotland were considerably delayed as compared with England, and to explain the paradox that this should occur in a country notable for contributions on the matters legislated for, requires an examination of attitudes in Scotland in the early part of the 19th century.

In the 18th century the success of Scottish intellectual life, and medical teaching in particular, had been undoubted. It had flourished in a time when parliament interfered little with the life of the nation, and in Scotland this support for unfettered private enterprise was strong, the greatest exponent of the theory and practice of *laissez-faire* being Adam Smith. In the early 19th century, Scotland could still consider herself to be at the centre of intellectual affairs. Edinburgh basked in the success of the *Edinburgh Review* which, starting in 1802, was the most successful British 19th century literary journal. The *Edinburgh Medical and Surgical Journal* started in 1805, had a similar format and had a similar authority in medical circles. The key to understanding the Scottish situation was that while Scotland and Edinburgh still considered themselves to be an important intellectual centre and the pacemaking area in Britain, in reality the power had passed to London and parliament. In denying or failing to recognise that reform in most matters now required parliament, the legislature and government money, Scottish affairs, isolated by the separate legal system and distance from parliament, went through a period of hesitation and confusion during which they were badly neglected.

Parliament could say with some justification that this neglect (which included health matters) was the result of the leaders of Scotland's lack of interest in practical politics, their hostility to the entry of government into the control of the Poor Law and public health and their opposition to London control in public health. The leaders of Scottish medical opinion could complain in their turn of a lack of consultation on early 19th century legislation affecting Scotland, like the Anatomy Act and the Apothecaries Act. There were also hints that the quality of the Scottish members of parliament did not impress the Scottish leaders of opinion and that they considered Scottish affairs were too important to be left in the hands of this members of parliament.

It was in the pages of the *Edinburgh Review* and *Blackwoods Magazine* that the first signs of the growth of power of central government in health matters can be seen. These Edinburgh periodicals contained the debate on the new legislation for the English Poor Law, and a complacent attitude to reform was encouraged by English criticism of their new legislation and compliments given by these critics to the old Scottish Poor Law. In reality, England was grappling with the problems of industrialism and the necessary intervention of government in the problems of poverty and unemployment, while Scotland, whose industrialisation had proceeded slightly slower than in England, and whose Poor Law had been run more cheaply than England, could graciously accept the admiration of those who opposed the necessary reform in England.

However, as disease and destitution worsened in the Scottish towns legislation in Scotland became necessary. In particular, criticism of the old Poor Law became stronger and the case for reform was made by William Pulteney Alison (1790–1859) the Edinburgh physician.[1] Alison had been influenced, as had a number of other reformers including Palmerston, by the Edinburgh teaching of Professor Dugald Stewart of the chair of Moral Philosphy. The other influence on Alison was his work in the New Town Dispensary in Edinburgh and he knew at first hand the real conditions of the poor in the towns, recognising clearly the links between poverty and disease. He was able to point out the known problems of the Poor Law, namely that the money raised was not enough, the administration was poor and that provision was not related to the needs of the community but to the sum available, and that all of these factors encouraged begging. He also brought forward statistics to show that Scotland's expenditure was low when compared with other European nations. He could also point to the success of the English Poor Law reform of 1834 in abolishing vagrancy. He marshalled the evidence in his pamphlet *Observations on the Management of the Poor in Scotland, and its effects on the Health of the Great Towns* (1840). In describing the health of the poor, he drew on comments from all over Scotland and hammered home the point that much disease came from poverty, and that disease caused poverty. He even reported that deaths from starvation had occurred in Edinburgh in patients dismissed from the hospital. Dr Alison also collected numerous testimonies to the amount of free medical assistance given by doctors to the poor, and constantly returned to the theme that the poor and starving were more prone to disease. Mr Forrest, surgeon in Stirling, commented that he had seen no cases of fever in persons who had a sufficiently nourishing diet.

Dr Alison also described difficulties in getting help for the poor in the towns and quoted a case of a man who had worked in Glasgow for eight years, but had lived as a lodger and hence had no legal rights as a resident. He had been injured and his leg had been amputated: he was unable to get work thereafter.

> His furniture, which was exceedingly neat and respectable, had been disposed of piecemeal until one evening his wife told me they were utterly reduced. The last thing was the coat, or rather the suit, in which he had been married. I applied to the Town's Hospital for a little temporary aid for him but it was in vain. He had only been a lodger. I corresponded with his native parish but they knew nothing of him as he had left it when a boy.

Nor were the doctors well treated by the Poor Law. Dr William Gibson commented that he had practised in Dumfries for twenty-eight years and during that time he had visited the poor regularly. In that time, he had never received more than a shilling a year for this work from the Kirk Session. Moreover

> during sickness, the poor would starve if I did not personally apply to individual landowners for help with a nutritious diet for the sick.

In Glasgow there was support from some medical men for Alison's campaign and occasionally it came with surprising vigour. Andrew Buchanan, professor of materia medica in Anderson's College, describing the condition of Glasgow in 1830 said

> that many of the poor in this city die of starvation . . . I have described the minds of these poor people as in a state of torpor. That torpor ought, perhaps, to be accounted a blessing, as it prevents them from speculating on the causes of their own misery.[2]

Robert Perry, President of the Faculty of Physicians and Surgeons, also wondered why there had been no revolution when

> a fourth part of the earnings of the industrious poor is taken from them to keep up the landlords' rents, the wealth of the sugar lords, and an expensive army of civil and military officers to keep them in order . . .[3]

He called for compulsory taxation and adequate spending on health care for the poor.

But there was determined opposition to taxation in any form. The General Assembly of the Church of Scotland had regularly declared against compulsory taxation and a state-run system of poor relief and could point to the new English Poor Law's bureaucratic problems and waste of money. Dr Alison therefore had to start a great debate on the principle of reform of the Poor Law. The churches, who had administered the system up to this time, had an energetic advocate in Dr Thomas Chalmers, the Glasgow minister, who held that the Poor Law should continue to be the responsibility of the Church. To back up this view he conducted a bold experiment in his own parish of St John's in Glasgow, and he and the elders of his church ran an economical poor relief system which was reported to be able to meet their needs. Though it took Dr Chalmers' enthusiasm to run such a system – it was not achieved elsewhere – his eloquence delayed the reform of the Poor Law in Scotland.

The alternative view that the state should step in where the Church had failed, was adopted as a result of a Royal Commission in 1844. The resulting Poor Law Amendment (Scotland) Act of 1845 placed the task of helping the poor in the hands of a lay Parochial Board, later to be called the Parish Council, who had powers to raise the necessary funds. The first weeks of the new law were chaotic and an account by one of the early Poor Law administrators, one sympathetic to Dr Chalmers' views, describes the events.

> In Glasgow, the advent of the new Act caused a great upheaval. Poor people of all kinds thought they were now provided for life. One thousand to thirteen hundred individuals besieged the office each day of the week, demanding relief, hundreds of them waiting till midnight before their cases could be examined. The sight of such a multitude was deplorable, consisting as it did of all kinds of characters – the aged, the infirm, the drunkard and idler, children in arms and at the feet, all mixed up in one motley multitude. Pauperism in the city increased at the rate of 10,000 a year, and this at a time when employment was good, provisions cheap, and the general health quite ordinary. This lapse from the principle of independence and self-reliance was greatly augmented by a rush of people from Ireland, who thought the new poor rate had turned Glasgow into an Eldorado.[4]

Eventually a reasonable level of application for relief resulted. The new Scottish Poor Law made little mention of medical services, and the English Act had made none at all. However a brief statement in the Scottish legislation made statutory provision for medical attention for the paupers both inside and outside the poorhouse. It was from this brief clause that the Poor Law medical services were to grow and which eventually gave rise to the state medical services of the 20th century. The medical services under the Poor Law will be described later, after considering the second great reform, that of public health.

Public health legislation

Scotland had a similarly slow start to the reform of public health. Legislation for Scotland was delayed even longer than in the case of the Poor Law and only in 1867 was the Public Health (Scotland) Act available, though some towns had taken advantage of local Police Acts and minor legislation to deal with 'nuisances'. The delay is surprising since at the start of the 19th century the Edinburgh doctors had a good grasp of the necessity for 'medical police' and writers like Pringle and Buchan in the 18th century had clearly established the need for sanitary measures. One of the first British texts on public health was written by John Roberton in Edinburgh – his *Treatise on Medical Police* of 1809. Scotland had made a remarkable start on the collection of figures on the health and welfare, particularly in large towns. Even the first use of 'statistics' had been by Sir John Sinclair the editor of *The Statistical Account of Scotland* 1791–99. Pioneer statisticians like Watt and Cleland in Glasgow had produced the first reliable data on disease and death in any large British population and shown that the public health problems of Glasgow were the worst in Britain. The delay in the Scottish legislation showed similarities to the delay in the Poor Law measures. Parliament was far away, and some of the early legislation did not fit the Scottish legal terminology.[5] Moreover, in the matter of public health, the Scottish views, again expressed by Alison in Edinburgh were different from those in England. The English reform was urged by the abrasive and intolerant reformer, Edwin Chadwick. Chadwick was a conspicuous supporter of the 'miasma' theory of disease and hence that the necessary action was to remove stagnant or polluted water or decaying material, regarding city graveyards as another possible threat to health. Chadwick's emphasis therefore was on grand schemes for improved water supply and sewage disposal. For Alison the priorities were different.[6] He was critical of the miasma theory without being totally convinced as a contagionist. His view was that infectious disease could spread from person to person in some way and that overcrowding and malnutrition were the main problems to be overcome. His campaign for the Poor Law reform in Scotland was also part of his solution to the health problem in the towns. While Alison had been held back by Chalmers in the Scottish campaign for Poor Law reform, his difference of opinion with Chadwick probably held back Scottish public health reform.

The legislation necessary to prevent the spread of infectious disease and epidemics required improved sanitation, a good water supply, a reduction in overcrowding, help for the destitute and starving, removal of dangers in food and a responsive democratic local government. The first legislation attempted was the Public Health (Scotland) Bill in 1848. The proposals were fairly simple, making permanent the short-lived Boards of Health, which had been set up from time to time to deal with epidemics, but the Bill never became law. It was the first major health Bill which would have treated Scotland simply as part of the United Kingdom. The legislation closely resembled the English Act, but more importantly, it suggested that the Scottish administration be supervised by a central Board of Health in London.

It produced in Scotland a response which was part of a growing expression at that time of remoteness from Westminster government, an attitude which was to intensify in the later 19th century and produce the office of Secretary for Scotland in 1885, later to be the Secretary of State. The Royal College of Physicians in Edinburgh boldly opposed the London control and suggested instead a General Board for Scotland 'conversant with the laws of Scotland'. The College's report continued:

> The Committee will take the liberty of adding that although they have a high respect for the individual members of the General Board of Health in London, the confident expression of opinion which the gentlemen have officially made on several important questions touching the diffusion of epidemic diseases, which the Committee regard as very difficult and doubtful – and on which they know that some of the most experienced practitioners in Scotland hold a very definite opinion – have by no means tended to increase their expectation of the efficiency of measures applicable to Scotland for restraining the diffusion of epidemics which may proceed from that source.[7]

In short, the College believed that Scottish doctors and local authorities were best equipped to deal with local problems. This attitude of the College may have been influenced by Chadwick's rather unhelpful attitude to the Edinburgh views expressed by Dr Alison on the spread of infectious disease, and the way the Edinburgh College's degrees were not recognised by some English authorities at the time.

Thus an Act for the whole of Scotland was delayed, but some towns – the 'big six' – including Glasgow, managed to get authority for their own improvements in housing and water supply, and other minor legislation was used elsewhere until the main Act appeared in 1867. Glasgow and Edinburgh had obtained early authority for an Officer of Health. The original suggestion was that the Officer would be a doctor and his duties would be merely to report on the numbers and causes of death in each district. By the time the legislation was passed, however, and in response to the Royal College of Physicians of Edinburgh's suggestion that the duties

> should be widened to a more general instruction to suggest from time to time such regulations as he may think fit for improving the sanitary conditions of his district

the Medical Officer of Health, as he was to be known, had aquired considerable statutory powers to inspect, report and use the law against individuals or groups threatening the health of the community. Such was the problem of the health of the towns and such was the power of the Medical Officer of Health, that these new posts, Edinburgh in 1862 and Glasgow in 1863, attracted some remarkable men whose social conscience was combined with considerable energy, and whose success in dealing with the serious problems made them considerable figures in the Scotland of that period.

The first Scottish Medical Officer of Health was Edinburgh's Henry Duncan Littlejohn (1826–1914). The initiative was taken in Edinburgh following a civic scandal in 1861. After the collapse of a tenement causing thirty-five deaths, it was found that one hundred persons had lived in the building, and measures against overcrowding had to be taken. Littlejohn moved carefully but decisively in Edinburgh, preparing the way with his classic contribution to public health literature *Report on the Sanitary Condition of the City of Edinburgh* (1865), and the reforms he desired were conceded.[8] His notable negotiating triumph was the introduction into Edinburgh in 1880 of the compulsory notification of infectious disease by the doctors, the first such law in Britain and one which eventually became a national measure. In this he was initially opposed by the Edinburgh doctors and the Royal College but in the end he won the argument and the Medical Officer of Health could thus acquire early warnings of dangerous disease and epidemics.

In Glasgow the problems were greater in quantity and quality, with overcrowding the greatest evil. Glasgow had the good fortune to have an enlightened chairman of the town's Sanitary Committee in John Ure, who had successfully steered the town's sanitary reform and who was determined to obtain a Medical Officer of Health for Glasgow. He wanted 'a man of enlarged view in sanitary science with a knowledge of infectious disease.' He had in mind the new professor of medicine in Glasgow, William Tennant Gairdner (1824–1907) and Gairdner accepted the part-time post in 1863.[9] Doubtless Gairdner's attitude to infectious disease was influenced by being a colleague of Joseph Lister in the Royal Infirmary at the time.

With Ure's firm support, Gairdner was provided with five full-time Medical Officers and a municipal Sanitary Department, a function served in other cities by a number of departments responsible to a number of committees. Dr Gairdner described himself as a

> Commander-in-chief newly appointed: an active enemy swarming all over the land, holding every strategic point, well found and well equipped.

To fight the battle he had to

> recruit, drill and equip his army and subsidise mercenaries

and he had, from the start, better municipal support than Edinburgh. The rise of these sanitary measures in Glasgow was not without its critics. The Glasgow doctors' journal, the noisy but conservative *Glasgow Medical Examiner* concluded that

> the sooner that the so-called sanitary office is closed the better, both in respect to our purse, our expectations and our peace of mind, for it is nothing but a specious pretension.[10]

In spite of these attacks the sanitary department prospered and a unique system of 'ticketing' was introduced during this collectivist phase in Glasgow's history, which was admired by other towns, if not by guardians of human rights. The Medical Officer of Health could limit the number of inhabitants in any dwelling simply by posting a notice on the outside of the house showing the upper limit of the number of inhabitants. The law was enforced by night-time raids by the police and the Medical Officers of Health, and in 1870 alone there were 47,163 raids of this kind in Glasgow. Gairdner, having accomplished much, resigned in 1871 at a time when the staff of his department had reached thirty-six, returning to his professorial post. Glasgow then appointed James B. Russell (1837–1904) as a full-time Medical Officer of Health.[11] He was also a pupil of Lister and had been in charge of one of Gairdner's most successful projects, the fever hospital in Parliamentary Road, Glasgow, the first of its kind in Scotland. He carried on the work of prosecuting sanitary offences, encouraging new legislation and, through his writings, became one of the best known and respected of the Medical Officers of Health. Medical Officers of Health had a broad range of legislative powers and they could deal with overcrowding, pollution, adulteration of food and drink and infectious disease carriers.

But one crucial improvement to Glasgow's health had occurred earlier – the provision of a pure water supply – which ensured that

Glasgow escaped the 1866 epidemic of cholera.[12] The Glasgow water scheme, which was greatly admired elsewhere, was brought in only after a struggle with conservative forces and commercial interests. In 1834 the first attempts to amalgamate the three private water companies were opposed in principle by the Glasgow Town Council on the grounds that it would remove competition. By 1852 the demand for a civic water supply was considerable and, after some alternative schemes had been considered, Loch Katrine was proposed as a source of supply for the town. The private water companies objected once more and there was a modest ratepayers' revolt against the cost. The opponents of the scheme managed to get the professor of chemistry at Glasgow to state that the Loch Katrine water was 'highly charged with lead' but, on further examination of this claim, the professor withdrew it and explained that he was merely quoting another vague opinion. Chemical analysis showed that the water was indeed of high purity. A more serious objection came from the Admiralty who alleged that this removal of the source of the water of the Teith would lead to silting up of the Firth of Forth and thus endanger the Navy's only anchorage north of the Humber. This objection carried enough weight to postpone the Loch Katrine scheme by a few years, but by 1855 the Admiralty conceded that their interests would not be harmed.

The drive against overcrowding in Glasgow met with opposition also. The reduction in overcrowding was thwarted initially by the landlords' opposition. Housing in central Glasgow, for instance, was controlled by a complex network of landlords and subletting, profitable at each step, and provost Blackie's radical proposal to deal with this problem by buying the worst area of overcrowded land and improving the housing was so unpopular with the owners and those who faced a 6p per pound assessment, that he was opposed and defeated in the election for the new Council in 1867. Nevertheless his schemes eventually were implemented by others.

In Edinburgh, bourgeois opposition focused instead on the provision of a pure water supply, and the controversy reached its peak in 1871, when the *Scotsman*, itself strongly against the plans was filled with letters in a ratio of 10:1 against the proposals.[13] But Edinburgh eventually obtained its water supply.

While the large towns in Scotland had pressed ahead with improvements, proudly using the legislation obtained for their town from parliament, the unsatisfactory national legislation for Scotland held back reform in the country towns and villages

> where only the closer proximity of the countryside sometimes made their insanitary horrors less horrific . . . the unlovely spectacle of late-Victorian Coatbridge, Motherwell, Blantyre and Port Glasgow . . .[14]

In Stirling, the struggle was a long one. The *Report on the Sanitary Condition of the Labouring Population of Scotland* in 1842 contained an analysis of the problems in Stirling written by Dr William Forrest, surgeon to the Stirling Dispensary, where he showed that the incidence of typhus in the town was worst in the overcrowded streets and where sanitation was poor. The problem and the solutions were clear: raising the money was difficult as the town had only a small separate income. While the Stirling inhabitants were prepared to respond to calls for occasional voluntary subscriptions to pave the streets or build a hospital during a cholera scare a permanent system of rating was quite another matter and was opposed by the inhabitants.[15] It was only achieved in stages. The case for a pure water supply was undeniable, but whether it should be by a private company or by municipal enterprise was the dominant issue in Stirling politics from 1844 to 1848. Eventually the principle of a compulsory rate for the water supply only was conceded. The ratepayers thereafter staged another revolt over plans for sewers, and fought the powers given in a new Police Act to the Town Council, with the effect that the new water supply exceeded the capacity of the old sewage system. By 1872 the ratepayers were prepared to part with another penny in the pound for the sewers, aided by some adverse comments on the town's sanitation during a visitation of the Board of Supervision. Thus, painfully and slowly, the town of Stirling was improved and local rates accepted grudgingly. None of the measures was forced on the town by government, but there was enlightened legislation there to be used and, if the town complied, funds from central government were available to increase the sum, a mechanism used thereafter by government to encourage reform and improvement. The last town in Scotland to deal with its sanitation was Forfar and the town became known for its determination to resist compulsory rates. Eventually government had to use its compulsory powers in 1877 to protect the inhabitants of the town from an unhealthy water supply and inadequate sewerage.[16] But above all it was in Glasgow that the sanitary measures could be seen to have worked: death rates and morbidity fell dramatically. The town's people valued it and were prepared to pay for it. The staff of the Sanitary Department in Glasgow rose from 90 in 1886 to 401 in 1914 and Glasgow could claim by then that the worst of the self-inflicted disease of the Industrial Revolution was past. By the mid-1870's, Glasgow crude death rate had declined from the peak of 56 per 1,000 in 1847 to regain the 22 per 1,000 rate of the 1820's and it steadily declined thereafter. Smallpox had become much less important and when cholera made a last appearance in Britain in 1866–67 Scotland was hardly affected. Many of the other problem diseases were declining rapidly – notably typhus, typhoid and scarlet fever, but measles, whooping cough and particularly tuberculosis were slower to go. Diseases of older age groups like cancer and heart disease inevitably increased. The birth rate also declined and the improved urban housing and rising real wages allowed an improved standard of living, which also must have helped reduced the incidence of disease. Glasgow's prosperity then allowed an enlightened local government to create almost unrivalled municipal services. The improved educational system of the second half of the 19th century spread ideas of hygiene and no longer did ratepayers fight the sanitary schemes of the councils nor did retailers rejoice in escaping prosecution for dangerous practices.[17] Though conventional medical practice contributed little to this general improvement in health, the doctors emerged with an enhanced status and power. This centred on the voluntary hospitals and other Victorian agencies then at the peak of their influence.

Doctors and medical education

The middle of the 19th century was a turning point for the doctors. Having been acknowleged as a professional group by the Medical Act of 1858, they left behind the struggles between the physicians and surgeons and the apothecaries. Though they succeeded in gaining their professional status in society, new problems developed. The first was that there were too many doctors being produced and success in private practice appeared harder and harder to attain and could only come after many years of difficulty. Private practice fees had not risen since the start of the century. With the output of large numbers of graduates from the Scottish medical schools, it must have been particularly difficult to become established in Glasgow or Edinburgh. As an alternative, the doctors were thrown back on the steadily growing number of salaried posts available from the State – Poor Law posts in the community or the poorhouses, Medical Officer of Health jobs with the large towns, salaried posts with the friendly societies and even in factories or prisons with a salary half that of the chaplain. And there was always the Army and Navy or work in the colonies. In all these positions, the doctors found themselves under lay control, whose interference was resented. The doctors fought an increasingly successful battle for freedom which was only completely accomplished by the middle of the 20th century. While the old divisions within the profession disappeared, a new cleavage appeared. The start of the 19th century saw the disappearance of the ancient separation between the physicians and surgeons, while the second part of the century saw a rise of as great a gulf between the general practitioner and the hospital consultant. In the second half of the century the hospitals became safer as a result of antisepsis, and the new skills of the hospital doctors marked them out as a separate caste. Moreover, the general practitioners complained that the hospital consultants were threatening their living, since the free out-patient dispensaries of the voluntary hospitals were treating patients who might afford the fees of a doctor, and people sent for an opinion to a hospital doctor might be lost as a private patient to the general practitioner for ever.

At the end of the century the differences in medical practice between Scotland and England which had previously existed were much less obvious. The reconciliation between the physicians and surgeons which had occurred first in Scotland was then repeated in England. England had also faithfully copied the Scottish medical schools and were teaching midwifery, medicine and surgery by the end of the century.

Though the Scottish university degrees were accepted throughout Britain after 1858, the universities had one or two battles to win in the middle of the century, a period known then as the 'thirty years war.' The first problem was a curious effect of the English Poor Law regulations which, to ensure a high standard of doctor, required all applicants to have qualifications in both medicine and surgery, just in the way that Scottish medical education had developed. Though the medical qualification could be from a university, the surgical diploma had to be from the London College of Surgeons, and the Scottish doctors had again to contemplate obtaining another English qualification. In the case of Scottish graduates, these regulations were unnecessary and obstructive, since both medicine and surgery had been taught. Eventually the weary Scottish universities and Colleges persuaded the Poor Law Commissioners that the regulation be waived. The second problem also arose from the insistence on a double qualification, this time in the regulations of the new General Medical Council stating that the Colleges of Physicians and Surgeons should give qualifications in both medicine and surgery. The corporations in Scotland had sensibly joined forces and formed a conjoint body to conduct examinations in both surgery and medicine, but the London Colleges had been dilatory. As a result, in 1871 the General Medical Council again had to propose a single U.K. examination to be sat prior to entry into practice. Lyon Playfair, M.P. for the Scottish Universities wrote to Principal Turner of Edinburgh University in 1871:

> I had hoped that you would make some arrangements [for a Board to run a national examination] in Scotland, which was not hostile to University interests. My own opinion is against these Conjoint Boards . . . but medical opinion in England and Parliamentary opinion is dead against us on this question and if you do not adjust your sails to the wind (which is not likely to change), you will find legislation go very injuriously to our interests.[18]

But he was wrong. Strong opposition to the plan appeared and a key debating point against the plan was the failure of a similar scheme in Germany – the *Staatsexamen*. In the face of this opposition, and helped by a change of government, the British single-portal scheme failed. The universities were still free to teach and examine their own students, and the doctors corporations could still license medical practitioners. But while the British universities had settled their internal differences, they faced a more serious challenge from outside.

Scotland and Europe

By the late 19th century the Scottish medical schools faced up to the reality that the continental medical schools were now the pioneers in medical research and education and particularly post-graduate education. The dominance of Germany is most clearly seen by the large number of British medical graduates who carried out post-graduate study in a German university. Even more revealing is the choice of the late 19th century American medical student for study in Europe rather than in Britain. The early American pioneers, like Benjamin Rush, John Morgan and William Shippen, had taken back their sophisticated Edinburgh education to America in the 18th century. There followed a period of rapid internal expansion in American and the rough and ready needs of the new frontiers and the fierce egalitarianism of American society led to minimal or even no training for their doctors. As in France during the Revolution, anyone could set up as a healer. By the end of the 19th century, however, America was ready for a return to conventional standards of training, but while their forbears a century earlier had looked to Edinburgh for this, they now travelled to Germany. The doctors who put American medicine on the course which would lead it to dominate 20th century medicine were trained at the great city universities of Germany or at the medical schools of the rural towns. A large number of Russian doctors also travelled to Germany, including Pavlov, and who, like the Americans, returned to introduce the new thinking to their homeland. Professor Gairdner of Glasgow reported in 1870 on his German travels:

> I came away convinced that medical science and scientific training are, unhappily, in danger of being starved in England and Scotland . . . the prospects for us are indeed rather gloomy unless we can succeed in rousing the public as well as ourselves to the idea that 'they manage these things better in Germany'. In almost all our medical schools we greatly need a physiological and pathological laboratory . . . I confess I do not know where to look at present for the liberal and wealthy citizen of Glasgow who would seek to immortalise himself . . .[19]

Gairdner's assumption that the money should come from philanthropic sources is interesting: for him to look to the government for aid was not clearly a possibility. To consider the intrusion of government into areas where there was no social crisis or threat to national security was intolerable to Victorian thought.[20] But Gairdner also hinted that the voluntary help for the laboratories, necessary to keep up with European medical science, would not be available. His concern was because the general public viewed both physiology and pathology with suspicion. The first because it meant vivisection was not favoured: the second because post mortem examination was reminiscent of the resurrectionists. Slowly the scientists started to press the government for support, and Lyon Playfair, the chemist trained at Anderson's College in Glasgow, was a crucial figure in this lobby which eventually led to the appearance of the Royal Commission on Scientific Instruction and also to the British Association for the Advancement of Science. Thus science in Victorian times stagnated: round the academic neck hung the millstone of the philosophy of individualism and self-help, and the attitude of the philanthropists was anti-science and hostile to medical research. In the short term the only hope was to raise voluntary subscriptions and Edinburgh University, who awarded an LL.D degree to Samuel Smiles, did manage by a remarkable effort to raise more than half of the £210,000 required for the new medical school in 1869 from private sources. Yet the assistant-less professors of the new school had to purchase their research equipment from their own pockets.

Some assistance did come from government after a Scottish Universities Commission of 1878. This followed the German example in not only increasing the number of salaried professors but also providing for salaried young assistants and for the first time the government provided money for laboratory equipment. In 1889 the University of Edinburgh abandoned its ancient system of paying fees directly to the professor, not without protest from defenders of the old ways. The Royal College of Physicians in Edinburgh opened a laboratory in 1887, though the proposal was initially turned down twice.[21]

The calm of the Edinburgh medical school, after the Medical Act of 1858, was interrupted by the increasing demands from women to study medicine. Although Elizabeth Garrett Anderson had managed to register as a doctor after a course of private instruction in London, the medical schools of Britain still excluded women. Medical reform gave the signal for women to start their fight for admission to the universities to train as doctors.[22] In 1869 Sophia Jex-Blake (1840–1912) applied to enter medical training in Edinburgh by enrolling in the classes of botany and natural history. The Senate considered the claim and allowed it, making Edinburgh the first medical school to admit women. But a small group including anatomy Professor W. Turner – later to be Principal – continued with their opposition. His case was that the presence of women would make discipline difficult, would be repulsive to the men and would make it impossible to teach anatomy. Jex-Blake, now joined by four others, asked the Senate to set up separate teaching classes. The Senate agreed and recommended the medical teachers to make the necessary arrangements. Some professors agreed to do so but a vocal minority were opposed to the change as were the male students and the Royal Infirmary managers. Proper teaching was impossible. The ladies took legal action to compel the University Court's decision to be put into action and won their case. On appeal, the decision was overturned and it was even ruled that the University constitution prevented the entry of women at all. The Edinburgh appeal judgement was applauded throughout the land:[23]

> Certain restless women have sought recognition as students, and especially have they pressed their claims on the University of Edinburgh and the General Medical Council. The former have said 'no' but the latter have opened the door to future trouble and have given grave offence to the profession.

Jex-Blake eventually graduated M.D. in 1876 in Switzerland where women were freely admitted and returned to practise in Edinburgh in 1878 and fight for the medical education of women, having also taken a registrable qualification in Ireland.

The Colleges of Physicians and Surgeons in Edinburgh allowed women to start studies in 1886, with clinical teaching at Leith Hospital but not the Royal Infirmary. Thus a small separate school of medicine for women was opened and the Universities (Scotland) Act 1889 opened the way for the admission of women with an equal status to men. Separate instruction was arranged and the number of women doctors practising in Scotland rose from 4 in 1881 to 60 in 1901. But it was World War I and the demand for doctors and the lack of young men that finally brought women their equal status. There was opposition to the last. In 1914 some Edinburgh women doctors raised funds and staff for the Scotish Women's Hospital but this offer to help was declined by the War Office. Instead, the doctors and nurses travelled to Europe and worked for the Russian, Serbian and Greek armies. They were led by one of Scotland's pioneer women doctors, Elsie Inglis.[24]

The voluntary movement

The later 19th century in Scotland saw the consolidation of the voluntary movement, and its hospitals missions and social work agencies made a major contribution to health care.[25] The new middle class created by the industrial revolution had an awareness of the social and health problems of 19th century society through their church work with the urban poor and they were dominant in the voluntary movement. The reward for the organisers of this voluntary work was thought to be largely a spiritual one plus the economic benefit of a healthy work force, but the prestige resulting from conspicuous charitable and social work gave opportunities to the middle class for social advance and contacts with the aristocracy.

Also important in the success of the voluntary hospital and dispensary movement was that for the doctors, success in private practice was assured following an appointment to one of the voluntary hospitals or to a lesser extent to one of the dispensaries. Thus the young doctors were prepared to spend their early years in the voluntary hospital posts on low salaries. Private means were often required to survive these early days, but on becoming a ward chief, those surviving would reap the rewards of private practice. Thus the voluntary hospitals were often the centre of feuds and tensions in the struggle for private practice. The voluntary movement was opposed to state control and taxation, and in this affluent period in Scotland it was particularly successful in slowing the growth of the state agencies. It mitigated poverty without changing society and gave opportunities for evangelism. In Scotland it was a notably protestant movement and members of the Roman Catholic community in Glasgow were usually excluded from the staff of the voluntary institutions: hence the Catholic churches often refused to support these charities.

There were a few additions to the number of Scottish voluntary hospitals in the late 19th century, notably Greenock in 1868 and Stirling in 1874. In Glasgow the building of the Western Infirmary (1874), the Victoria Infirmary (1890) and the Royal Hospital for Sick Children (1883) kept the ratio of beds to the population at about 1.6 per 1,000 persons. This figure was similar to other cities in Britain, though Edinburgh had the more favourable ratio of 3.1 beds per 1,000 persons. Even so, there was opposition to new projects in Glasgow, and the managers of the Royal Infirmary opposed not only the plan for the Western Infirmary but also for the children's hospital, on the grounds that no need existed and that the limited charitable support from the city would be split and hence reduced. In the event, both new hospitals were needed and the Western Infirmary, situated beside the University and carefully fostered by it, at last provided clinical status for the university staff. After 150 years of disputes with the Royal Infirmary, university teaching was possible and the students deserted the Royal. The plan for the Edinburgh Hospital for Sick Children (1860) was also opposed by the Edinburgh Royal Infirmary.

In addition to the large voluntary hospitals, the number of smaller specialist hospitals in Glasgow, Edinburgh and Aberdeen and Greenock increased, as the concept of specialisation in one type of disease was favoured. The maternity hospitals had come first, with the Glasgow University Lying-in Hospital of 1792. Venereal disease cases were excluded from some Scottish voluntary hospitals and for this reason a special Lock Hospital was subscribed to and erected in Glasgow in 1805, but it was not a favourite charity and needed grants from the parish authorities to keep it open. Edinburgh's Lock Hospital was even less well supported, and had a short life only from 1835–47. The treatment of eye disease also emerged early as a specialty, following the German lead, and the Glasgow Eye Infirmary appeared in 1824 and the Edinburgh Eye, Ear, Nose and Throat Hospital opened in 1834. From then on a large number of other small specialist hospitals opened throughout Scotland.

While the large hospitals were corporate collections of practitioners, these smaller hospitals were often the result of the enthusiasm of individuals who persuaded a philanthropist to raise a subscription for the erection of the building. Professional jealousy was acute in Victorian times, and the prospect of a practitioner making his name by means of his own hospital could irritate the other doctors, and the Glasgow medical scene was enlivened by a number of polemics against such new specialist institutions. One of these new hospitals in Glasgow caused this type of controversy in 1865. An eye specialist, Dr J.R. Wolfe, who later pioneered methods of skin and cornea grafting and had trained on the continent, arrived from Aberdeen and set up his Ophthalmic Institution, advertising free treatment to the poor between certain hours. The disgruntled *Glasgow Medical Examiner* commented:

> The varied phases of medical benevolence in our day is a subject well worthy of investigation. It may afford a theme to future cynics and historians . . . In two of the leading daily papers

> of this city . . . appears an egregious puff direct of yet another special institution for Glasgow; and in the name of our profession, which is by these means outraged, we enter our protest. . . notwithstanding Dr Wolfe's assertions to the contrary, he exacted fees during the hours advertised for gratis consultation . . . It is very true that with the skin, the chest, the ear and other dispensaries in view, Dr Wolfe might adopt a *tu quoque* argument; but the existence of one evil does not justify the formation of another.[26]

Apart from these polemics, more reasoned criticism of the voluntary movement existed. A comprehensive service might not be provided, since the philanthropists had their own priorities, and might favour emotionally charged appeals, rejecting less attractive problems like venereal disease, mental illness or the problems of chronic disease like tuberculosis and cancer. Secondly the philanthropists were not attracted to schemes for support of research or laboratories and hence in Scotland and Britain, hospital research and development lagged badly behind the efforts in France and Germany. Towards the end of the 19th century, the need for further major hospital projects faded and the energies of the voluntary movement and their philanthropists were instead directed into subscriptions for building cottage hospitals in the smaller towns, the development of convalescent homes, spreading the temperance movement and running the new nursing organisations.

Nursing

In the later 19th century the quality of nursing care also improved.[27] The pressure for this came from reformers like Florence Nightingale and doctors who saw the benefits of improved care and skills in managing surgical patients. The reform of nursing care was aided by royal patronage and the early feminist movement, and it became the first suitable occupation for women who earlier had been forced to remain idle at home. Reluctantly the managers of the Scottish voluntary hospitals found the money for the improved pay of the nurses and, for the first time, paid for the nurses food. Charitable bodies helped the hospitals by paying for the new nurses homes. The middle class also realised the need for expert nursing care and since all treatment for the well-to-do, even surgical operations, was carried out in their homes a number of private nursing agencies appeared in the Scottish cities. These agencies also did charitable work outside the hospital and funds were raised for nursing of the poor.

Dispensaries

The earliest dispensaries were founded in the 18th century but the urban crisis of the mid 19th century accelerated the growth of the dispensary movement. The early voluntary hospitals did not wish the financial burden of an out-patient department and preferred the appearance of separate charities which constructed and financed dispensaries. The original Edinburgh Royal Public Dispensary of 1776 has been described earlier, and it continued its work in the 19th century. The opening of a second dispensary in Edinburgh in 1815 – the New Town Dispensary – caused controversy, though the rivalry diminished after they agreed to divide the work of the town between them. The new dispensary pioneered home visitation of the poor. A third dispensary appeared in 1841, with its original aims that of evangelism and medical missionary work abroad, notably in China – the Edinburgh Medical Mission Society.[28] The founders however became aware that as much need existed in the slums of Edinburgh and that free medical treatment was highly successful in promoting evangelism. They therefore opened a free dispensary in 1859 in the Cowgate. Medical students were essential to the work of the Mission, and found the training useful. Those patients wishing to be seen gathered at a certain hour, a service was held and the patients then treated.

In Glasgow the dispensaries were more numerous, but less permanent, and many had a short life.[29] The first was the Glasgow Dispensary of 1801 which lasted fifteen years, and the Celtic Dispensary followed in 1837 with a life of about ten years. At about this time also the Western Public Dispensary had a short existence and at its peak its four medical officers were seeing 1,000 patients per year. There were also missionary dispensaries in Glasgow, copied from the Edinburgh example, such as the Glasgow Medical Mission, which dispensed advice, medicines and scripture. However there were no provident dispensaries on the English model, which led to anxiety in Glasgow that the poor were being too well served, and their initiative numbed. Dr Russell, Medical Officer of Health for Glasgow, calculated however that the main cities of Scotland provided less of a service through voluntary dispensaries than elsewhere.

While in Liverpool, 18.1% of the population were treated in a dispensary in 1874, the figures for Edinburgh (13.1%) and Glasgow (5.5%) were lower.

The reasons for this curious neglect in Glasgow is not clear. It is true that it was sometimes hard to raise the money for the dispensary and, since free medicines were given, the annual running costs were considerable. Certainly, the dispensaries came in for criticism over the number of patients seen in such a short time and the use of students in training. But the main inhibiting factor was probably opposition from the local doctors, notably those in general practice, who suspected that many of the patients attending the dispensaries could afford the doctor's fees. With the production of doctors by Glasgow and Edinburgh medical schools greatly in excess of local needs, doubtless many young graduates attempted to start practice in these towns and to them the dispensaries were probably a threat.

The problem of knowing who was genuinely poor was also an insoluble problem. The Perth Dispensary had opened in 1819 to vaccinate, give medicine and obstetric care when necessary to the poor. Until 1832, about 304 patients were treated annually in this way. But there was concern in Perth that not all the patients were really deserving of this charity and the directors of the Dispensary, sensitive to the attitudes of the subscribers, made one of the few Scottish attempts at a provident dispensary, the Perth Self-supporting Dispensary to treat those who were regular wage earners. Medical care was given in return for a subscription of one penny a week, and this new institution opened in 1834. In the next three years, however, the number of workers contributing to this experimental institution numbered 31, 9 and lastly only 4, while the original free dispensary increased its work. The debate on the principle of self-help in Perth went no further, since the Royal Infirmary opened in 1838 and the two dispensaries closed.[30]

The work of the independent dispensaries waned towards the end of the 19th century, as the voluntary hospitals' own dispensaries and their out-patient departments increased their work. These departments could admit the patient for treatment inside the hospital and hence were attractive to patients. The staff of the hospitals were increasingly discarding their general practice and were glad to have this flow of new cases. They also could afford to ignore the protests of those doctors outside the hospital in general practice who knew that well-off patients were now going directly to the hospitals.

Mental hospitals

By the time of the first Scottish inquiry into the care of the insane – the Royal Commission on Lunacy in Scotland appointed in 1855 – there was a total of seven large mental hospitals.[31] The great demand for mental care had also led to the appearance of a number of private mental hospitals housing about twenty-five patients on average, and about one quarter of all mentally ill patients were thus housed. Doctors were also prepared to take paying patients into their own homes. The Royal Commission found much to criticise and indeed the inquiry had been stimulated by criticism of Scottish conditions, notably by an American, Dorothea Lynde Dix, who had visited Scotland in 1855. There was evidence of neglect and ill-treatment of the patients and profiteering by the private homes. The trussing and restraint used in all types of accommodation was criticised and the use of these methods during transport of the patients on the long journeys to the mental hospitals was the cause of physical injury. After the Report, facilities improved under the 1857 Lunacy (Scotland) Act which was more liberal than the corresponding English legislation in allowing for boarding out and admission of voluntary patients. Because of the difficulty in getting support for this work through the voluntary movement the new mental hospitals were run by the state, as part of the Poor Law, and administered by the parish. In the fifty years from 1860, 19 such asylums were built, the first being for Argyll and Bute in 1863.

Temperance movement

While this organisation was primarily a moral crusade, its success must have resulted in a modest improvement in the health both of the poor, at whom it was directed, and of those middle class imbibers also converted to its views.[32] The temperance movement started in Greenock in 1829. Numerous factors joined to produce the rapid rise in Scotland of this moral and political campaign. Until the middle of the 18th century the Scottish national drinks were ale for the poor and claret for the rich, but the Highlanders coming south after the 1745 rebellion and later after the Highland clearances spread the use of whisky to the Lowlands. Greenock, the point of arrival for many

Highlanders, became a problem area for drunkenness and alcoholism. These assertions can be backed up by statistical evidence, since by 1840 there was one liquor licence for every hundred persons in Greenock and every third or fourth house was some sort of pub. Between 1815 and 1840 the consumption of distilled spirits in Scotland increased four times. This was helped by a cut in liquor tax, a measure designed to stamp out illicit distilling and smuggling.

The rise in the temperance movement was explosive and brought forth a huge amount of literature in Scotland. The leaders combined a sincere concern for social welfare with a hard-headed assessment that alcohol interfered with industrial production and drove working men and their families for help to the Poor Law and charities, money which ultimately had to come from middle class incomes. From Greenock the cause was taken up by the publisher William Collins, and he spread the movement through Britain. Within four years there were four hundred temperance societies in Scotland.

The first political success of the temperance movement was in 1853 under the Forbes MacKenzie Act which introduced shorter opening hours and, above all, Sunday closing of the pubs, legislation which was limited to Scotland. Benefit from the Act was claimed by the temperance movement, since in the year following the Act, they claimed a 20% reduction in spirit consumption had occurred in Scotland, but a 10% rise occurred in England, where there was no similar legislation. A fall in arrests for drunkenness also occurred in Scotland. The temperance movement continued to expand and it sensibly provided counter-attractions to pubs, notably coffee houses and reading rooms, and the Band of Hope specialised in children's entertainment. The second piece of legislation forced by the temperance movement was the Temperance (Scotland) Act of 1913, the main provision of which was for local districts to be able to opt to be 'dry' or 'wet'. In the first poll in Greenock the vote in the whole town was very close – 11,221 votes for licensing of public houses and 10,504 against. Only the eighth ward, which was the largest, went 'dry', thus shutting thirteen public houses in that area. The temperance movement again claimed that statistics showed benefit from this Act, notably a fall in crime in Greenock. Even tougher legislation was suggested in an earlier report of 1909, which ominously stated that 'public opinion is ripe for the adoption of methods which formerly were held by many to invade the liberty of the individual'.[33]

The report had in mind compulsory internment in State Inebriate Reformatories, of which a few had been set up in the 1890's, but since those persons sent to the Reformatories simply ran away, the pressure for more penal measures grew.[34] However, the hard times of the World War I and afterwards led to reduced alcohol consumption. Thereafter, the temperance movement lost its vigour.

Medical missions

Though the lives and work of the Scottish missionary doctors in Africa are well known, an assessment of the contribution to the early medical care in Africa by them and also by the lay doctors of the civil service and trading companies has not been made.[35] The early medical missionary work in Africa had a considerable Scottish contribution, largely from the Free Church and the Church of Scotland, but also from the Roman Catholic Church in Scotland. All the money was raised by contributions from the churches.

The medical and lay missionary movement in Africa was greatly stimulated by David Livingstone's work and lonely death there and the return of his body to Britain. Livingstone (1817–73) was trained in medicine at the Anderson's College extramural medical school in Glasgow. He took the licence of the Faculty of Physicians and Surgeons of Glasgow and then under the administration of a London-based missionary organisation, travelled to Africa. He was primarily an explorer and evangelist, and secondly a doctor.

His death was the event which boosted the voluntary medical missionary movement in Scotland. Though this effort was widely known and admired, it had continuous financial difficulties and shortages of staff. Of the African enterprises, that in Nyasaland (now Malawi) was the special object of Scottish endeavour and in that country in the years up to 1900, twenty-seven of the thirty-one medical missionaries were from Scotland. The main stations in Nyasaland were Blantyre, run by the Church of Scotland, and Livingstonia, run by the Free Church of Scotland.

In the early days of the missions, medical care was restricted to the Europeans, and the Africans received only evangelism: only later did the missionaries take on the health care of the Africans. This task was begun in 1896 by Dr Neil Macvicar who started the African recapitulation of the development of British health care by starting systematic vaccination for smallpox. These missionaries in Nyasaland also started the education of local Africans to help in medical treatment and raised a corps of 'dispensers', many of whom moved into neighbouring Tanganyika and Northern Rhodesia. One of these early dispensers joined John Chilembwe's rising against colonial rule in 1915, and the Free Church Mission was accused of 'over-educating' the natives. Thereafter, it has been suggested that the Scottish presence in these countries may also have helped the political moves towards independence: certainly the missionary movement was an independent source of advice and information to those in Britain interested in the independence debate.

Medical practice

The methods of the physicians made steady progress in the later 19th century through the elimination of the older methods, notably the disappearance of blood-letting from routine practice. This ancient practice is thought to have been finally terminated in Scotland by the publication of John H. Bennett's *The Restorative Treatment of Pneumonia* in Edinburgh in 1865 which employed statistical methods of comparison which were being used in Europe and which were to lead to improved medical investigation from then on. He showed that cases not treated by blood-letting did better than those so treated. This pamphlet seems to have ended the argument in Scotland, though distinguished physicians including W.P. Alison, had argued for blood-letting until the last. The physicians methods thereafter became simple and supportive. The newer chemical methods from the continent also enabled drugs like morphine to be extracted from opium, and quinine from cinchona bark.

But in surgery the progress was more dramatic and Scotland made two crucial contributions. Anaesthesia with ether had first been demonstrated to be effective in Boston in 1846. It is generally held that Liston, later that year, was first to use ether in Britain but there is some evidence that a Scottish ship's surgeon sailing from Boston took the news back to his native Dumfries and that an operation using ether was carried out there two days before Liston's use of the agent in London.[36] The use of chloroform, which was to rival ether, was introduced by Sir J.Y. Simpson in Edinburgh in 1847, after a famous experiment carried out by him and his colleagues on themselves.[37] Thereafter the relative merits of ether and chloroform were the subject of a long debate, though in Scotland chloroform was the favoured agent. There were cases of death after chloroform which made many users cautious and strengthened the case of opponents.

But ether and chloroform themselves did not immediately produce a major change in surgery. The limiting factor to surgical progress was not anaesthesia but the appalling sepsis rate and death after surgery in the hospitals of the mid-nineteenth century: this was not an old problem, it was a new one.

The death rate from all causes including surgery seems to have been about 10–15% in most hospitals in the early 19th century, though there were occasional allegations from disaffected local factions that the true figure was higher. Certainly, a low figure could be obtained by omitting those dying within 24 hours of admission, or by discharging those who were dying. This practice was hinted at in the Annual Report for Dundee Royal Infirmary of 1841–42 which claimed only a 3% death rate.

> This has not arisen in the slightest degree from any exclusion of patients in consequence of their being incurable nor from any urging of patients to leave the House when they were approaching a fatal termination, a mode by which a medical attendant of a hospital may at any time bring the mortality within a convenient ratio.[38]

But the mortality rate in the Scottish voluntary hospitals by the middle of the 19th century was rising. Edinburgh Royal Infirmary reported in 1846 that amputations had become 'alarmingly fatal', with a 60% death rate, and it related this to the overcrowding of the hospital with fever cases. The deaths after surgery were the result of fulminating wound infections followed by septicaemia – the feared hospital gangrene.[39] The term 'hospitalism' was used for this new problem, particularly as a careful study of British surgery by Edinburgh's Sir J.Y. Simpson showed that in 1869 there was a 41% death rate in patients undergoing amputation in the voluntary hospitals and only an 11% death rate in those operated on in their own homes.

The problem was solved, in Glasgow appropriately enough, and the methods used led to a new era of surgery. Joseph Lister (1827–1912) was a Quaker and hence could not study medicine at the older English Universities.[40] Instead he could train at the relatively new University College Medical School in London, which was open to nonconformists, and had imported a largely Scottish professoriate.

After qualification these links led him to travel to Edinburgh for further surgical training, and from there he was promoted in 1860 to the regius chair of surgery in Glasgow. There the hostility between the university and the Glasgow medical profession still existed, and it was fifteen months before he obtained wards in the Glasgow Royal Infirmary. Initially he continued his earlier research on blood clotting but then changed direction in response to the challenge of the infection in his surgical wards. The local professor of chemistry, Thomas Anderson, told him of Pasteur's discovery of the microorganisms responsible for fermentation, and Lister argued that carbolic acid dressings or spray might combat similar airborne infection in his wards, and he patiently recorded his experience and success with these methods. Lister met opposition from scientists and surgeons. His claims to be the first to use the methods were disputed and even the need for them questioned.[41] Mr John Borland, surgeon at Kilmarnock near Glasgow, did not use antiseptics and recorded a much lower death rate in his amputations than Lister. He suggested that Lister's methods were only required in the special and temporary circumstances of the overcrowded and insanitary Glasgow Royal Infirmary.[42] The managers of the Royal Infirmary claimed that the high death rates noted by Lister in the cases not treated by his methods were exceptional and were caused by the temporary overcrowding of the hospital by fever cases. The methods worked however and, perhaps helped by a reduction in hospital overcrowding and improving nutritional standards in the community, there was a remarkable expansion of surgical practice. The number of operations carried out in the years after Lister in Glasgow's Royal Infirmary can be seen in Table 6:1. In this expansion the work of William Macewen (1848–1924) at the Royal Infirmary was important since he took the methods of Lister and extended them into the aseptic method which allowed a new range of surgical operations to be attempted.[43] Thus a fall in death rate occurred in spite of increasingly complex surgery of a type which would not have been attempted before.

The parallel between Lister's methods and the public health measures being introduced into Glasgow at the same time is very close. Both were necessary as a result of the 19th century urban and hospital overcrowding and cross-infection, and both succeeded by the end of the century not only in banishing the self-inflicted disease but also in setting new standards for bacteria-free environment in hospital and town. Lister's methods had another effect. The reputation of the voluntary hospitals in the community rose as a result of this new safety and the successful treatment. Annual reports now commented that the poor fled less often from their treatment.

Table 6:1
Operations and mortality at Glasgow Royal Infirmary 1851–1910

Years	*Operations*	*Post-operative mortality*
1851–60	2,014	10.8%
1861–70	3,403	12.4%
1871–80	5,257	8.6%
1881–90	9,741	6.4%
1891–1900	16,749	7.2%
1901–10	36,729	5.1%

Source: Pennington[44]

These famous individualistic innovations by Simpson and Lister conceal however serious defects in the support of Scottish and English medical science and its lack of organisational structure. Lister had no laboratory, little equipment and no research assistants. His modest research costs were paid personally, since they could be met in no other way.

Medical care

The Medical Act had simplified the recognition of medical men as a profession and the effectiveness of medical therapy also improved. Towards the later part of the century medical care became available to an increasing number of the population, though it was dispensed through a complex variety of agencies. The officially designated poor were looked after by the poor law medical officers and pauper patients might be sent to the hospital section of the poorhouse for in-patient care of chronic disease. The working class could obtain health insurance through the growing number of friendly societies or get treatment from cut-rate doctors or attend the increasing number of dispensaries. In cases of serious illness, admission to the voluntary hospitals was possible. Patients with infectious disease were treated in a third type of hospital, neither charity nor poor law, namely the municipal fever hospitals. Lastly, the quacks had not disappeared, but changed into the rich sellers of patent medicines by post or retail outlets.

But before considering these agencies for health care it is worth looking briefly at the most mysterious and least well described of these aspects of health care – private medical practice. Although the majority of the medical men derived all their income from this source and spent most of their professional life attempting to achieve success in this area, we have little knowledge of day-to-day private practice.[45] Lister's letters briefly mention some success in private practice, but biographers of other practitioners are silent on this subject. Certainly all the private practice was done in the home of the patient or doctor and even major surgery was invariably carried out there. Nor were any nurses available for home care until the end of the century when the improved training in the voluntary hospitals led to the appearance of private nursing agencies outside.

While in the early 19th century, society was fairly clearly divided into those who could afford the fees of the physicians and surgeons and those who could not, by the late 19th century the industrial revolution had produced a new class of skilled working men who acknowledged the new medical skills and who could afford the fees of the doctor, if a system of insurance was available. This need was met by the growth of the friendly societies, and to a lesser extent by commercial organisations.[46] Indeed, the friendly societies were eventually to become so strong that they became an important political force in early 20th century medical politics. By 1892 there were 1,320 societies in Scotland with 280,000 members and £1.25 million funds.

The earliest friendly society in Britain was formed near Edinburgh. The Bo'ness United General Sea Box was started in 1634, and like the others to follow, it enrolled members who if they were found to be fit and healthy could for a regular payment obtain benefits in times of unemployment and ill health. These societies were selective of members and disqualified those who defaulted in payment. Those in dangerous trades were not taken on and the full benefit was only given for the first 3–6 months, with the rate falling thereafter. If the disability persisted, payment was stopped. The societies, who had charismatic and confident names, grew rapidly in the later 19th century and eventually could employ their own doctors, not only to examine new members but also to treat them in time of illness. To be a doctor to a friendly society also brought other income for the doctor since he might be called in to see the members of the family who were not insured. There is more than a hint that the doctors were chosen by these societies for a helpful attitude towards an early return to work, thus conserving the society's funds. By the end of the century the friendly societies had acquired a reputation also of being bad employers, since the doctors were taken on only for short contracts and were badly paid, and the great production of doctors in the later 19th century permitted the friendly societies to be tight-fisted. To deal with these problems with the friendly societies and the Poor Law, the doctors became the first professional group to become organised, using the body now known as the British Medical Association.

For the working class not covered by friendly society insurance, there were an increasing number of possibilities for medical help in the late 19th century. For hospital treatment there were the voluntary hospitals, and a subclass of '6d doctors' who saw large numbers of patients and did obstetrics at cut price rates often consulting patients in batches of three and offering only an unchanging bottle of medicine as treatment.[47] Lastly, particularly in the Highlands, there were local 'clubs' where for an annual fee the services of the doctor were available.

Finally, there were the quacks who still worked in public in the early part of the century but who later in the century found it more convenient to advertise their cheap and infallible wares in the growing number of popular newspapers.

Patent medicine sellers

The Medical Act of 1858, though ostensibly aimed at the need to abolish quackery, was in reality a liberal plan to remedy the confused state of orthodox medical qualifications. It did not outlaw the quacks: they merely could no longer take the title 'Dr'. They had in any case disappeared from the streets, and instead of the old uncomfortable peripatetic life, they now sold single nostrums by post or through retailers, and from some of these highly successful enterprises grew the later ethical drug firms. Most of the 19th century 'patent' medicines were used to move the bowels, correct anaemia, relieve pain, or 'quieten' babies.

The growth of the patent medicine industry in the later nineteenth century was phenomenal. It had a large turnover and great success, and the popular patent aperient medicines in Scotland were Morrisons Pills and Holloways Pills. There were Cockles Pills for biliousness and liver conditions and it almost daily vied in the columns of the *Glasgow News* with Beechams Pills 'worth a guinea a box'. The American patent medicines were skillfully advertised, notably Carters Little Liver Pills. There was Bells Fairy Cure for pain relief, of which the advertiser said there is 'nothing else like it', and like many other patent and orthodox remedies it contained the dangerous but potent compounds acetanilide and phenacetin.[48] The need for a government stamp on the label gave added authority to these preparations. The patent medicine manufacturers were mostly based in London but imported American remedies were highly regarded. There were a small number of Scottish manufacturers notably that of Dr Collie whose ointment was highly thought of, and Rollos Remedy for Piles which on analysis showed 99 percent fat and a 'small quantity of very dark stuff'.

The cost of advertising these cures and distributing them by post was considerable but the profit margin on the materials used was still substantial. Even so, they were a cheap alternative to seeking doctors advice. Kearsleys Original Widow Welchs Female Pills – iron sulphate estimated to cost one-twentieth of a penny for the box – sold at one shilling and one and a half pence, but this was still cheaper than a doctor's consultation and prescription. Dr Collie's Ointment sold at one shilling and nine pence but the material cost only one penny. These patent medicines and their sellers remained the only serious challenge to the monopoly of the doctors, and it was not until the 20th century that the doctors could limit the activities of the patent medicine industry, by successfully objecting to the sale of potentially dangerous drugs by lay persons. The doctors directed skilful propaganda against the profit margins and the ordinariness of the constituents. The activities of the patent medicine sellers were then restricted.

Poor Law

Though the new Poor Law legislation in 1845 had allowed for medical care for the paupers – those declared officially destitute – the details were vague and the Poor Law medical services slowly evolved over the rest of the century. The poor obtained the benefit of the new, effective therapy and nursing of the later 19th century and perhaps they were lucky to have missed much of the earlier therapy inflicted on the rich. The medical services of the Poor Law were controlled by the Board of Supervision in Edinburgh who allowed the local organisations to have some independence. Only later in the century when central direction was more acceptable did the Central Board begin to flex its legislative muscle. The progress made in developing the medical services under the Poor Law came slowly with the Central Board in Edinburgh offering money to parishes which complied with their suggestions. When the Board clashed with local authorities, the cost of litigation usually made the local parish climb down and the Board won the day. The most notable example of this permissive legislation was the ruling that each parish should have a medical officer. The original Poor Law Act had been vague when describing the arrangements for the sick poor, but subsequent decisions by the Board of Supervision made matters clearer, and their decision that it was desirable that a medical officer should be appointed was an important one. But what was ideal for the large cities was not necessarily suitable for the small parishes and the ruling was not made compulsory. It was eventually a condition of the receipt of central government money for medical poor relief that the parish appoint such an officer, and the parishes could decide to opt in or not.

Another feature of the Scottish system was that workhouses on the English model did not exist initially. The English workhouses were numerous and were a determined effort to deal with unemployed able-bodied persons. Anyone who was fit but claimed relief was admitted to the workhouse and put to work, a mechanism which deterred many from using the system. In Scotland, this system was not in use and the poorhouses continued to admit only the old, feeble, and sick. Not until the end of the century was any help given to the unemployed and only at this later time were some unemployed persons admitted for a short period to the poorhouse to check their sincerity and their destitution. Thus the number of poorhouses in Scotland was less than the number of workhouses for the population in England. By 1868 there were sixty poorhouses in Scotland and one person in every twenty-four of the Scottish population was receiving poor relief: only one in fourteen of these was in a poorhouse. Towards the end of the century, however, the poorhouses became increasingly used as a test of poverty and by 1894 the Board of Supervision proudly claimed that the incidence of pauperism had fallen to one in forty-four of the population.

The early arrangement of the poor law medical help was deliberately bureaucratic and awkward. It was generally agreed by the taxpayers and the poor law authorities that medical help should not be easily available to the poor and while the doctors occasionally suggested that the poor might directly call on their services, this expensive suggestion by the doctors was easily thwarted by the apprehensive parish authorities. The poor therefore had to go through the slow and uncertain process of calling first on the Relieving Officer, who in a country parish might be many miles away, and having got authority to use the doctor's services, yet another long journey was undertaken to the doctor. These obstacles were regarded as an essential feature of the medical services under the new Poor Law. In the middle of the 19th century home treatment was probably satisfactory and admission to hospital was only requested on social grounds. However, towards the end of the century as medical therapy improved and better nursing in the poor law hospitals appeared, admission of the sick poor to the poorhouse for medical reasons became a routine, where they mixed with the paupers. By the end of the century, however, deterrent was not thought to be a suitable method of running the service for the sick poor and many of the stigmata of relief under the Poor Law, notably the loss of a vote, were removed from those who were merely sick. Another rather surprising piece of compassion towards the sick poor was the refusal of the poor law authorities to allow the teaching of medical students in the poorhouses, and not until well into the 20th century did teaching of students in these hospitals appear, whereas teaching of students in the voluntary hospitals had always been allowed. This sensitivity was the result of the poor's ancient fear of experimentation by the doctors.

The new Poor Law resulted in a number of new posts for doctors. Before the legislation of 1845, a few salaried posts had existed, paid for by the parishes for the medical care of their poor. The new law encouraged all parishes to appoint a doctor, but many were slow to do so, and the Parliament of 1847–8 voted an extra sum of £10,000 to be spent on medical relief of the poor in Scotland under the Poor Law Act.[49] The incentives offered to the parish by government were familiar ones – the parish had to spend a minimum amount of its own money, and the government would match it with a grant, provided also that a salaried medical officer was appointed. By 1849 only half the parishes in Scotland had taken up the offer of a grant: but by 1902 only 79 out of the 874 parishes were still outside the scheme. In these, when a doctor's services were required for the poor, his services were paid for by the parish for each visit. These non-participating parishes were all in the rich agricultural area of the Lowlands, outside of the towns. In the towns, the poor law medical funds were welcome and in the Highlands or Borders this money was even more useful and indeed the government grant was the only way of attracting a doctor into the area. In Glasgow in 1847 there were twenty-five parish doctors, and in Edinburgh in the same year there were fifteen. Dundee and Aberdeen had seven each. There was no bar to private practice by the poor law doctor, and the salary given was adjusted to take into account the earnings expected from fee-paying patients. These posts in the city were popular with the newly qualified doctors, who obtained some security while attempting to obtain a reputation in private practice. Moreover, these posts gave the essential introductions to the prominent citizens associated with the Poor Law Boards. The jobs were sufficiently popular for the parish to be tight-fisted in their dealings with the doctors and by the end of the century poor law appointments in Britain gained a reputation for parsimony and insecurity, since the parish council could hire and fire without reason, an attitude shared by the friendly societies. However, relationships may have been warmer in Scotland, and the only dismissal of a Poor Law doctor, which caused a protest, was in 1859 when Dr J. Henderson carried out a post-mortem examination on a Fordoun poorhouse inmate. Dr Henderson was reappointed on appeal. In the Highlands, the Poor Law reforms were successful in bringing a doctor for the first time to many parishes but the posts were not attractive since there was little chance of success in private practice locally or promotion out of the post. Indeed there were complaints about the type of doctor attracted. The other salaried positions available were the medical officers appointed to the poorhouses.

Part of the medical care of the parish poor was provided by the poorhouses, and they were regarded with dread.[50] In Scotland, the largest was the Barnhill poorhouse in the Barony Parish of Glasgow (later Foresthall Hospital). Built in 1854 for 2,000 inmates, it was the largest inhabited building in Scotland and in 1914 there were still 1,619 persons being maintained at a cost of 1/10¼d each per week. Life was bleak and discipline was prominent. The sexes were segregated and movement out of the house was restricted. There were separate courtyards for the exercise of the inmates, one yard each for men, women, boys and girls. Each group within the building was recognised by the colour of the tartan scarf worn. The Govan Combination Poorhouse (later called the Southern General Hospital) was built in a more spacious pavilion style, and the term combination referred to the mixture of poor, sick and mentally ill. This mixture was unpopular and eventually a separate asylum was built for the mentally ill – the splendid Hawkhead Asylum, later called Leverndale Hospital, erected in 1896.

Until local government took over these huge institutions in 1930, they were run by parish committees with the Inspector of Poor as the executive officer. The pressure on this organisation was considerable since the great need and the lack of facilities for the poor called for increased expenditure, and reforming groups agitated for better conditions. On the other hand, the parochial boards obtained their funds from a levy on the local inhabitants, and those paying the tax were suspicious of any increases and were vigilant in looking for waste or any suggestion of support given to idlers.

The doctors of the poorhouses were hard pressed and were often young graduates for whom these salaried posts gave security at the start of their careers. Later the poorhouses were first to employ women doctors. The ratio of doctors was 1:300 poorhouse patients, and the work was particularly hard. Many of these doctors knew that malnutrition was the cause of much of the disease seen and they knew that even inside the poorhouse the basic diet – whose cost was vigilantly watched by the authorities – was inadequate. The doctors often took the bold step of prescribing a nutritious diet as part of the treatment.

The formal links with the Church had been broken with the amended Poor Law of 1845, but the informal ties continued, and the ministers of the Barony Church of Glasgow, a fashionable charge, were the chaplains to Barnhill. The opportunities for charitable work by the members of the Church among the poor continued through these links. One poorhouse inmate, John Young, wrote an account of life in the Barnhill Poorhouse. He became unemployed when his father's family business was sold and eventually could no longer support the family. In Barnhill, he turned to writing and eventually earned enough to gain his release. He spoke charitably of the work of the staff and the visitors:

> To deal fu' gently wi' the puir, and win
> that crown o' moral beauty,
> Summ'd up in this wee word – duty.

Occasional reactionary thoughts occurred however:

> Noo, doctor, bout yon pills ye sent
> Yer pardon, gif ye please,
> They dune him guid tho' be it kent,
> Say wad as mony peas.

Nursing in the poorhouses was originally undertaken by the inmates themselves, thus saving money but, as elementary nursing skills became required, nurses were appointed to the poorhouses. Though Glasgow was early to do this, Scotland lagged behind England. Even in 1866 the Glasgow Medical Officer of Health, J.B. Russell, described nursing as

> the last resort of female adversity – slatternly widows, runaway wives, servants out of place, women bankrupt of fame and fortune.

The Glasgow poorhouses took quite energetic steps to improve matters and in 1879, after visiting hospitals throughout Britain, the administrators of Barnhill Poorhouse advertised the post of Lady Superintendent, and from thirty trained applicants they appointed Miss Pigott from Guy's Hospital. Thereafter, the training of nurses proceeded rapidly at the poorhouse, though they lagged behind the voluntary hospitals.[51]

As the amount of destitution fell steadily in the later part of the century and as wages rose and social benefits increased, people were sent less frequently to the poorhouses; but as the number of paupers in the poorhouses fell, the proportion of sick rose, and the poorhouses slowly turned into hospitals and the stigma of poor law relief was removed from those in need of medical treatment. Thus in 1862 15% of Barnhill's occupants were sick, but by 1924 the proportion had risen to 37%. Soon thereafter, the poorhouses were taken over as local authority hospitals as part of local government reform.

The relationship between the poorhouse medical care and the

services of the voluntary hospitals were initially fairly clear but became blurred as time went on. The early poorhouses took in the officially designated paupers – those certified poor and destitute by the parish authorities. The voluntary hospitals took only those in regular work and those who could support themselves after discharge. Circumstances served to blur this distinction since, with the rise of successful surgery after the introduction of anaesthesia and Lister's antiseptic methods, surgical cases, notably accident cases, among the poor were taken to the special skills in the voluntary hospitals. There the emerging hospital specialists of the 19th century were keen to admit any interesting case, and began to ignore the distinction between the poor and the pauper. However, the managers of the voluntary hospitals required quick turnover of cases, and could discharge those whose illness became chronic. These patients, though not destitute, were taken to the poorhouse, and it was estimated that about one patient each week was transferred in this way from Glasgow's Royal Infirmary at the end of the century.

The century ended with a new concern for the working class and their health. This was not a new humanitarian impulse but a fear of a national decline as evidenced by military defeats in South Africa. The consequences of this concern were to make health and health care a political issue and to bring the state even further into the provision of health care and social welfare.

7

The rise of the state 20th century

The start of the century saw a national crisis of confidence which caused a radical rethinking of the attitudes of the 19th century to the social services and led to a restructuring of the provisions for welfare and health care. This loss of nerve followed the military reverses in the Boer War, and realisation of the growing strength of other European nations, notably Germany. This fear of national decline became a major political issue after studies of the physique of army recruits suggested a decline in the heights and weights of the working class, and government was now prepared to listen attentively to criticism of Britain's attitude to social problems. Whereas the policy of self-help, individualism and philanthropy had been the essential features of Victorian social policy, these were now abandoned in the face of national disaster. The necessary legislation was passed by the Liberal governments of 1906–14 and Lloyd George's health insurance scheme, which closely resembled its German equivalent, was the most notable of these innovations. In this new atmosphere the long struggle by the scientists and the universities to obtain government support was also acceded to.

This reluctant growth in the power of central government necessarily meant the loss of local individualism within Britain. Though a separate Scottish approach to the practice of medicine and medical education can still be identified in the early part of the century, the post-World War II NHS legislation removed any important decision-making from Scotland. The old numerical dominance of British medicine by the Scottish schools also slowly disappeared, since the new medical schools, funded by government money, were placed to ensure a fairer geographical distribution of teaching centres. A sturdy independence remained in the Scottish colleges, which showed a remarkable revival as a result of the popularity of their post-graduate degrees. But Scottish health care became part of British health care, and British medicine part of an increasingly successful international effort for the improvement of medical and surgical treatment.

In considering the health of the nation a continuous reduction in the incidence and mortality of infectious disease was the striking feature of the 20th century. By the middle of the century these major killing diseases had become negligible in their impact, though tuberculosis proved slower to go than the rest. The major killers instead became heart disease and cancer, and Scotland, having suffered badly from the old problems, also had a greater than expected incidence of the new ones.

The reduction in infectious disease was the result of many improvements – public health legislation, better housing and sanitation, adequate nutrition and better medical services and drugs: the parts played by these various factors in the general improvement cannot be unravelled. This improvement in health – measured in detail by an increasing flood of statistics – was gratifying, but the health of Scotland did not improve as rapidly as in England and Wales, and the British figures were less than satisfactory when compared with Europe.

The century was later dominated by the increasing attempts to identify and remedy all kinds of problems of inequality in society, and government and other agencies became increasingly dependent on statistical and social indices and comparisons with other countries and between regions. In medical practice these statistical approaches were also used in new sophisticated methods of preventing bias in judging the effectiveness of new and old treatments of which an increasing number were shown to be valueless. Though this made the adoption of new methods more sure it also led to a perceptible cynicism about the effectiveness of medical care and a modest revival in fringe medicine.

The voluntary hospital movement reached the peak of its power and influence early in the century, but by 1948 it was facing a major financial crisis, which made it easy for the NHS to take over both the voluntary and old poor law hospitals. The NHS in Scotland was perhaps more successful than that in England and won the more whole-hearted support of those employed by it. The private health care sector in Scotland, which had looked after the health needs of the middle class until 1948, was almost extinguished by the state service. However, by the 1970's the brave 'cradle to grave' offer of health care by the NHS was less confident. Firstly, the NHS manifestly could not give a preventative service for the new wave of disease and secondly, as Britain's economic strength declined and the cost of health care escalated, the NHS funds became insufficient to maintain the service. It is convenient to describe first the period up to the introduction of the NHS in 1948 looking first at the changes in disease incidence.

Health in the early 20th century

The striking change in health in the 20th century was the wide ranging decline in all forms of infectious disease and a steady improvement in many other measurements of health.[1] The most widely used is the infant mortality rate (IMR), which can be used as a sensitive index of health, health care and social conditions. The rate increased in Scotland during the last half of the 19th century and by 1900 had reached 129 deaths under the age of one year for every 1,000 live births. It started its downward trend exactly on the turn of the century, reaching 17 by 1978. The decline in mortality from typhus and diphtheria had started in the 1860s, but the fall in deaths from measles and whooping cough was delayed until the turn of the century and tuberculosis was even slower to decline. The improvement in health statistics was most striking in the towns, though they had most room for improvement. By the start of the 20th century the mortality figures for the cities showed that the health of the towns had approached the figures of the rural areas. Both town and country improved in tandem after that.

The factors producing this improvement were multiple. The public health measures contributed considerably, as did earlier detection and the availability of health care to all sections of the community. The appearance of specific measures of immunisation and newer methods of treatment such as the antibiotics also helped. The slow improvement in housing gave better health by lessening the chances of infection and better nutrition raised the immune mechanisms to combat disease. The parts played by these different factors can hardly be disentangled.

Much use of the infant mortality rate is made as an index not only of child health but also of health care and social conditions. At the turn of the century, the Scottish IMR was lower than England and Wales. However, the Scottish figure declined much more slowly than in England in the early part of the century, and was slow to decline thereafter, always lagging behind many European countries who had a lower IMR than either U.K. or Scotland. Glasgow's IMR continued to be higher than the rest of Scotland, largely as a result of the social deprivation found in west-central Scotland.

By the turn of the century the battle of the municipal health authorities over the more spectacular infectious diseases had largely been won, although measles and whooping cough remained serious threats to child life. As already observed, recruitment for the Boer War revealed major defects in the physique of recruits and this led to development of the personal health services, of which the first was the School Medical Service instituted in 1908 under the school boards. Notification of births, at first a voluntary measure in 1907 but made compulsory in 1915, led to the evolution of maternal and infant welfare which were placed in the hands of local health authorities. Venereal disease caused concern during World War I and clinics were set up. Some attention was paid by the larger municipal health authorities to dental health and the welfare of the mentally handicapped. Inspection of food supplies and of animals became the responsibility of sanitary and veterinary departments of local authorities. Thus the early decades of the present century saw great developments and expansion in the work of local health authorities.

In 1929 local government reform led to local authorities assuming control of poorhouses and their associated hospitals and so to the development of municipal hospital services in addition to the infectious disease hospitals already administered by most major local authorities. The problem of tuberculosis, however, remained a major challenge. Developments in Scotland in the control of this infectious disease were largely due to the pioneer work of Dr (later Sir) Robert Philip of Edinburgh. He persuaded Edinburgh to introduce voluntary notification of tuberculosis of the lungs in 1903, made compulsory locally in 1907, but it was not until 1912 that it was made compulsorily notifiable nationally. He instituted the dispensary system, sanatorium and hospital treatment and finally, a farm colony for the rehabilitation of healed cases, a system which became copied internationally. By 1939 tuberculosis had declined in Scotland but there was a set-back during World War II when notifications rose alarmingly. It was not until 1955 that control was once more established by the use of the new drugs and public drives for the detection of the disease.

Health care

The three levels of health care noted in the 19th century – private practice, the Poor Law and the variety of services for the working class – underwent great and rapid changes and by 1948 virtually all sections of the community used the same state health service.

For the well-off in the first part of the century, medical care was provided by private practice. Self-sufficiency was a virtue and insurance against medical costs was rare. Though doctors' bills might be considerable, the other fees were not high, and most illness was treated at home, including surgical operations.

About this time, however, the advantages of hospital treatment even for the well-off became clear. The voluntary hospitals were pioneering increasingly skilled methods of nursing, anaesthesia and surgery. The tradition of being nursed in the home and of childbirth in the home or even surgery on the kitchen table looked increasingly old-fashioned and risky. The wealthy would not contemplate admission to the voluntary hospital for in-patient care, and hence a new type of small hospital grew up – the nursing home. These were to reach the peak of their popularity around the 1930's: the number in Scotland on one list were Glasgow (47), Edinburgh (27), Dundee (8), Ayr (4), Dunfermline (3), Perth (2), Paisley (2), Dumbarton (2) and one each in Wick, Dumfries, Stonehaven, Airdrie, Elgin and Stirling. Doubtless many other smaller homes did not appear on published lists.[3] These nursing homes were usually small, and did not necessarily have single rooms for all patients. They were usually run by a nurse who had been trained, and the home may have been owned by a company or a doctor. These little nursing homes in the large towns were grouped together in fashionable areas and often the successful practitioners had their houses and consulting rooms nearby.[4] The nursing homes lasted till the World War II, when, with the relative fall in middle class income and the rise of the voluntary hospitals and their advanced methods, both the private patients and their doctors agreed that the small nursing homes were not to continue. The remaining need for private care in Scotland was met by a small number of larger nursing homes funded by national private medical insurance agencies. Thus the nursing home movement rose and fell entirely in the first half of the 20th century.

The official poor in the 20th century dwindled as rising standards of living, secure and fuller employment and insurance against the accidents of life abolished the pauper. The poorhouses were already changing into hospitals at the turn of the century, and this metamorphosis was completed when they were taken over as local authority hospitals in the reforms of 1929. The final upgrading of fabric and standards came in 1948 when these hospitals joined the NHS on the same basis as the voluntary hospitals. Even before this, in Glasgow and Edinburgh the teaching of students and the growth of academic units had started in the municipal hospitals.

In the era before the NHS these hospitals had been staffed by younger doctors hoping to return to the voluntary hospitals and success in private practice. The appointment to the staff in the Poor Law days and later was made by lay committees and the uncertainties of this and the canvassing required gave the doctors a lasting dislike of municipal control.[5] However in one area the non-voluntary sector was progressive since it did not share the old religious and other prejudices found in the voluntary hospitals. It was quick, for instance, to employ women doctors at the start of the 20th century.

For hospital treatment, working men were taken into the voluntary hospitals. The Scottish voluntary hospitals were financially stable in the early 20th century and were reasonable secure when taken over by the NHS in 1948. However, elsewhere the voluntary hospitals had been having increasing problems with finance, and in 1920 many London hospitals faced the prospect of closure and were only rescued by introducing a new scheme of hospital payment for those with modest incomes and who took out insurance. This was the second period of crisis for the London hospitals, since in the period 1881–1896 a similar lack of money had forced the closure of some wards in the voluntary hospitals. The problem was solved at St Thomas's and Guy's hospitals by admitting private fee-paying patients to these beds. Thus started the private wings and pay-beds of the London hospitals. The Scottish hospitals appear not to have had this severity of problem though in 1856 the Glasgow Royal Infirmary shut beds and considered the acceptance of funds from the Poor Law to treat paupers, but the crisis was solved without assistance. The Western Infirmary in Glasgow had financial shortfalls in the late 19th century, but these were easily made up by prompt responses to public appeals.[6] Thus private wings and paybeds were not usually found in the Scottish hospitals. The standards of care in the voluntary hospitals remained high and they were the pacesetters for innovation in treatment. In the doctors' professional life the voluntary hospitals dominated training and promotion after graduation. The hospital service was a long, hard struggle for promotion to the higher levels at which a private practice was gained.

Thus the hospital care of the working class remained unchanged during the 20th century. What did change considerably was the care of the working class by general practitioners in the community. At the start of the century this was unsatisfactory. The best treatment was probably given by the doctors of the friendly societies, but for those not covered by this type of insurance there was only the out-patient departments of the voluntary hospitals or cut rate general practitioners. It was this unsatisfactory community care together with the political concern over 'physical deterioration' that led to the proposals for national health insurance.

Nutrition and health

At the start of the 20th century, concern arose that Britain might be entering a period of national decline as a result of physical deterioration. The reverses suffered by the British army in the Boer war at the hands of a few Dutch farmers and the knowledge that an increasing number of recruits – as many as 2 out of 5 – were being turned down as unfit for the army (although the minimum height had been reduced) confirmed anxieties that Britain was entering a period of physical decline which would lead to a national decline. Lord Rosebery was first to sense this issue of national efficiency as an important one, and his statement in 1900 that 'health of mind and body exalt a nation in the competition of the universe' was to start a great national debate.[7] Fear of losing the Empire through inferiority of the army was the main reason for the pressure for something to be done. There was now admiration of the German system of national health insurance and their medical education, and fears that Germany might attempt to dominate Europe were never far away. A further factor in the new governmental concern was the growing power of the working class, who had obtained the vote in the reforms of 1885. Some riots in England and Scotland were a reminder to government of the lack of social insurance and health care for that class, a group who also provided the bulk of the soldiers for the forces. Scotland was in particular a highly successful recruiting ground for the Army, and within Scotland the Highlands were the most responsive area.

The first statistical evidence on the inferior physique of the working class came from Scotland. The reasons for establishing the Royal Commission on Physical Training in Scotland of 1903 are not clear, but its comments on health and physique were the first of their kind in Britain.[8] The report suggested that there was a marked difference in height and weight between well-off children and poorer ones. A more detailed study in Glasgow confirmed this in 1905.[9] The problem had by then become a political one – the Government had already been prodded into a further study of 'physical deterioration' by the report of an Interdepartmental Committee of civil servants in 1904 who reaffirmed the inferior physique of working class children.[10] The report discussed the possible explanations of these facts. Firstly 'racial deterioration' as the result of inbreeding was considered and on the basis of these data some otherwise respectable socialists advised the 'sterilisation of failures' and hinted that medical science was preserving the unfit from an early death. A second explanation was that the poorer children merely required more exercise, and since this was an attractive explanation to the politicians, the enduring idea was put about that physical jerks for undersized school children was beneficial. The third explanation was more serious and politically sensitive, namely that the poorer children were underfed and that this was the result of poverty.[11] The Committee discarded this explanation, suggesting that any underfeeding was the result of the mother's fecklessness. By 1906, however, a reluctant government accepted that underfeeding did exist, and Parliament with a heavy heart agreed in 1906 that free school meals and milk should be provided. In 1907 medical inspection of school children was also proposed and subsequently undertaken, moves which were fiercely opposed by conservative critics. Middle class parents refused to have their children inspected and the doctors' organisations complained that the children who were discovered at the inspections to have defects were being sent for free treatment to the poor law or voluntary hospitals instead of to private practitioners. The doctors' successful protest led to the Schools Medical Service being set up. Thereafter both school inspection and school meals became routine.

Controversy over nutrition did not end in 1906 since the difference in height and weight between the social classes persisted. The problem reappeared in the 1930's when two kinds of measurement could be made by the scientists, namely the energy contained in the food eaten by a person and the energy required in their work. These types of study were favoured by the British physiologists – possibly as an alternative to animal experiments to which much hostility remained. The Scottish nutritionists were particularly active. Through this work, the basic requirements for food became known. A government committee was again set up to look at the question of food intake in relation to income. The matter proved so sensitive that the committee was disbanded and Aberdeen's John Orr – later Lord Boyd Orr – the activist of the committee, carried on with the gathering of statistics and, like Chadwick before him and Beveridge after him, published the controversial report *Food, Health and Income* under his own name.[12] The book caused a stir at the time, which Orr did not discourage, and his claim that one third of the population was underfed was aimed at a wide audience. The controversy continued until the 1939–45 war, when new concern over the physique of the British army compared with the German youth led to the views of nutritionists being accepted in their entirety. The rations allowed during the ensuing war were based on the principles established by Orr and others.

National Health Insurance

Thus the pressure for the reform of the health services at the start of the 20th century came from a new government concern for the physique of the working class and from working class pressure for reform through their new political power. The free school meals and school medical inspection mentioned above were the first benefits to be introduced and they were followed in 1911 by Lloyd George's scheme for National Health Insurance.[18] This was not a comprehensive medical scheme as it did not provide hospital treatment and only affected men in regular work: it was primarily designed to support a working man during illness and return him quickly to work, thus saving him from poverty and hence being a charge on the state. Workmen contributed 4d a week, the employers added 3d and the government contributed 2d thus giving, in the Chancellor's famous phrase, 'ninepence for fourpence'. The doctor was to be paid an annual fee for each patient. While the friendly societies paid only about 3–5/- a year for each patient, during the tense negotiations with Lloyd George the doctors had managed to have the offer raised to 7/- for each patient plus 1/6d for drugs. Only the relatively less well off were allowed to participate in the Scheme, and the upper income limit was £160: by 1948 this had risen to £420. A small fund was to be set aside for research: this was the origin of the Medical Research Council.

Lloyd George faced opposition from two sources – the numerous large and small friendly societies who were already in the health insurance work and the doctors. The doctors had already had experience of working for the medical insurance clubs and societies and these were not always popular since the doctors had experienced excessive demands on their time, low pay and the humiliation of having to be re-elected annually. To the doctors, Lloyd George's insurance scheme looked as if it would not only demean the doctor and perpetuate these problems, but might give benefits to some reasonably well-off working people who would normally have been paying patients. However, others in favour of the scheme argued that it would greatly increase the income of doctors in practice in working class areas, as proved to be the case.

The debate on the proposals became increasingly bitter and increasingly rigid attitudes were taken up. The British Medical Association (BMA) contended it would ruin the British worker and so tax the manufacturer that foreign imports would be subsidised. A less successful debating point was the allegation by the doctors that it would cause tension between servants and mistresses since the mistresses would have to buy the insurance stamps and attach them to the insurance card. Nevertheless, Lloyd George (like Bevan later) pressed on in the face of opposition. Opposition to the insurance scheme in Scotland was less strident than in England and Wales. The large areas of Scottish urban and rural poverty and ill-health made the scheme attractive to both patient and doctor. Moreover, fewer doctors were involved in private practice in Scotland than in London. Nevertheless the Scottish doctors joined in the anti-government rhetoric of the BMA and the Scottish BMA passed on to their members the militant messages of their London leaders. In November 1912 the chairman of the Scottish Medical Insurance Council (a body set up by the BMA and the Scottish colleges to oppose the Scheme) claimed that Lloyd George's new proposals were a trap –

> the hook has had an extra worm put on it. But it is not a real one, but a phantom. The Act means degradation and servitude of a section of the profession.[14]

Further attempts were made, exhorting the profession to unity and solidarity against the Scheme, and on December 10th at the eleventh hour, a meeting of Glasgow doctors decided not to work under the Act.

The crucial nationwide doctors vote on December 14th showed a remarkable result. When the votes of the individual medical district organisations throughout England, Wales and Scotland were recorded, it showed that in England only 2 out of 88 BMA divisions favoured the Scheme.[15] In Scotland however, 8 out of 16 divisions voted for it, and substantial majorities for the Scheme were recorded in Ayrshire and Dundee. Glasgow was only narrowly against the Scheme, but Edinburgh, Perth and the Borders were strongly opposed. The vote thus corresponded to the amount of industrial practice carried out by the doctors.

It was a confusing time for the doctors in Scotland. If many doctors joined the Scheme any doctors left ouside would not survive since they would have no patients. There were pleas from the BMA to boycott the Scheme, yet the doctors in Scotland had virtually voted for it. An editorial in the *Glasgow Herald* on 23 December 1912 commented on this difference, and hinted that there would be little doubt that most districts would succeed in getting sufficient number of doctors to join the Scheme. An announcement by the Scottish Insurance Commissioners on 26 December showed that in response to their invitation, 70 doctors in Glasgow were willing to work the Scheme. This caused a shift of opinion, and when the Glasgow doctors met again, they voted 144–144 on a motion to join the Scheme. The Chairman cast his vote in favour. With relief, the doctors all joined up and rushed to sign up patients. The doctors of many other Scottish towns joined in, but in Edinburgh and Aberdeen they held out stoutly into 1913.

The first months of the Scheme were difficult and in London there was bad-tempered picketing by doctors and allegations were made of the death of doctors from overwork. Another wild tale was of busloads of Scottish doctors arriving in Lymington to take over the work there. After the Scheme had been going for three weeks, the BMA conceded defeat and at the last meeting the doctors sang 'Rule Britannia' and dispersed. Though the doctors conceded defeat, there were a number of major problems. It was the biggest governmental administrative mechanism ever set up and in its early period the organisation was close to breakdown. This, together with the continuing hostility from some doctors, made the first year a troublesome period. The separate administration set up for Scotland and Wales was of benefit since in these countries the Scheme was going well, and the English problems were thus bearable.[16] In Scotland some resistance remained. Edinburgh held out for the longest time, helped by the fact that Edinburgh's largely middle class population favoured private practice. A Medical Guild was formed in Edinburgh to rally the forces against the Act, consisting of all practitioners who had not joined up. It was in good heart in February 1913 when it alleged that only 122 out of 372 of the doctors in the Edinburgh and Leith district had joined the Scheme,

> and it is believed that a certain number will give up the scheme at the end of three months, as some of them have already had enough of it.[17]

However, the Guild disappeared shortly afterwards.

The Scheme was beset with problems, not the least of which were over the benefits allowed. Of these the most interesting was a hitch which appeared immediately. The insured working men could now choose a doctor from a panel of names (hence the lasting term – panel doctor) and from whom, for the first time, they were entitled to free treatment. Before the Scheme many patients had been accustomed to going to the voluntary hospitals for medical treatment and their employers had often contributed to these hospital funds. With the Scheme, this outpatient work was supposed to stop, and there were incidents when injured workers were turned away from the voluntary hospitals.[18] The Royal Northern Infirmary, Inverness decided against the outpatient treatment of any insured persons, but the Royal Infirmary of Edinburgh, having turned away an employee of the London Road Foundry, were told that the firm would no longer contribute to the Infirmary. The managers considered the problem and allowed outpatient treatment to continue.

Overall the Scheme was a great success in Scotland. It guaranteed a salary for a doctor, and made possible rewarding medical practice in the poorest areas. For the patient, it meant less fear about possible illness, a concern further reduced by the introduction of unemployment relief. Moreover the friendly societies and the commercial insurance societies were also happy, since the final decision allowed them to administer the Scheme. Though they made no profit from it, their army of insurance salesmen had the chance to sell other policies to the contributors and their families notably for covering burial expenses.

But the Scheme did not provide complete cover. It was restricted to those earning a wage and the medical cover was not complete. It did not cover hospital treatment, nor did it provide dental care, dentures or spectacles, unless the friendly society involved had a surplus to expend: the free spectacles and dentures provided in 1948 by the NHS were its greatest novelty. Moreover the Scheme did not apply to the Highlands.

Highlands and Islands Medical Scheme

Only the working man or woman with regular income could join the National Health Insurance Scheme. These regulations therefore excluded the crofting community in the Highlands just at a time when there was mounting concern about medical conditions and the health of the area. Moreover there had been unrest in the Highlands at the end of the 19th century and the government were well aware of the need to recruit soldiers in the Highlands. The crofters survived on tiny patches of land given to them after the clearances and they lived at barely subsistence levels with such an irregular income that they could not join the insurance scheme. Much of the crofters financial dealings were done by barter, and payment for services such as the doctors' were often made in kind. The supply of doctors to the Highlands and Islands was also patchy and there was concern at the quality of the doctors. This was not surprising as the only inducement to the Highlands and Islands for a professional man was private practice (which was rare and seasonal) and a few poor law patients. Moreover not only was the doctor's income low, but his travel expenses were high and the journeys could be long and arduous. Under pressure from M.P's from Highland areas who realised that the Insurance Scheme would not bring any benefits to the Highlands, a committee was set up and reported in 1912.[19] The report of the Dewar Committee was a radical one and proposed a scheme, the

Highlands and Island Medical Scheme (HIMS), which was to anticipate the comprehensive health service to be set up in 1948. Whereas the debate on the national Insurance Scheme had been bitter, discussion on the HIMS was good-tempered. A closer examination shows that the HIMS was, at its origin, a more radical and interesting plan than it was eventually allowed to be. Successful though it was, its original concept had been more ambitious.

The full report is still a remarkable social document. Sir John Dewar (later Lord Forteviot), M.P. for Inverness was chairman and included in his committee were Dr Leslie Mackenzie, a socialist and friend of the Webbs, and the Marchioness of Tullibardine, the wife of the future Duke of Atholl, who was to be Scotland's first woman M.P. Her appointment was a shrewd one since on paper at least she would represent the interests of the gentry.

The meetings held throughout the Highlands of Scotland were followed with great interest and were described both in the Scottish press and the *British Medical Journal*. When complete, the report confirmed that the health and medical services of the Highlands and Islands were at unacceptably low levels. The quality of doctor was also thought to be poor. The basic health service was provided by the Poor Law, which obliged each parish to provide a small salary for a doctor to attend the paupers on the roll. This was often the only way in which a doctor could be attracted into the Highlands, and he would hope to pick up some extra income from the occasional private consultations by the gentry or their summer visitors. There were also informal, unsatisfactory and short-lived 'clubs' whereby the crofters paid an annual fee to the doctor and were entitled to free treatment. It was common for some members to renegue, yet be treated, and the club would then collapse. The report records a visit to a Highland doctor and the committee were outraged to find him with 'his sleeves up, cooking his own dinner'. His income was £40 a year, and it was commented that the ministers of the numerous presbyterian churches in the area, an area which could support only one doctor, lived in much greater style. There were also many testimonials to the amount of free medical attention and devotion to the crofters that the doctors were prepared to give. But there was a limit to what could be provided free, since travelling expenses were considerable.

The report found that the nursing services were hardly better and were even more fragmented. The voluntary principle was still strong in the crofting area and was highly regarded. This held that the gentry (or rather, their wives) had an obligation to provide for the deserving poor by the organisation of voluntary contributions for nurses for their area. This voluntary organisation meant that services only existed where there was enthusiasm, so the nursing services were patchy. Lastly, the report had factual evidence which gave an accurate and detached picture of medical practice in the area through the incidence of uncertified deaths in the crofting community. An uncertified death was (and is) one in which the doctor is unwilling to sign a death certificate, as the patient was not seen by a doctor during the last illness and the cause of death was therefore unknown. The committee found that while an uncertified death was a rarity in urban Scotland there were numerous such deaths in the Highlands. On the west coast in parishes such as Farr and Ullapool, the uncertified death rate was 40% and could reach 90% at times in the parishes of Kilchoan and Coigach in Ardnamurchan. High rates of uncertified deaths could even exist when a doctor was in the parish, showing that little help for the community could exist, other than through private practice.

After studying the facts of medical care in the Highlands and Islands, the report was clear in its conclusions. The medical services and the health of the people were so bad as to be unacceptable – 'That such conditions can exist within twenty-four hours of Westminster is scarcely credible. Nor is it creditable,' said the report.

Nevertheless the committee must have had some problems in framing their recommendations. It was suggested to them that the crofters were lazy and congenitally prone to disease. To provide free medical services for one part of Britain would establish a dangerous new precedent, and the principle of 'from each according to his ability and to each according to his needs' must have been novel thinking even for the Left on the Dewar Committee. Moreover, the voluntary principle was highly regarded and it was argued that a government grant would simply switch off this private source of medical and nursing help and provoke a downward spiral. But everything that the committee had found spoke against the provision of medical care either by private practice or as a patchy dispensation from the nobility. In the main recommendations of the report, the thistle was grasped firmly and it was acknowledged that access to health care was a basic human right. The recommendations were clear and decisive. For the doctors, the report proposed that a minimum salary be introduced, thus guaranteeing a reasonable income for doctors in the area. Since travel costs were the main problem, the report recommended that the travel of the doctor to all patients should be paid by the state and grants for the doctors and nurses to obtain a car or a buggy, bicycle or boat should be available. The doctor would be free to try and obtain a fee of 5/- for the first visit to a patient (about a quarter of the usual charge) thus attempting to reduce frivolous calls. Private practice was encouraged to supplement the doctor's income. The nursing services would be expanded and made available throughout the area.

But this was not all. The report also envisaged a comprehensive scheme with hospices for simple health care together with a house for the nurse and funds to improve the telephone system. To administer the scheme, a central body in Edinburgh with a local district committee was recommended. On commenting on this part of the plan the report makes a historic remark. 'It is not desirable to multiply authorities without necessity, and in the Highlands and Islands, on account of the difficulties of attending meetings, this principle deserves special consideration'. In the event the pragmatists who ran the HIMS found they could dispense even with the local tier and run it from Edinburgh. It was, in later NHS terminology, a one-tiered system

The report met with a favourable public reception and the *British Medical Journal* commented that the existence of 'such conditions of medical practice in the present day may be difficult to believe. It is well that such a reproach to our administrative methods has been brought to our notice'.[20] No opposition to the introduction of the recommendations of the report can be found, a surprising finding in view of the degree of government intervention involved. Perhaps because of the government awareness of their dependence on the Highland regiments, or memories of the 19th century Highland disturbances or even because the burden of poor law medical services had fallen heavily on the lairds, the recommendations were accepted without complaint by the government. The scheme was allowed to proceed, and the new body proved to be a successful one, since the direct simple relationship between the doctors and the administration in Edinburgh was always cordial. The independent Board set up to run the HIMS had Sir John Dewar as Chairman, Sir Donald MacAlister (Principal of Glasgow University and the President of the General Medical Council) and Mackenzie and McVail from the Dewar Committee on the Board.

The first problem was that though the Board had clear objectives, the cost had not been calculated. The Board, therefore, sent out questionaires to the local government authorities for assessment of the needs of each community. The response was enthusiastic and the request for the county of Sutherland was typical:

Table 7:1
Expenditure requested for HIMS in Sutherland

To:	Doctors house at Laxford	£900
	Ambulance at Lairg	£250
	Nurses Houses (7) and extension to Lawson Memorial Hospital at Golspie	£4560
	General Practitioners Grants (Travel and Salary)	£1230
	Nursing Salaries	£400
	General	£60

The board added up the proposals for each county and then submitted a final sum. The Lords of the Treasury graciously, and apparently without quibble, conceded the entire amount – £42,000. The HIMS seemed to be on the point of revolutionising the medical services of the crofting area.

But it was to be ten years before some of the proposals were even considered : by 1929 only three of the seven nurses' houses for Sutherland had been built. The ambulance was never purchased and it was not until 1938 that the extension to the hospital at Golspie was started. The problem was that just as the HIMS was starting World War I broke out and severe restrictions on all expenditure were enforced. Life in the north of Scotland was disrupted even more than elsewhere by the great exodus of local men, doctors and nurses to join the forces. Moreover, inflation was a new national problem. Though the amount of money available at the beginning of the war was adequate for the plans of the HIMS, by the end of the war, expenditure on doctors salaries and travel had risen so much as the result of inflation, that it was taking almost all the HIMS budget. Only half of the expenditure approved in 1914 for the HIMS was designed for salaries, yet by the end of the war the entire amount was being spent on the doctors salaries and travel expenses. When peace was restored and the HIMS might have expected an increase in the budget to cover inflation and to get the other plans started, new financial problems appeared and in the period of the depression, all non-essential government expenditure was frozen. Any plans that the HIMS might have had about building houses or laying telephone lines had to be forgotten and indeed the only expenditure, other than payments to the doctors, was one for urgent repairs and modifications to the Belford hospital in Fort William. Even then special Treasury permission had to be obtained. The final irony was that the HIMS had been allowed to keep any unspent money from the lean years of the war and they now had accumulated a fund of £129,000 representing all the unbuilt houses and non-appointed nurses. Because of government policy this money could not be spent on houses, ambulances and hospitals, and the HIMS had, during the 20's, to watch this healthy fund disappear slowly as the doctors salaries and travel rose to meet and exceed the annual grant. Even then however, the HIMS, truncated as it was, had revolutionised medical practice, and there were for the first time adequate numbers of good doctors in the crofting areas.

With economic health of a kind returning to the nation in the later 30's the HIMS made a successful application to the Treasury for more money. In granting this, the Treasury were not prepared to make any open-ended commitment to a comprehensive health service, although this was the intention of the Dewar Report. The records show that the Treasury suggested that before they would give the money 'the Board should consider if the time had come for the Scheme to be devolved to the local authorities'. This was certainly a device to remove central government from responsibility for the central administration of the scheme, but it was also a method of limiting expenditure, since the HIMS would be relegated to a limited fund to which the local authorities could apply for support. The HIMS administrators had no option but to accede to this strong hint from the Lords of the Treasury. All the schemes of the HIMS were obediently handed over to the new local government organisation, and the Treasury doubled the grant to the HIMS.

This fund, in spite of its new and less radical role, was to do remarkable work. Even in the 20's it had revolutionised medical care in the Highlands and brought health care within the reach of the entire community. In the 30's the flexibility of the scheme was its most valuable feature and even with a second authority now involved, decisions seemed to be quick and personal. Numerous improvements to the hospitals were made, notably at Stornoway, Wick, Lerwick, Golspie and Fort William. The fund was also able to provide the first consultant surgeons for Stornoway and Lerwick and a consultant physician for Inverness. With the rise of hospital-based medicine, the Fund gave money for a postal laboratory service at Inverness to serve the Highlands and Islands. The scheme also caught the public imagination, by giving health care to the inhabitants of St Kilda and by launching the Air Ambulance to the Western Highlands in 1935 which proved invaluable in ferrying ill patients from the Western Isles to Glasgow.

The end of the HIMS came in 1948 when the fund was fused with the common fund for the NHS in Scotland. Commentators at the time remarked that the health services in the Highlands were absorbed more easily into the NHS than elsewhere. The reason was simply that the principle of a centrally run health service had been conceded many years previously.[21]

Plans for the NHS

By the end of the World War I Scotland had a number of agencies responsible for health, notably the HIMS, the National Health Insurance Schemes, municipal health authorities and the Poor Law. In 1919 administrative simplification was introduced which put these main agencies and the smaller ones under a Scottish Board of Health. This Board was not directly under political control, but the Secretary of State was in charge as the President. After the war, the National Health Insurance Scheme started to broaden its intervention in health care and to extend its benefits to the community. This was done against the post-war background of inflation and unemployment and the legislation was encouraged by industrial unrest, though inhibited by the economic problems.

At this time a preliminary plan for a health care service in England and Wales was produced by the Dawson Committee.[22] It was intended to be an interim report to the Minister by the Consultative

Council on Medical and Allied Services and the intention clearly was to proceed to a more detailed report on a comprehensive health service. The economic climate of the 20's prevented this and the consultative council dispersed and did not meet again regularly.

In Scotland a similar but shorter interim report was produced by Sir Donald MacAlister and his committee in 1920.[23] The interesting feature of both the reports was their emphasis on the general practitoner as the key figure in the health services. This emphasis was against the trend of events in Britain and elsewhere, where a move towards specialism was occurring. Both reports wanted 'whole-person' medicine. As the Scottish report remarked, 'It is not for disease in the abstract that provision has to be made, but for persons liable to or suffering from disease'. Both reports suggest that family doctors were to be grouped together in health centres supported by laboratories, dispensaries, physiotherapists, operating rooms and X-ray facilities. The aim, said the Scottish report, was 'the continuous safe-guarding of the family health rather than the occasional treatment of individual illnesses'. As regards payment, the Scottish report was a little coy:

> 'a complete and adequate medical service should be brought within the reach of every member of the community. We do not contemplate that such a service should be provided for all at public expense or that it should be furnished to all by a body of state or civic officials and practitioners'.

In the hospital service (awkwardly renamed 'secondary health centres') consultants would see patients referred by the general practitioners and in Scotland this meant an extension to all the hospitals of the out-patient clinics of the voluntary hospitals. The Scottish report hoped that the teaching hospitals would not be deprived of cases and predicted correctly that this proposal would mean that all the city hospitals would become involved in teaching. Emphasis was placed on convalescence in the Scottish report, reflecting the mood of the day. Convalescent homes would be available, not only in the recovery phase from illness, but as a form of rest and rejuvenation in times of physical or mental decline. This part of the scheme, clearly inspired by the health services in post-revolution Russia, was never introduced.

Though England and Wales never issued a later version of the Dawson plan, in Scotland the planning committee continued to meet and produced a full plan – the Cathcart report of 1936.[24] The Cathcart report emphasised again the role of the family doctor. Without him, said the report,

> as the principal liaison between the homes of the people and the statutory medical services these services cannot in modern conditions function to their full extent as part of a comprehensive policy for promoting and safe-guarding the health of the people.

The Cathcart report had the benefit of enlightened support from the Scottish BMA. The Scottish BMA's evidence argued from the theme that

> if health is a matter of the reaction of an individual to his environment it follows that the person who is to give him expert advice on health should be one who, to the greatest possible extent, is familiar both with him and his environment and that such a one is to be found in the person of the family doctor.

Even the Royal Colleges in Scotland argued that the family doctor was the key person in the health services. As to the form of the health service, only the Corporation of Glasgow and the Scottish Trade Union Council put forward the case for a whole-time salaried service. The Scottish BMA proposed special health boards grouped round the hospitals and suggested the integration of the public health sector with the curative services. The Cathcart committee did not accept these proposals fully but did suggest that the general practitioner and the hospital should be under one administration (a proposal which was ignored in 1947 and was not enacted until 1974). Worse still, by the time the NHS was set up the emphasis was on hospitals and the consultant. The concept of the general practitioner and the health centre, so clearly supported by both Dawson and Cathcart, almost perished in the post-war 'big hospital' medicine. The general practitioner did disappear in other countries.[25]

Once again, however, the Cathcart report and the planners of the 30's were overtaken by events and the war prevented any legislation on a health service. It was however a temporary postponement, and as the war turned in favour of the Allies, thinking could turn again towards the health services at the end of the war. The fraternal spirit of wartime, the Beveridge report, the utopian hopes for a new world at the end of the war, the success of central planning during war, all contributed to a consensus on the need for a centrally funded comprehensive health service. However those who were to co-operate during the war were to feud after it. In 1948 the disputes between the doctors and the government were similar to those in 1912 and uncanny similarities can be seen in the events and language used.

Before describing these events however, a description of the health services in Scotland during World War II is of interest as they set a pattern and the mood for the post-war era, and explain some features of the hospital services in Scotland which persisted long afterwards.

Emergency Medical Service

The medical services in Scotland during World War II were supplemented by an Emergency Medical Service (EMS), a scheme primarily designed to deal with the consequences of the war, but also cleverly used by the Secretary of State to bolster the existing services. On his appointment to this office in 1941 Tom Johnston recalls:

> I ticked off in my mind several of the things I was certain I could do – even during a war. I wondered how far the inadequate sleeping and housing conditions pre-war were responsible for the fact that the young recruits to the Argyll and Sutherland Highlanders were adding nine pounds to their weight in sixteen weeks at Stirling Castle. And I had ideas about hospitals . . . which I was certain might be operated without legislation.[26]

Tom Johnston succeeded in all his plans and used brilliantly the power given to him in wartime. Scotland had, in 1939, been short of hospital beds compared with England and waiting lists in the voluntary hospitals were long. The reason for this was clear. Though Scotland had many voluntary hospitals, there were few municipal hospitals, since the Poor Law administration in Scotland had for a century opposed the introduction of poorhouses.

Scotland was an ideal place to receive large scale troop or civilian casualties from England and Wales, and was therefore allowed to build hospitals though of a temporary type of construction, and to make annexes to existing hospitals and take over hotels as hospitals. These hospitals were deliberately built outside of the main towns and can still be found today at Law, Ballochmyle, Killearn, Peel, Bridge of Earn, Stracathro and Raigmore. These new hospitals had 7,038 beds, and numerous annexes to existing hospitals were also built, bringing a further 8,526 beds into use. The great hotels at Gleneagles and Turnberry were turned into convalescent homes. Tom Johnston doubtless was also amused at the previous take-over of many large country houses as hospitals which provided 3,426 hospital beds. In addition, other nations built hospital accommodation for their troops in Scotland. The United States built Cowglen hospital in Glasgow and the Poles had the Paderewski Hospital, formerly a childrens' home, in Edinburgh. The Norwegians had a unit in Edinburgh's Southern General Hospital, the French had units at both Quothquhan and Knockderry and the Canadian navy constructed the Smithston Hospital at Greenock.[28]

These hospitals were built rapidly but the expected military and civil disasters never occured. The threatened invasion of England never came, and the bombing of Clydeside gave the only major mobilisation of the EMS. The blitz on London did produce some evacuees and the Turnberry Hotel was briefly taken over by the staff of a London hospital. The only other occasion when the Scottish EMS had to deal with a large number of patients was when a large Australian convoy arrived in the Clyde in June 1940, and 170 cases of mumps were taken to Robroyston Hospital, 93 cases of mumps were taken to Knightswood Hospital and 209 other cases, including chicken pox, to Hairmyres. Gradually, as the threat of invasion faded, Tom Johnston was able to offer the services of his efficient, modern and unused hospital service to the old voluntary hospital system, now under great pressure and with long waiting lists. Tom Johnston opened the EMS hospitals firstly to civilians involved in the war effort, and then widened this definition to include almost all the citizens of Scotland. Johnston offered to take patients from the waiting list of the voluntary hospitals and with a typical gesture, he extracted thirty shillings from the voluntary hospitals for each patient treated. It was calculated that 40,000 civilians in wartime Scotland were eventually treated in the EMS hospitals. Moreover, these hospitals were used for an imaginative rehabilitation scheme for ill workmen – the Clyde Basin Scheme.[29]

There were two other features of the EMS in Scotland which are of interest. The first was the stimulus that it gave to specialist surgery and medicine. In pre-war Scotland hospital doctors were heavily dependent on private practice for their livelihood and hence specialism was resisted, since it might limit the doctors earning capacity from private cases by limiting the type of case treated. Nor did the doctors encourage specialism in others since the new specialist might take cases away from colleagues. Under the EMS, however, these constraints did not apply and specialist units were set up easily to deal with war injuries – fractures, burns, head and hand injuries. Anaesthetics, radiology and pathology were also encouraged, and while few hospitals had specialist units before the war in orthopaedics, few lacked this specialty after the war. Brain surgery and plastic surgery, little developed in 1939, were encouraged in the EMS, and the Burns Unit of the Glasgow Royal Infirmary encouraged the scientific study of shock and tissue transplantation. These effects of war on the pattern of the health service in Scotland were to benefit not only the practice of medicine, but also teaching and research for decades.

The other success of the EMS was that a state run hospital service could work at all; in England the EMS had not attempted to do this. Relations in Scotland between the administrators and the administered were good and the voluntary hospitals found they fitted surprisingly easily into the scheme. The contacts made with the municipal hospitals allowed their deficiencies to be noted. The result was that when a national health service was proposed for Scotland there was less resistance to it than in England, and under the Scottish Bill, all the hospitals were brought easily together under one local administration, usually centred on a university, a move which resulted in great benefit for the teaching and specialist services in Scotland. It was not until 1974 that the teaching hospitals in England conceded the necessity of working in harmony with their non-teaching neighbours. The official historian of the EMS in Scotland said it was

> the story of how the hospital and medical services in Scotland were transformed under the force of circumstances of the war from a heterogeneous collection of independent units into a homogeneous organisation which undertook the task of underwriting all the medical risks associated with war as well as the normal risks of ordinary life.

Lastly, and most importantly, these extra wartime hospital beds became indispensable to Scotland during the war, and, as Tom Johnston had planned, they were not given up after it finished. Thus while Scotland at the start of the war had 35,331 beds (21,248 in voluntary and 14,083 in local authority hospitals) by the end of the war 12,970 beds more had been built and were kept in use.[30] The extra beds brought in by the EMS gave Scotland a remarkable hospital service, based on specialism and which, in the towns, helped strengthen traditions of clinical medicine and the teaching of medicine and in the country gave comprehensive hospital care for the first time. The other effect of the EMS was that when the NHS was set up in 1948, the extra expenditure necessary to maintain these beds in Scotland had to be conceded, with the result that the NHS expenditure in Scotland was generous.

National Health Service

As can be seen above, planning for a centrally directed comprehensive health service had existed since the 1920s but had been delayed by the inter-war economic problems and World War II. The medical profession had been interested and co-operative, notably so in Scotland.[31] In the wartime atmosphere this enthusiasm for a new service after the war was rekindled and planning proceeded amicably. The Beveridge report appeared, and government and doctors accepted the principle that there should be a comprehensive health and rehabilitation service available to all members of the community. In 1942 the interim report of the Medical Planning Commission, an influential body set up by the BMA in collaboration with the colleges of physicians and surgeons, also supported an extension of the Insurance Scheme to cover the whole population. It was obvious that the voluntary hospitals were facing problems and would require help. Moreover the middle class were becoming less and less happy at paying for the National Health Insurance Scheme and getting nothing back for themselves. However, the wartime harmony on the need for reform did not last. In 1943, the Minister of Health, Ernest Brown, made his first proposals, which involved a salaried general practitioner service with local authority control.

These were rejected by the BMA. A ballot organised by the BMA showed a notable split on the proposals, since the younger doctors and the hospital doctors tended to favour the proposals but the older members and most of the general practitioners were against it. Many of their objections were real, notably the doctor's longstanding dislike of control by local authorities, as experienced under the Poor Law, and some were imaginary, namely that private practice would be eliminated. The next Minister of Health, Henry Willink, modified the Bill, but before it could be introduced, the General Election of 1945 took place, and the Labour government with a crusading

Minister of Health, Aneurin Bevan, was in command. The scene was set for another monumental struggle between government and the doctors. On one side was the BMA who adopted increasingly rigid attitudes as a result of emotional representative meetings of the doctors. On the other side was Bevan, one of the toughest yet charming negotiators ever produced by the Labour Party. The BMA took up more and more extreme stances against a National Health Service, while Bevan took the view that the will of Parliament must prevail. He also conducted private discussions with the presidents of the London colleges, notably Lord Moran. Bevan had a view of health and health care which was simple: it had to be removed from the market place and from charitable effort. The state had to provide the necessary services and he was opposed to the voluntary principle. He confessed to Michael Foot that

> a patchwork quilt of local paternalism is the enemy of intelligent planning. It is repugnant to a civilized community for hospitals to have to rely on private charity. I have always felt a shudder of revulsion when I have seen nurses and sisters who ought to be about their work, and students who ought to be at theirs, going about the streets collecting money for the hospitals.

He was also unashamedly against devolution of power and regarded separate Scottish legislation as a nuisance. Even during the inaugural Welsh Day debate in the House of Commons in October 1944, Bevan denounced the new arrangements as a farce: 'My colleagues', he said, 'have no special solution for the Welsh coal industry which is not a solution for the whole of the mining industry of Great Britain. There is no Welsh problem'. Small hospitals also met with his disapproval. 'I would rather be kept alive in the efficient if cold altruism of a large hospital than expire in a gush of warm sympathy in a small one.'[32]

While the BMA were opposed to the whole scheme, Bevan's strategy for the hospital consultants was successful. They were to be given salaries for their work. This alone was a major new departure, as the voluntary hospitals had always relied on the unpaid help of the consultants in return for the prestige the hospitals offered them. Bevan proposed to pay them for what had previously been done free. Bevan also made two important concessions to the consultants which won them over to the NHS and split the ranks of the BMA. Firstly he allowed the consultants to treat private patients in the

NHS hospitals and that pay-beds should be set aside for the purpose. Secondly he conceded a merit award system to reward consultants for major contributions to the NHS. The awards were to be secret to prevent the label of merit being publicly displayed, thus giving the owner advantages in private practice For the general practitioners, Bevan proposed a free choice of doctors, a basic salary and fees according to the number of patients on the doctor's list. The plan was revealed to the BMA in January 1946 and they were surprised to see these major concessions on the choice of doctor, and the absence of local authority control. The BMA then split. The basic mood was of opposition in the hope of further concessions, but the hospital doctors, led by Webb-Johnston favoured co-operation. The official BMA line became more and more intransigent, influenced by angry correspondence in the *British Medical Journal* and by support from Tory politicians and the Conservative press. A letter to the *British Medical Journal* could say that the health service was 'the first step, and a big one, towards national socialism as practised in Germany'. Nevertheless Bevan won the argument and got his Bill through Parliament. The BMA were meeting simultaneously at a special conference and by a colossal vote opposed the scheme. With the Bill now through Parliament, there was concern that the doctors would not co-operate. In Scotland, Arthur Woodburn, the Secretary of State for Scotland could say sadly that

> 'prior to the time the Scottish doctors became associated with the BMA there was every indication that the Scottish doctors were willing to co-operate with us, but a conflict of loyalties seemed to have arisen'.

In May the last plebiscite of the doctors was called and the Scottish doctors showed approval of the NHS but England and Wales did not. The votes for and against the NHS are shown in Table 7:2. The BMA judged that the opposition was not enough and gave in. They accepted the useful concessions but the general practitioners, who fought to the death, took years to catch up with the consultants in conditions of service, though they had won an 'independent contractor' status.

When the NHS (Scotland) Bill was studied, only small differences between the legislation in Scotland and England could be seen.[33] Perhaps the biggest of these differences in the Bills (and one which was to give a different atmosphere to the hospital service and medical education in Scotland) was that all hospitals in an area were to come under their own Board of Managment. Thus the famous voluntary teaching hospitals, and municipal hospitals nearby, were to be jointly administered under the NHS. In England this had been resisted by the teaching hospitals, with the consequence that in England the teaching hospitals maintained an aloofness which was to handicap them later, since without a full range of modern specialities, the teaching of students and the training of staff and even the research effort were handicapped.

Table 7:2

Voting of British doctors on the NHS proposals

	General Practitioners		Full-time hospital consultants		Part-time hospital consultants		Totals	
	For	*Against*	*For*	*Against*	*For*	*Against*	*For*	*Against*
Scotland	1050	736	161	42	234	197	1893	1341
England	6586	7757	916	360	1347	2148	10,906	12,550

Note: the 'Total' column includes some doctors not entered in the categories listed.

Source: *British Medical Journal*[34]

Other small legislative variations in Scotland were that the endowments of the hospitals were to be held by the Board of Management (not by the hospitals) and that health centres were to be provided by the Secretary of State. The ambulance service was to be run as a centrally directed service. Bevan was concerned that these slightly more radical proposals for the Scottish hospitals might give him problems and wrote to the Secretary of State requesting that the publication of the Scottish Bill be delayed since these 'points might embarrass us if they were to be known publicly before our Bill has been dealt with in the Commons. Some amendments may be forced on us.' Clearly the unification of the administration of the hospitals proposed for Scotland had also been hoped for by some in England, but had been given up as part of the compromise to get the hospital service into the NHS. Bevan was obviously not prepared to see the debate on the London teaching hospitals re-opened by letting the M.P.s see that the matter had been successfully arranged in Scotland. Another of the compromises in England was to give trouble in Scotland. The pay-beds had been allowed as a concession to the

English profession and the Scottish Bill also contained this provision. No pay-beds existed in Scotland (the Edinburgh Royal Infirmary's charter even forbade the presence of private patients) and it looked as if these beds would have to be created by converting some of the existing public beds to private use. Though the Scottish doctors lobbied for this, the M.P.s objected, and a compromise was agreed that allowed for any new hospital beds to be considered for use as pay-beds. In the event few new beds appeared, and pay-beds were rare thereafter in Scotland.

The debate on the NHS (Scotland) Bill contains some interesting points, some of which have become more interesting as the years pass. Conservative amendments were put forward to keep the Scottish teaching hospitals separate from the other local hospitals: this was successfully resisted. The case for the merger was given eloquently by the Secretary of State and he predicted correctly that the bigger group of hospitals would eliminate the old difference in prestige between the two types of hospitals and that the standard of the municipal hospitals would rise. He also pointed out correctly that the children's hospitals, psychiatric hospitals, infectious disease hospitals and maternity hospitals, being brought in as part of one hospital group would increase the service given, and increase the reputation and quality of the teaching in the medical schools. Conservative amendments also sought to allow any doctor to have access to the private beds in hospital. This interesting amendment touched on the principle of whether a general practitioner could treat his own patient in the hospitals. It was lost, thus denying the general practitioner access to hospital beds.

Reaction to the NHS Bill in Scotland was muted. The older doctors realised that the Cathcart committee's view that the general practitioner was the key to the health service was not incorporated in the Bill, and the lowly place of general practice was a particular disappointment in Scotland. Another principle in the Cathcart report was that a co-ordinated service was necessary, but the NHS was being set up with a split between general practice, the hospital service and the local authority services, with only passing references being made to the need for liaison between the services. The Secretary of the Scottish BMA, recalling the original Cathcart proposal, said that

> it seems to be considered necessary with our present legislative

> machinery that a Scottish Act of Parliament must so closely resemble its English counterpart as to be distinguishable only by the faint Caledonian flavour of its language. There is little doubt in my mind that it was principally conceived in the minds of Whitehall. I think I can detect – and this is rather curious – a definite flavour of Harley Street.[35]

Administratively the NHS started smoothly, and without the incidents seen at the time of the introduction of the National Health Insurance Scheme. One feature caught the public imagination – the 'free' spectacles and teeth, since one deficiency of National Health Insurance had been that only the more successful societies provided free dentures or spectacles. When the NHS started, there was a rush to obtain these items.

The introduction of the NHS was a unique innovation in the western world, and owed nothing to previous experiments in Europe. Only in the aftermath of war was such a step possible, but it was the logical outcome of a century of extension of health care from the wealthy to all classes of society. It encouraged altruism in the staff and endless patience was shown by the users. There was also a great simplicity about the NHS, since its funds were collected cheaply and no form-filling was required during the giving or acceptance of treatment. The salaried part of the service was also administratively easy to run. But above all, it was free. Indeed so sacred and precious was Bevan's principle that there should be no extra or hidden charges that the charges introduced later for dentures and spectacles was an emotive political issue for decades to come. The central funding and direction of the NHS at a stroke allowed its resources to be allocated to the places where they were most needed. Private practice had tended to concentrate doctors in the affluent parts of the towns and the voluntary movement had also produced a patchy hospital service. The NHS was able to allocate buildings, doctors and services where the need existed, a benefit keenly felt in Scotland, and prevent costly duplication of facilities. Central design of buildings and equipment could ensure the best buy and the most suitable design. The facility for paying doctors a salary, irrespective of the speciality or geographical place of work, had benefits in staffing the unfashionable specialities and in giving a general and specialist service in rural areas. Only the NHS could raise the necessary capital for the building of a modern hospital service which, by the end of the war had been beyond the means of private enterprise and the voluntary effort of previous generations.

But the NHS had problems in doing so. The original philosophy of meeting all the needs was upheld as far as possible in the expenditure budget, but no capital was released for new building until 1955. Thereafter the provision of costly general hospital facilities was maintained as long as possible leaving poor facilities in other parts of the NHS. Britain's poor economic performance and a lower allocation of Gross National Product to health than in many other countries in Europe led first to the reintroduction of charges for prescriptions, spectacles and dentures and the ultimate admission that resources for running the NHS were not unlimited. By the 1970's the NHS was having to pioneer how to ration health care, an endeavour which all advanced countries watched closely.[36] Waiting lists grew, aggravated by industrial unrest in the NHS, and the private insurance schemes, to their surprise, showed a revival. A new philanthropy appeared and the NHS was glad to fall back on charitable gifts of kidney machines. The second problem in the NHS was that it proved to be a bad employer, and though the doctors quickly realised that militancy was required, others like the nurses and low-paid staff were slow to realise this. Lastly, the central direction of the NHS, though appropriate in the post-war atmosphere, looked increasingly authoritarian in a society wishing to see the devolution of power to more local agencies, and the obsession with bureaucratic management both in nursing and administration, coupled with the deteriorating NHS service, caused protests. In 1974 the NHS took a further step which, if not mistaken, came at the wrong time. During the earlier period of increasing public expenditure a complex new administrative structure was designed for the NHS and a three or four layer system of management devised. By the time it was introduced, public spending was being cut back and the expensive and eventually suspect new management system became widely criticised.[37] Though the scheme was designed to improve management it led to management failures and increased the exasperation with the NHS. This discontent coincided with moves towards devolution of political control of health care back to Scotland and brought into prominence the odd and unique system of government of Scotland and the control of the NHS within Scotland.

Politics of health care

The political control of health care in Scotland in the 20th century can only be understood by tracing its development over almost a century. The office of Secretary of State for Scotland and his curious system of government in Scotland started with the establishment of the office of the Secretary for Scotland in 1885.[38] This office was only set up after prolonged controversy and debate and the failure of numerous earlier Bills to establish it, events repeated in the debate on devolution to Scotland in the 1970s.

The idea of a Secretary for Scotland can be traced even further back to 1709 when, after the Union of the Parliaments, the Westminster parliament established a third Secretary of State whose responsibilities included Scotland. Even this idea was controversial and Daniel Defoe, the pro-Union activist, protested that the office would become

> the centre of the hungry solicitations natural to a poor, cravening and importunate people and would prevent the union from becoming a reality.

The office, he said correctly, 'would keep up a faction in Scotland.' After the '45 Rebellion, the office lapsed, but by the middle of the 19th century, events led to irresistible pressure for restoration of Scottish representation in the government. The earlier pressure had come from the neglect of Scottish legislation, but a later factor in moulding Scottish opinion had been the growth in Scotland of many independent 'Boards' as a result of the reluctant but steadily increasing government intervention in the life of the nation.[39] While in England responsibility for these new functions were given to ministers, in Scotland an independent board was set up. The best example was the increasing power of the English Poor Law Commissioners (called the 'three kings of Somerset house') and they were eventually taken into the mechanism of government and put under a minister of the Crown. The Scottish Poor Law Commissioners were, however, left as an independent Board.

A similar series of events took place in public health legislation and the College of Physicians in Edinburgh had been prominent in fighting successfully for retention of Scottish control of health, again under a devolved board. The same pattern evolved in the other functions of government in Scotland, and by the middle of the 19th century Scotland was the least governed nation in Europe, by reason of this growth of these semi-autonomous boards, responsible to the Home Secretary or Lord Advocate, but only at a great distance. The maximum power of the boards was in the period up to 1855 (though after 1906 the increasing complexity of government yet again allowed the boards to grow), and the necessity for the Scottish boards to have parliamentary accountability and control was realised. Since public opinion (articulated by the Society for the Vindication of Scottish Rights) was against the placing of the boards under Westminster control, a Secretary for Scotland was proposed.

The resistance to the office of Secretary of State for Scotland was considerable and was led by the MPs for the Scottish Universities, Sir Lyon Playfair and J.A. Campbell. In particular they were concerned about the devolution of control of Scottish education to the Secretary for Scotland, and Playfair argued

> this Bill was intended to accentuate the differences between England and Scotland for the future and in my opinion it will tend to convert Scotland into a province with the narrower peculiarities of provincial existence. No country can less afford than Scotland to narrow the ambition of its educated classes, or to parochialize its institutions.[40]

After prolonged debate on a succession of Bills, a Scottish Secretary was set up in 1892 and took his place in the cabinet with responsibility for the activities of government in Scotland. The Scottish boards were slowly taken under his wing and a substantial Board of Health for Scotland was formed in 1919, taking over the problems of poor relief, national health insurance, housing and the Highlands and Islands Medical Scheme. This involved a great simplification, since public health in Scotland had been run by 204 Burgh Councils and 107 District Committees, the Poor Law medical services were run by 876 Parish Councils and the inspection of school children by 947 School Boards. Thus the size of the new department was considerable and an Under-Secretary for Health was soon required to share the work of the Secretary for Scotland. In 1926 another change of name occurred and the Scottish Secretary became a Secretary of State. In 1939 the devolution process continued with the erection of St Andrew's House in Edinburgh to contain all the functions of government in Scotland after their transfer from Dover House in London.[41] In Parliament an increasing number of Committees were necessary for dealing with Scottish

Bills. Legislation on health matters in Scotland was carried out under separate Acts and was debated by the Scottish MPs together as a separate committee. This political devolution was obscured by the fact that this separate system operated so closely in harmony with the England and Wales legislation that its existence was not obvious. The system should not have worked but it did, in spite of the fact that the political problems arose in Scotland and those who were in charge and sensitive to democratic pressures – the MPs and ministers – were in London. Worse still, the ministers in London were separated from their files and civil servants in Edinburgh. A major failing of the system was that the users and the commentators were so baffled that the system was left to run itself and was never driven to act separately by pressure from Scotland. So inscrutable and complex was the government of Scotland, that pressure groups seldom arose to challenge the separate Scottish legislation as it went through. The devolution proposals of the 1970's would have simplified this system by adding political devolution to the existing administrative devolution, but the Scotland Bill met considerable political opposition and was abandoned after the fall of the Labour government in 1979.

Health and health care after 1948

After 1948, the indices of health such as the infant mortality rate showed a steady fall, and the remaining morbidity from infectious disease declined even further.[42] But in Scotland the infectious diseases proved harder to eradicate than elsewhere, and tuberculosis was still a major problem in the 1950's. Not only did Scotland not participate fully in the decline of the old health problems, but was then markedly affected by the 'new wave' of disease, notably lung cancer and heart disease – mainly coronary artery disease. In particular the smoking-related diseases – lung cancer, chronic bronchitis, heart disease and some of the complications of pregnancy – rose to be very important in Scotland.[43] While the smoking of cigarettes reached a peak in Britain in 1960 and then declined in England, the Scottish consumption remained unchanged. By 1976 the Scottish consumption of cigarettes was 30% higher than England and Wales. Scotland also reached the highest rate of lung cancer in the world, a record held by a convincing margin, the male annual death rate (per 100,000) being 349 for Scotland, 310 for England and Wales, 281 for the Netherlands and 271 for Finland. Smoking also played a part in the high incidence of coronary heart disease in Scotland.

Alcohol abuse, always an important cause of illness in Scotland, became important again later in the 20th century and had wide ramifications in the community, being not only responsible for psychiatric disease and social problems but also for much self-injury and hospital admissions with fractures, bumps and bruises as well as injury to others by the battering of wives, children and grannies. Almost invariably, murders and road traffic accidents had alcohol as a major contributing factor, and a revival in the temperance movement occurred not through the voluntary bodies but as an official government drive using the media. Dental health in Scotland failed to improve even with a dental service which, though no longer free, was certainly cheap.

It is impossible to attempt to determine the role played by the NHS in these successes and failures: the interaction of too many factors exists – housing, income, nutrition, and cultural attitudes as well as health care.[44] But there was one surprising failure of the NHS and that was the failure to abolish regional and class differences in disease indices. In 1948 there was a 2.5 times greater infant mortality in social class 5 compared with social class 1 and the differences in the deaths of infants in the first year of life were even higher. By 1975 these ratios were unchanged. Heights and weights of children in social class 5 remained lower than in social class 1 and dental health was poorer and immunisation rates lower. Interestingly no difference in visual acuity between the social classes existed – a faculty not affected by environment.[45]

After 1948 the role of the Medical Officer of Health in dealing with infectious disease and the environmental hazards was contracting, largely through the success of their own efforts. But two problems of the old type remained – tuberculosis (TB) and smoke pollution. Until the appearance of drug treatment for TB in 1955 there was a shortage of sanatorium beds in Scotland and in 1951 an imaginative scheme was devised whereby patients were flown to Switzerland for sanatorium treatment, where 70 beds in the Sanatorium Wolfgang in Leysin and a further 80 beds in the Sanatorium du Mont Blanc were paid for by Scotland. By 1955, 770 patients had been successfully treated in Switzerland. In that year, with the arrival of successful drug treatment for TB, the waiting list for treatment in Scotland fell considerably and the termination of the Swiss scheme was announced. This closure, though justified, proved to be a sensitive issue. In the General Election two months after the announcement, the ruling Conservative party were put on the defensive in Scotland by Hector McNeil, the Labour former Secretary of State, who had set up the scheme and who made it an election issue in Greenock. At the same time, a major drive was launched for the detection of TB by Mass Miniature Radiography in which the public responded and became greatly involved. In a preliminary drive in Motherwell a door-to-door canvass was carried out by volunteers and 8 out of 10 cinemas had shown propaganda for the TB drive. Most shops displayed a banner and one out of five lamp posts bore a poster. One of the radiography units claimed a record number of 1,033 chest X-rays taken in one single day.[46]

The last public health measure of a kind reminiscent of the old pioneering days of public health came in 1956 when the Clean Air Act (later strengthened in 1968) made a major improvement in the problem of chest diseases provoked by the pollution of the cities, particularly by the lethal winter 'smog' – the toxic fog forming in still cold air in winter.[47] The problem had been a chronic one in Scotland and had been a favourite complaint of the Medical Officers of Health who had had a running battle with the worst industrial offenders. Some measures were taken before 1939, but the pall of smoke over the industrial cities during the war was an effective protection against air raids and smoke abatement was abandoned during this time. After the war, the problem was agreed to be soluble and the deaths in the London smog of 1952 accelerated the appearance of legislation, helped by the arrival of smokeless fuel and a less charitable view of unrestricted industry.

By 1974 it was judged that the separate public health service was no longer necessary, and it was taken from the local government authorities and fused with the NHS in the reorganisation. The medical officers of health became community medicine specialists but without the intrusive power given to the founders of the public health movement, they had few weapons with which to attack the new wave of disease.

Medical practice and education

By the 1950's and 60's the hospital sector of the NHS reached the highest point of its esteem and influence. New technology made possible heart surgery, the artificial kidney and transplantation; effective new drugs, notably the antibiotics, made possible dramatic cures of previously fatal diseases. In this science-based expansion, Scotland had a number of unexpected and unplanned advantages within the NHS, and while in the pre-war period Scottish medical science had lagged behind since the staff had to earn money through private practice and lacked assistants and laboratories, in the post-war period these defects were remedied. Firstly the NHS administrative areas in Scotland often centred round a university, and the specialist units still existed after the war. Secondly the relative absence of private practice in Scotland made the consultants income similar to the new full-time university salaries which started in 1946, making an academic career as attractive as a purely clinical one. The results of this were impressive: career medical scientists were produced in large numbers in Scotland, and after an essential period of study in America, these doctors took on many important posts in Britain and elsewhere.

In the 1970's a reaction against hospital-based medicine occurred. It was extremely expensive and made huge demands on an increasingly hard-pressed budget. Moreover the success of the post-war curative medicine and improved social conditions was resulting in an increasingly older population and the new social and medical problems of the degenerative diseases were baffling to the health services. The result was, not for the first time in Scottish medical history, the appearance of cynicism about the powers of the medical men, and a return to Hippocratic methods of regulation of diet and exercise, and health farms appeared to take on the role of the ancient water cures. These methods of self-help were encouraged by the poverty-stricken NHS.

At the start of the 20th century the considerable reputation of Scottish medical education was easily explained. The momentum established by the great era of the Edinburgh medical school in the 18th century gave Scotland a remarkable reputation for medical education. The 19th century medical education had consisted largely of lectures and since no limit on the numbers of students was placed, the earlier 18th century reputation for quality was added to by a 19th century reputation for the quantity of graduates produced. However, all was not well in Scottish medical education at the start of the 20th century.[48] The new English medical schools had equalled the quality of Scotland and Edinburgh in particular, and it was generally conceded that the German postgraduate education was superior. Painfully, the Scots acknowledged that the old ways were no longer working.

The nation which learnt most from Germany was America and the dramatic rise of their medical education and research was one of the main features of the 20th century.[49] The American expansion's most notable event was the new Johns Hopkins medical school which sought to tempt Macewen from Glasgow to be their first professor of surgery, and on his declining to go, they offered, in the manner to be familiar later, to employ all his hospital staff as well. With the destruction of Germany's lead in education by World War I, America took over as the centre for postgraduate study, a change noticed early by Scotland, and by Edinburgh staff first.

In the 20th century the output of Scottish graduates relative to England declined for several reasons. Firstly, the medical course itself became more complicated and, to copy the German example, practical work was necessary and the teaching of students in small groups at the bedside became favoured. Thus a practical limit to the number of students who could be taught in any one university arose and the universities began to limit the numbers taken in. Secondly, the appearance of new medical schools in England reduced the Scottish dominance. Central Government now had an increasing say in medical education and it was reasonable to plan a fairer geographical spread of medical schools. A further reduction in the Scottish output occurred when the extramural medical schools in Scotland – Anderson's College and the St Mungo College in Glasgow and the School of Medicine of the Royal Colleges of Edinburgh, were also closed after the World War II in favour of teaching in the universities only.[50] The numbers of graduates from Scotland as a proportion of the British total is shown in Table 7:3.

These figures show that the proportion of medical students within the U.K. being educated in Scotland have steadily fallen since 1935. Prior to this there had been an even higher Scottish proportion in the 19th century. The proportion of female medical students rose considerably and in Glasgow and St Andrews the admission rate of women approached 50% in some years. The fall in the number of overseas students became progressive and the universities increasingly concerned themselves with local applicants.

Table 7:3

Scottish medical students as a percentage of U.K. total and percentage of overseas and female medical students in Scotland.

	% U.K. Total	% Women students in Scotland	% Overseas students in Scotland
1935	35.1	15.8	Not known
1965	22.7	26.6	9.0
1972	22.9	38.7	2.1
1976	17.4	37.4	2.5

Source: Royal Commission on Medical Education[51]

During World War II Scotland's internationalism was acknowledged and strengthened by the setting up of the Polish Medical School in Edinburgh, from which 228 doctors graduated and 33 completed their studies elsewhere.[52] Though the medical school was planned as a means of restoring the Polish health services after the war, only a few graduates chose to return on closure of the school in 1949 though many of their Polish teachers did so. An earlier international link had been the training of American Jewish medical students in Scotland, since they were not admitted to their own universities. The old tradition of supplying doctors for other countries was revived in Scotland, but in a new and less praiseworthy form, since in the 1960's a marked exodus of Scottish graduates in medicine started, mainly to Canada, a loss which made all calculations of medical 'personpower' unreliable, estimates which central government never managed to get right. The loss of doctors by emigration was the result of less attractive salaries and prospects in the U.K. than elsewhere, and Britain's poor economic performance. This considerable loss did not produce a crisis in the running of the health service, as there was a new wave of immigrant doctors into Britain, largely from the medical schools of India and Pakistan, set up to provide the Empire with their own doctors. They now rescued the NHS and filled the vacant posts, vacancies made greater by a mistaken cut in the number of medical students being trained. Britain joined the European Economic Community in 1973 but the expected exodus of doctors did not occur, though it was detectable in those specialties in which language was less of a barrier to such a move.

It might be said that Scottish medical education, made famous by the innovative sparkle which gave it its original reputation, had now lost its numerical preponderance in the 20th century. This is not to say that Scottish medical education completely lost an identity. Firstly a slightly broader range of social class of student was taken into the Scottish medical schools. This was the result of the traditions of the Carnegie Trust for the Universities of Scotland which, starting in 1901, assisted less well-off students to pay the fees in pre-war times.[53] The trust paid the fees of 59,029 Scottish students of all faculties up till the time when, with lower fees and local authority grants, higher education came within the reach of all.

Lastly the 20th century was marked by a remarkable revival in the Scottish doctors' corporations, whose survival in a time of marked standardisation and centralised control might seem surprising. This success was the result of the Colleges of Physicians and Surgeons in Scotland diversifying their interests into postgraduate education and their higher diplomas in medicine and surgery became obligatory for promotion in a hospital career. So successful was the introduction of these diplomas that huge numbers of overseas graduates sought them enthusiastically. Edinburgh took the lead in this new phase of the Colleges' activities and the Glasgow College, after an indolent half century, revived after World War II and shared in this lucrative, if precarious, postgraduate activity.

This rise of the Colleges was a remarkable reminder of the great days of Scottish medicine. Just as the Scottish undergraduate medical schools triumphed in an age of unfettered competition and without government money, expensive buildings or equipment, so the 20th century Colleges thrived in the competitive world of postgraduate teaching and licensing, where no laboratory instruction or public money was required, and as many as presented themselves could be accommodated. Adam Smith would have been proud of them.

Bibliography and references

BIBLIOGRAPHY

Primary Sources

The earliest records of Scotland were carefully studied and used for J.D. Comrie's *History of Scottish Medicine* London 1932 and the early records of the doctor's corporations and the older voluntary hospitals have been used by the historians of these institutions (see below for details). Other records relevant to health care are being only slowly exploited, and much must remain in the records of government, Town Councils, Kirk Sessions and the voluntary bodies. Even major collections of material such as the Royal Commissions into the universities in Scotland and the workings of the Poor Law or the health of towns have only slowly been investigated. Three studies however have used extensively such primary sources – C.L. Pennington *Mortality, Public Health and Medical Improvements in Glasgow 1855–1911*, unpublished Ph.D. thesis University of Stirling 1977, M. Flinn (ed) *Scottish Population History* Cambridge 1978 and O. Checkland *Philanthropy in Victorian Scotland: Social Welfare and the Voluntary Principle* Edinburgh 1980.

Scotland until the mid 19th century was rich in medical journals of high quality. The *Edinburgh Medical and Surgical Journal* of the early 19th century (1805–55) was the best of its kind in Britain, though the later *Edinburgh Medical Journal* (1855–1954) and the *Glasgow Medical Journal* (1828–1833 and 1853–1955) are also helpful. The disgruntled *Glasgow Medical Examiner* (1829–30 and 1876–78) had a shorter life, as had the cheerful *Sanitary Journal for Scotland* – later the *Sanitary Journal* (1876–1902). The earlier Scottish medical periodicals of the 18th century are described in W.R. Lefanu 'British periodicals of medicine' *Bull. Med. Hist.* (1937) 5,735–761 and 827–855. In the early 19th century *The Lancet* was particularly attentive to Scottish matters. In the 20th century the *Health Bulletin* (1941–), produced by the Scottish Home and Health Department, is devoted to Scottish health matters, and the *Scottish Medical Journal* arose in 1956 from the fusion of the *Glasgow Medical Journal* and the *Edinburgh Medical Journal*. The *Caledonian Medical Journal* (1891–1948) has much of interest to the medical historian of the Highlands and Islands.

Secondary Sources

The history of medicine in Scotland to the end of the 19th century is well covered by J.D. Comrie's classical work of reference, *History of Scottish Medicine* London 1932. T. Ferguson's books, *The Dawn of Scottish Social Welfare* London 1948 and *Scottish Social Welfare 1864–1914* Edinburgh 1958 are primarily concerned with public health, but also have much other data. Scattered information is to be found in the histories of the universities, colleges and hospitals, but most of these works do not extend beyond the end of the 19th century. Two other works are invaluable in the study of Scottish medicine, T.C. Smout's *A History of the Scottish People 1560–1830* London 1969 gives splendid account of the social history of Scotland, and all available health statistics for Scotland are collected in M. Flinn (ed) *Scottish Population History* Cambridge 1977, which also has a valuable narrative. All the epidemics in Scotland are described in C. Creighton *A History of Epidemics in Britain* Cambridge 1894. G.M. Howe *Man, Environment and Disease in Britain* London 1972 has much related material of interest. Of the general histories of medicine the social historian is best served by R.H. Shryock *The Development of Modern Medicine* London 1948.

Up to 1800

For medieval times see A. I. Dunlop *The Life and Times of James Kennedy, Bishop of St Andrews* Edinburgh 1950. For general studies of 17th and 18th centuries, readable accounts are given in H.G. Graham *The Social Life of Scotland in the Eighteenth Century* Edinburgh 1899 and M. Plant *The Domestic Life of Scotland in the Eighteenth Century* Edinburgh 1952. For medical practice, there is much in the histories of the colleges and hospitals (listed below) and also in E.A. Underwood *Boerhaave's Men at Leyden and After* Edinburgh 1977,

R.E. Wright-St Clair *Doctors Monro: a medical saga* London 1964 and E.H.B. Rodger *Aberdeen Doctors at Home and Abroad* Edinburgh 1893. For an account of Scottish health and health care in this period, see J.H.F. Brotherston *Observations on the Early Public Health Movement in Scotland* London 1952. Folk medicine and the healing wells are covered in J.G. Dalyell *The Darker Superstitions of Scotland* Edinburgh 1834 and J.M. McPherson *Primitive Beliefs in the North-East of Scotland* London 1929.

Medical teaching and research in the Enlightenment is covered in A.C. Chitnis *The Scottish Enlightenment* London 1976, A.L. Donovan *Philosophical Chemistry in the Scottish Enlightenment* Edinburgh 1975, A. Hook *Scotland and America 1750–1835* Glasgow 1975, A. Kent (ed) *An Eighteenth Century Lectureship in Chemistry* Glasgow 1950, N.T. Phillipson and R. Mitchison (eds) *Scotland in the Age of Improvement* Edinburgh 1970 and J. Gray *History of the Royal Medical Society 1737–1937* Edinburgh 1952. Three important articles in *History of Science* vol 12, 81–141 deal with this period, as does G. McLachlan (ed) *Medical Education and Medical Care: a Scottish-American Symposium* London 1977, R.G.W. Anderson and A.D.C. Simpson (eds) *Symposium on the Early Years of the Edinburgh Medical School* Edinburgh 1976 and the Scottish Society of the History of Medicine Symposium on *Edinburgh's Infirmary* Edinburgh 1979.

Important biographies covering this period are *The Autobiography of Sir Robert Sibbald, Kt, M.D.* Edinburgh 1833, J. Glaister *Dr William Smellie and his Contemporaries* Glasgow 1894, L.H. Roddis *James Lind, Founder of Nautical Medicine* New York 1950, A.G. Stewart *The Academic Gregories* Edinburgh 1901, C.F.W. Illingworth *The Story of William Hunter* Edinburgh 1967, Jessie Dobson *John Hunter* Edinburgh 1969, G.W. Corner (ed) *The Autobiography of Benjamin Rush* Princeton 1948, W. Ramsay *The Life and Letters of Joseph Black* London 1918, J. Thomson *An Account of the Life, Letters and Writings of William Cullen M.D.* Edinburgh 1832, and R.K. French *Robert Whytt, the Soul, and Medicine* London 1969.

For the use of Scottish medicine in fiction, the works of Sir Walter Scott can be consulted for details of folk medicine and occasional glimpses of medical education. More direct use of 18th century medicine was made by Tobias Smollet in his works, notably in *Humphrey Clinker*.

19th and 20th Centuries

There are a few separate studies on Scottish medicine of the 19th and 20th centuries, but T. Ferguson *Scottish Social Welfare 1864–1914* Edinburgh 1958, A.K. Chalmers *The Health of Glasgow 1818–1925* Glasgow 1930 and H.P. Tait *A Doctor and Two Policemen* Edinburgh 1974 cover public health. Surgery is dealt with by A.J. Youngson *The Scientific Revolution in Victorian Medicine* London 1979 and J.A. Ross *The Edinburgh School of Surgery after Lister* Edinburgh 1978. Some material of Scottish interest is found in F.B. Smith *The People's Health 1830–1910* London 1979 and M.J. Peterson *The Medical Profession in Mid-Victorian London* London 1978, but the recent interest in the social history of medicine has largely ignored Scotland.

Social conditions and the health of the Highlands are dealt with in J. Hunter's *The Making of the Crofting Community* Edinburgh 1976. The Lowlands are dealt with in the neglected work L.J. Saunders *Scottish Democracy 1815–1840* Edinburgh 1950. Scottish medicine in the 20th century has been neglected, though W.S. Craig *History of the Royal College of Physicians of Edinburgh* Oxford 1976, gives some information. Also the recent revival of interest in Scottish affairs has produced a number of collected essays which include a discussion of Scottish medicine. These are G. Brown (ed) *The Red Paper on Scotland* Edinburgh 1975, R. Underwood (ed) *The Future of Scotland* London 1977 and G. Kennedy (ed) *The Radical Approach* Edinburgh 1976. Reviews of aspects of health care in Scotland are also found in the annual *Scottish Government Yearbook* edited by H.M. Drucker and M.G. Clarke.

Important biographies covering the 19th century are J. Muir *John Anderson, Pioneer of Technical Education and the College he Founded* Glasgow 1950, A.M.W. Thomson *The Life and Times of Dr William MacKenzie: Founder of the Glasgow Eye Infiramry* Glasgow 1973, W.S. Craig *John Thomson: Pioneer and Father of Scottish Paediatrics 1856–1926* Edinburgh 1968, I.Rae *Knox, the Anatomist* Edinburgh 1964, R.B. Fisher *Joseph Lister 1827–1912* London 1977, J.A. Shepherd *Simpson and Syme of Edinburgh* Edinburgh 1969, A.L. Turner *Sir William Turner: a Chapter in Medical History* Edinburgh 1919, R. Christison *The Life of Sir Robert Christison* Edinburgh 1885, J. McGrigor *The Autobiography and Services of Sir J. McGrigor* London 1861, C.A. Gibson *The Life of Sir William Tennant Gairdner* Glasgow 1912, P. Manson-Bahr *The Life and Work of Sir Patrick Manson*

London 1927, J. Chiene *Looking Back: 1907–1860* Edinburgh 1908, Conan Doyle *Memoirs and Adventures*.

For fictional accounts of 19th century Scottish medicine, see the works based on the Knox scandal, notably James Bridie *The Anatomist*. *Jamie Simpson* London 1935 by Laurence Oliver deals with Sir J.Y. Simpson. For a terrible kailyard medical classic see Ian MacLaren *A Doctor of the Old School*.

Medical biographies of the 20th century are few as yet, but include A.K. Bowman *The Life and Teaching of Sir William Macewen* Glasgow 1942, Lord Boyd Orr *As I Recall* London 1966, E.F.B. MacAlister *Sir Donald MacAlister of Tarbert* London 1935 and James Bridie *One Way of Living* London 1939.

For fictional works describing 20th century Scottish medicine see the novels of A.J. Cronin, particularly *Adventures in Two Worlds* and the Colin Douglas Edinburgh novels *The Houseman's Tale* (1975), *The Greatest Breakthrough Since Lunchtime* (1977) and *Bleeders Come First* (1979).

College, University and Hospital histories

The older works college histories are C.H. Creswell *The Royal College of Surgeons of Edinburgh* Edinburgh 1926 and A. Duncan *Memorials of the Faculty of Physicians and Surgeons of Glasgow* Glasgow 1896. More recent is W.S. Craig *History of the Royal College of Physicians of Edinburgh* Oxford 1976. Other sources are J.B. Tennent *Records of the Incorporation of Barbers, Glasgow* Glasgow 1899 and R. Peel Ritchie *The Early Days of the Royall Colledge of Phisitians, Edinburgh* Edinburgh 1899.

There are a number of early histories of Edinburgh University, of which the most readable is A. Bower *The History of the University of Edinburgh* Edinburgh 1817. More recent accounts are A.L. Turner *History of the University of Edinburgh 1883–1933* Edinburgh 1933 and D.B. Horn *A Short History of the University of Edinburgh 1556–1889* Edinburgh 1967. Much of the history of Edinburgh medicine is also found in J. Gray *History of the Royal Medical Society 1737–1937* Edinburgh 1952. Glasgow has probably the best written of this genre – J. Coutts *A History of the University of Glasgow* Glasgow 1909. Glasgow is also described in the collection of essays *Fortuna Domus* Glasgow 1952, in D. Murray *Memories of the Old College of Glasgow* Glasgow 1927 and in J.D. Mackie *The University of Glasgow*

1451–1951 Glasgow 1954. For Aberdeen University, see J.M. Bulloch *History of the University of Aberdeen 1495–1895* London 1895, W.D. Simpson (ed) *The Fusion of 1860* Aberdeen, 1963, E.H.B. Rodger *Aberdeen Doctors at Home and Abroad* Edinburgh 1893 and R.S. Rait *The Universities of Aberdeen: a History* Aberdeen 1895. For St Andrews/Dundee see D. Douglas *Practitioner* (1972) vol 209, 103–109 and R.G. Cant *The University of St Andrews: a Short History* Edinburgh 1970. See also F.N.L. Poynter *The Evolution of Medical Practice in Britain* London 1961 and A.R. Cunningham *Aspects of Medical Education in Britain in the Seventeenth and early Eighteenth Centuries:* unpublished Ph.D. thesis, University College London 1974.

Hospital histories have to record the skill and wisdom of the past and present staff and often have little space left for matters of historical interest. However, the best of a large number of such works are A.L. Turner *Story of a Great Hospital: The Royal Infirmary of Edinburgh 1729–1929* Edinburgh 1937, H.J.C. Gibson *Dundee Royal Infirmary 1798–1948* Dundee 1948, M.S. Buchanan *History of the Glasgow Royal Infirmary* Glasgow 1832, J.M. Cowan *Some Yesterdays* Glasgow 1949, O.M. Watt *Stobhill Hospital: The First Seventy Years* Glasgow 1971, L. MacQueen and A.B. Kerr *The Western Infirmary 1874–1974* Glasgow 1974, A.M.W. Thomson *The History of the Glasgow Eye Infirmary 1824–1962* Glasgow 1963, D. Guthrie *The Royal Hospital for Sick Children Edinburgh*, T.C. MacKenzie *The Royal Northern Infirmary, Inverness* Inverness 1946, I. Murray *The Victoria Infirmary of Glasgow*, Glasgow 1967 and J. Patrick *A Short History of the Glasgow Royal Infirmary* Glasgow 1940. See also James Carmont *The Crichton Royal Institution*, Leicester 1896 and J. Ferrier *Greenock Royal Infirmary 1806–1968*, Greenock 1968. For general accounts of the voluntary and other hospitals see O. Checkland *Philanthropy of Victorian Scotland: Social Welfare and the Voluntary Principle* Edinburgh 1980, J. Woodward *To Do the Sick No Harm* London 1974 and F.N.L. Poynter (ed) *The Evolution of Hospitals in Britain* London 1964.

REFERENCES

Chapter 1: The dark ages

1. For an account of these early peoples see A.A.M. Duncan *Scotland: the Making of the Kingdom* Edinburgh 1975.
2. Scottish Bronze Age injuries are described in D. Waterston 'A stone cist and its contents found at Piekie Farm' *Proc. Soc. Ant. Scot.* (1926) 61, 30–44.
3. Dental decay in skulls of all periods of Scottish history is detailed in D.A. Lunt 'The prevalence of dental caries in the permanent dentition of Scottish prehistoric and medieval populations' *Arch. Oral Biol.* (1974) 19, 431–437.
4. The Rothesay skull is described by J.W. Parry 'The art of trephining among prehistoric and primitive people' *J. Brit. Arch. Ass.* (1916) 22, 33–69.
5. Possible Scottish surgical instruments are mentioned in J. Anderson *Scotland in Pagan Times* Edinburgh 1883. Discussion of trepanning in ancient and modern times is found in R. Munro 'Notes on prehistoric trepanning in the old and new worlds' *Proc. Soc. Ant. Scot.* (1896) 32, 220–235.
6. Trephining in Skye in the 17th century is mentioned by M. Martin *A Description of the Western Isles* 1699, p198.
7. The presence of Druids in Scotland is discussed in J.D. Comrie *History of Scottish Medicine* London 1932, p 29. Further details are given in A. MacGregor *Highland Superstitions* Stirling 1922.
8. Pliny: *Natural History* Book 30, sect. 13 describes the medicine men and the human sacrifices.
9. Columba's brushes with the Magi are described in W. Huyshe (ed) *Adamnan's Life of St. Columba* London 1905, pp 144, 146.
10. Comrie (ref 7) p 29.
11. J.Y. Simpson *Was the Roman Army supplied with Medical Officers?* Edinburgh 1856.
12. The National Museum of Antiquities of Scotland in Edinburgh holds a number of Roman medical finds but not all are Scottish in origin. The medicine spoon is described in L. Dopson 'Pharmaceutical antiquities at Edinburgh' *Apprentice or Student (Chemist and Druggist)* (1961) 50, 4–5.
13. Both Hadrian's Wall and the Antonine Wall are well described in J. Forde-Johnston *Hadrian's Wall* London 1978.
14. A.P. Forbes *Lifes of St. Ninian and St. Kentigern* Edinburgh 1874.
15. For Columba's life see Huyshe (ref 9). Attempts to reconstruct Columba's real life and works have been made in W.D. Simpson *The Historical St. Columba* Edinburgh 1963 and A. MacBain *Trans. Gaelic Soc. Inver.* (1884) 11, 137–166.
16. Huyshe (ref 9) p 50.
17. The English leech books of the 10th century are mentioned in Comrie (ref 7) p 55 and contain some 'Scottish' cures.
18. Huyshe (ref 9) p 107.
19. *The Life of St. Cuthbert* Surtees Society Edinburgh 1891, p 93.
20. Comrie (ref 7) p 31 and P.W. Joyce *Social History of Ancient Ireland* London 1903 vol 1, p 597.

21. Comrie (ref 7) p 45 lists many of the holy wells and others are described in Dom Michael Barrett *A Calendar of Scottish Saints* Fort Augustus 1919. For a discussion on the holy healing wells see J.M. MacKinlay *The Folklore of Scottish Lochs and Streams* Glasgow 1893, and E.B. Simpson *Folklore in Lowland Scotland* London 1908, p 33.
22. Two possible pagan water-shrines have been described. A shrine to the Roman god Coventina is mentioned in J. Clayton 'Description of Roman remains discovered near to Procolitia, a station on the wall of Hadrian' *Arch. Ael.*(1879) 8, 1–48. Votive offerings to a water god are suggested in S. Piggot 'Three metal-work hoards of the Roman period from southern Scotland' *Proc. Soc. Ant. Scot.* (1952) 87, 1–50.
23. L. Wright *Clean and Decent* London 1960, p 2.
24. A well in Barra (Cille Bharra) still has a modest reputation for spiritual healing.
25. C. Creighton *A History of Epidemics in Britain* London 1894, Vol 1 p 4. and G.M. Howe *Man Environment and Disease in Britain* London 1972, p 89.
26. W.F. Skene *John of Fordun's Chronica Gentis Scotorum* Edinburgh 1871. Quoted by T. Ferguson *The Dawn of Scottish Social Welfare* London 1948, p 47.
27. D. Laing *Cronykil of Andrew of Wyntoun* Edinburgh 1872, vol 2 p 482.

Chapter 2: The middle ages 1100–1600

1. For accounts of early Scotland by travellers see P. Hume Brown *Early Travellers in Scotland* Edinburgh 1891, and M. Lindsay *The Discovery of Scotland* London 1964.
2. For descriptions of violence in Scottish society see T.C. Smout *A History of the Scottish People* London 1969, p 103 and details of the devastation in the Borders at the time of the 'Rough Wooing' are found in W. Croft Dickinson (ed) *A Source Book of Scottish History* London 1953, vol 2 p 132. Physical violence rather than poisoning was preferred by the ruling class, but the use of poison is reviewed in A.F. Steuart 'Poisoning in Scotland to the year 1625' *Ed. Med. J.* (1905) 17, 68–481. Steuart also describes an early judicial post-mortem in 1579.
3. S.G.E. Lythe *The Economy of Scotland in its European Setting* Edinburgh 1960, 17–23. and M. Flinn (ed) *Scottish Population History* Cambridge 1977 p 109.
4. D. Laing (ed) *Cronykil of Andrew of Wyntoun* Edinburgh 1871, vol 2 p 454.
5. P. Hume Brown *Scotland before 1700 from Contemporary Documents* Edinburgh 1893, pp xv, 19 and 24; T. Ferguson *The Dawn of Scottish Social Welfare* London 1948, pp 15, 16.
6. See C. Creighton *A History of Epidemics in Britain* London 1894, G.M. Howe *Man Environment and Disease in Britain* London 1972 p 93 and J.F.D. Shrewsbury *A History of the Bubonic Plague in Britain* Cambridge 1970 p 45.
7. W.F. Skene (ed) *John of Fordun's Chronicle of the Scottish Nation* Edinburgh 1871, vol 2 p 359.
8. Laing (ref 4) vol 2 p 482.
9. The rarer pneumonic and septicaemic forms of the plague were even more rapidly fatal, but caused less pain.
10. J. Michon quoted in P. Ziegler *The Black Death* London 1969 p 30.
11. The disease causing an epidemic in medieval times is seldom clearly identifiable: see works listed in ref 6.

12. C. Elliott (ed) *Robert Henryson: Poems* Oxford 1963, p 122.

13. G. Eyre-Todd *Mediaeval Scottish Poetry* Glasgow 1892 p 187.

14. For early ideas of disease spreading like a cloud see W. Huyshe (ed) *The Life of St. Columba, by Adamnan,* London 1905, p 103 and A. McKerral *Kintyre in the Seventeenth Century* Edinburgh 1948, p 74.

15. T. Ferguson (ref 5) p 107 describes these moves. The Aberdeen evacuation is mentioned by E.H.B. Rodger *Aberdeen Doctors at Home and Abroad* Aberdeen 1893, p 4.

16. A.I. Dunlop *The Life and Times of James Kennedy Bishop of St Andrews* Edinburgh 1950, p 380.

17. For favourable comments on the Scottish regulations see C.F. Mullet 'Plague policy in Scotland, 16th–17th centuries' *Osiris* (1950) 9, 435–456.

18. For further details of the plague regulations see J.D. Comrie *History of Scottish Medicine* London 1932, p 202 and J. Ritchie 'Quarantine for the plague in Scotland' *Ed. Med. J.* (1948) 55, 691–701. There is little evidence that the severe penalties were enforced.

19. Henrysoun's life is described by J. Ritchie 'James Henrysoun: chirurgian to the poore' *Med. Hist.* (1960) 4, 70–79.

20. This account of leprosy in Scotland is based on three scholarly articles by J.Y. Simpson *Ed. Med. Surg. J.* 56, 301–330 and vol 57 pp 121 and 394. The leper hospitals are listed in I.B. Cowan and D.E. Easson *Medieval Religious Houses* London 1976, p 162.

21. *Acts of the Scottish Parliament 1124–1423*, vol 1 p 344.

22. J.Y. Simpson (ref 20) vol 57 p 395 gives details of the occupants.

23. J.Y. Simpson (ref 20) vol 57 p 150.

24. Eyre-Todd (ref 13) p 115.

25. R.S. Morton 'Some aspects of the early history of syphilis in Scotland' *Brit. J. Vener. Dis.* (1962) 38, 175–180. See also Comrie (ref 18) p 199 and J.Y. Simpson *Archeological Essays* Edinburgh 1872 vol 2.

26. *Extracts from the Council Register of the Burgh of Aberdeen 1398–1570* Spalding Club 1844, p 425.

27. Aberdeen Register quoted in Morton (ref 25) p 177.

28. Pitcairn *Criminal Trials* Edinburgh 1833, vol 1, pt 1 p 110.

29. This account is taken from Cowan and Easson (ref 20) and J. Durkan 'Care of the poor: pre-Reformation hospitals' *Innes Review* (1959) 10, 268–280. Comrie (ref 18) p 105 also describes the hospitals.

30. E.A. Hammond 'Physicians in medieval religious houses' *Bull. Med. Hist.* (1958) 32 105–120.

31. G. Chalmers *Caledonia* Paisley 1887, vol 2, p 768, and D.E.R. Watt *A Biographical Dictionary of Scottish Graduates to A.D. 1410* Oxford 1977.

32. Dunlop (ref 16) p 417.

33. For accounts of the Scots students abroad see A.I. Dunlop 'Scots abroad in the 15th century' *Historical Association Publication No. 124*, London 1942; A.F. Steuart 'The Scottish "Nation" at the university of Padua' *Scot. Hist. Rev.* (1906) 3, 53–62.

34. D.E.R. Watt 'University graduates in Scottish benefices before 1410' *Recs. Scot. Church Hist. Soc.* (1964) 15, 77–88.

35. For a general account of European medical education see L.C. MacKinney 'Medical education in the Middle Ages' *J. World Hist.* (1955) 2, 835–861.
36. Wood Brown's *Life and Legend of Michael Scot* Edinburgh 1897, is added to in Comrie (ref 18) p 58. Scots place as an early alchemist is discussed by J. Small 'Sketches of the early Scottish alchemists' *Proc. Soc. Antiq. Scot.* (1875) 11, 179–197 and his reputation as a scientist is defended by J. Read 'Michael Scot, a Scottish pioneer of science' *Scientia* (1938) 64, 190–197. A recent biography is Lynn Thorndike *Michael Scot* London 1965, and bibliographical details of his work are found in *Records of the Glasgow Bibliographical Society* (1931) 9, 73–100.
37. Holdings of medical books in medieval Scottish libraries is described in J. Durkan and A. Ross 'Early Scottish libraries' *Innes Review* (1958) 9, 5–178.
38. Comrie (ref 18) p 83.
39. Comrie (ref 18) p 184.
40. R. Nicholson *Scotland: the Later Middle Ages* Edinburgh 1974, p 300, describes some of the visitors as do J. Durkan and J. Kirk *The University of Glasgow 1451–1577* Glasgow 1977, p 173.
41. J. Tweedy 'The deterrent effect of social and legal restrictions on the medical thought and practice' *Trans. Medico-legal Soc.* (1911) 3, 1–8.
42. Comrie (ref 18) p 152.
43. D. Guthrie 'King James the Fourth of Scotland: his influence on medicine and science' *Bull. Hist. Med.* (1947) 21, 173–193.
44. Comrie (ref 18) p 151.
45. The early Scottish alchemists were distinguished enough to merit several studies: J. Small (ref 36); J. Read 'Alchemy in Scotland' *Chemist and Druggist* (1938) 128, 742–745 and J. Read *Through Alchemy to Chemistry* London 1957.
46. Comrie (ref 18) p 154.
47. Eyre-Todd (ref 13) p 199.
48. For the Scots doctors in Europe see E.H.B Rodger *Aberdeen Doctors* Edinburgh 1893, J.H. Burton *The Scot Abroad* Edinburgh 1881 p 303 and J. Robertson (ed) *The Book of Bon Accord* Aberdeen 1839 p 305.
49. W. McWilliam 'Early Scottish Medicine to the 18th century' *Cal. Med. J.* (1929) 14, 366–392.
50. Seton is described in Read (ref 45) and Kinloch in R.C. Buist 'David Kinloch (Kynalochus) 1559–1617' *Brit. Med. J.* (1926) i, 793.
51. D. McDonald *Surgeons Twoe and a Barber* London 1950 p 27.
52. This poem is omitted from the standard works on Henryson but is quoted in McWilliam (ref 49) p 373.
53. Comrie (ref 18) p 146.
54. D. Waterson 'Bishop James Kennedy: an anthropological study of his remains' *Trans. Roy. Soc. Ed.* (1934) 58, 75–112.
55. C.H. Creswell *The Royal College of Surgeons of Edinburgh* Edinburgh 1926, p 6.
56. R.C. Buist 'Dundee doctors in the sixteenth century' *Ed. Med. J.* (1930) 37, pp 293 and 357. Other cases are found in the Dundee Burgh and Head Court Book held in the Dundee archives.
57. P.W. Joyce *A Social History of Ancient Ireland* London 1903, p 597, and D.A. Binchy 'Bretha Déin Chécht' *Erui* (1966) 20, 1–65.

58. Healing stones and charms are dealt with by G.F. Black 'Scottish charms and amulets' *Proc. Soc. Ant. Scot.* (1892) 27, 433–526.

59. For details of the holy wells see Chapt 1, ref 21.

60. A.M. Fraser 'A mysterious cure' *Scot. Hist. Rev.* (1972) 51, p 241.

61. W. Barclay *Callirhoe, Commonly called the Well of Spa* Aberdeen 1615 p 21.

62. This account is based on D.S. Thomson 'Gaelic learned orders and literati in Scotland' *Scottish Studies* (1968) 12, 57–78, and A. Nicholson 'The McBeths – hereditary physicians of the highlands' *Trans. Gaelic Soc. Glasg.* (1958) 5, 94–111. See also McWilliam (ref 49) and M.M. Whittet 'Historical aspects of celtic medicine' *Proc. Roy. Soc. Med.* (1964) 57, 429–436.

63. The manuscripts are described in detail by Comrie (ref 18) p 64, and for further details see G. MacKay 'Ancient gaelic medical manuscripts' *Cal. Med. J.* (1904) 6, 34–45, and J. MacKechnie *Catalogue of Gaelic Manuscripts in Selected Libraries* Boston 1973. See also H.C. Gillies *Regimen Sanitatis: the Rule of Health* Glasgow 1911.

64. Smout (ref 2) p 94.

65. W. Croft Dickinson (ed) *John Knox's History of the Reformation in Scotland* London 1949, vol 2 appendix 8, gives the social and education policy of the Church.

66. D. Laing (ed) *The Works of John Knox* Edinburgh 1895 vol 2 p 211.

67. These important points are taken from A.R. Cunningham *Aspects of medical education in Britain in the seventeenth and early eighteenth centuries*; unpublished Ph.D. thesis University College London 1974.

68. D. McRoberts (ed) *Essays on the Scottish Reformation 1513–1625* Glasgow 1962, p 385.

69. A.L Turner *Story of a Great Hospital: the Royal Infirmary of Edinburgh* Edinburgh 1937, p 78.

Chapter 3: The troubled years: 17th century

1. For social conditions in Scotland in the 17th century see T.C. Smout *A History of the Scottish People* London 1969 p 119.

2. T. Johnston *The History of the Working Class in Scotland* London 1946, p 290.

3. The sequence of war, famine and disease is carefully analysed by M. Flinn (ed) *Scottish Population History* Cambridge 1977, and the ultimate loss of life is termed a 'mortality crisis'.

4. J.G. Dalyell *The Darker Superstitions of Scotland* Glasgow 1834 p 657.

5. *Chronicle of Perth* quoted in Flinn (ref 3) p 120.

6. Sir W. Brereton quoted in M. Lindsay *The Discovery of Scotland* London 1964, p 55.

7. Lindsay (ref 6) p 57.

8. Flinn (ref 3) p 119 has detailed studies of the burial records of the period.

9. D. Calderwood *The History of the Kirk of Scotland* Wodrow Society (1845) vol 7 p 514.

10. Flinn (ref 3) p 123.

11. Flinn (ref 3) p 124.

12. R. Sibbald *Provision for the Poor in Time of Dearth and Scarcity* 1699, p 2.
13. C.F. Mullet 'Plague policy in Scotland, 16th–17th centuries' *Osiris* (1950) 9, 435–456. See also J.F.D. Shrewsbury *A History of the Bubonic Plague in Britain* Cambridge 1970.
14. The Leith Session Clerk in 1645 was excused from writing up the Parish Minutes as he had been confined to his house as a plague suspect: T. Burns *Old Scottish Communion Plate* Edinburgh 1892, p 216.
15. *Extracts from the Records of the Burgh of Aberdeen* p 81, quoted in J.D. Comrie *History of Scottish Medicine* London 1932 p 218.
16. G.A.G Mitchell 'The medical history of Aberdeen and its Universities' *Aberdeen University Review* (1958) 37, 225–250.
17. T. Ferguson *Scottish Social Welfare 1864–1914* Edinburgh 1958 p 371.
18. These regulations against the plague were much stronger than those enforced against cholera in the 19th century.
19. *Register of the Privy Council of Scotland* XIII, p 836–38.
20. P. Hume Brown *Scotland before 1700 from Contemporary Documents* Edinburgh 1893, p 289.
21. In Scotland the word 'hospital' thereafter was used in connection with the poor house or similar charitable foundations (e.g. Glasgow's Hutchesons Hospital), and the term 'infirmary' was later used for the new institutions for the sick. In England the terms were used in the opposite sense.
22. J.M. MacPherson *The Kirks Care of the Poor* Aberdeen n.d. (?1945) p 130. Much other material must exist in other parish records. For early child welfare see J. Ritchie 'The beginnings of child welfare in Scotland before 1800' *Health Bulletin* (1954) 12, 45–47.
23. *The Diary of Mr. John Lamont 1649–1671* Maitland Club Edinburgh 1830 p 21.
24. A. Duncan *Memorials of the Faculty of Physicians and Surgeons* Glasgow 1896 p 54.
25. This account is taken from A.R. Cunningham *Aspects of medical education in Britain in the seventeenth and early eighteenth centuries*: unpublished Ph.D. thesis University College London 1974.
26. An occasional student was taught at Aberdeen and Edinburgh started some teaching under Pitcairne – see C.P. Finlayson 'Two Highland proteges of Dr. Archibald Pitcairne' *Ed. Med. J.* (1953) 60, 52–60.
27. L. Jolley 'A. Pitcairne' *Ed. Med. J.* (1953) 60, 39–51. Pitcairne's philosophy is described by W. Coleman 'Mechanical philosophy and hypothetical physiology' *Texas Quarterly* (1967) 10, 259–269. Pitcairne's period at Leyden is covered in G.A. Lindeboom 'Pitcairne's Leyden interlude described from the documents' *Ann. Sci.* (1963) 19, 273–284. The Edinburgh troubles are described in W.B. Howie 'Sir Archibald Stevenson, his ancestry and the riot in the College of Physicians at Edinburgh' *Med. Hist.* (1967) 11, 269–283.
28. Comrie (ref 15) p 270: A Cunningham 'Sir Robert Sibbald and medical education, Edinburgh 1706' *Clio Medica* (1978) 13, 135–161: *The Autobiography of Sir Robert Sibbald, Knt, M.D.* Edinburgh 1833, and F.P. Hett (ed) *The Memoirs of Sir Robert Sibbald (1641–1722)* London 1932.
29. Finlayson (ref 26) p 53 describes methods of uroscopy.

30. Pitcairne's postal practice is described by Jolley (ref 27). For other examples of postal consultations see M. Clough 'Material of medical interest in the Cromartie papers' *Med. Hist.* (1973) 17, 185–188. Cullen's 18th century postal advice is analysed in G.B. Risse 'Dr. William Cullen, Physician, Edinburgh' *Bull. Hist. Med.* (1974) 48, 338–351.

31. D.L. Cowen 'The Edinburgh Pharmacopoeia' *Med. Hist.* (1957) 1, 123–139.

32. These methods were later satirised by Robert Burns in his poem *Death and Dr Hornbook*, and for the therapeutic torments inflicted during the last days of the life of the 'Marquesse of Douglass', see C.G. Drummond 'Thomas Borthwick 1617–75, the first surgeon apothecary in Scotland' *Chemist and Druggist* (1962) 177, 736–738.

33. Comrie (ref 15) p 229.

34. Duncan (ref 24) p 240 describes a Paisley apothecary who was to receive prescriptions in 'Scots Languadge because he hes no uyr Languadge'.

35. The early history of the apothecaries in Edinburgh is given by C.G. Drummond 'Pharmacy and medicine in old and new Edinburgh' *Scottish Genealogist* (1965) 12, i, 1–10.

36. A number of surgeon-apothecary's bills are found in collections of 17th century papers. For published examples see Drummond (ref 32) and *Cal. Med. J.* (1914), 10, 27–33.

37. J. Stuart (ed) *List of Pollable Persons within the Shire of Aberdeen 1696*, Spalding Club Aberdeen 1844; M. Wood (ed) *Edinburgh Poll Tax Returns for 1694* Scottish Records Society Edinburgh 1951.

38. Duncan (ref 24) p 200 and J. Finlayson *Dr. Sylvester Rattray, author of the treatise on sympathy and antipathy* Glasgow 1900. Rattray's work was the first medical text written in Glasgow.

39. See the introduction by J.Y. Simpson to C. Innes *The Ledger of A. Halyburn and the Book of Customs 1612* Edinburgh 1867.

40. J.G. Wallace-James 'A Haddington Surgeon's Account' *Scot. Hist. Rev.* (1905) 2, p 102.

41. For an early account of the problem of bladder stones see R. Smith 'A statistical enquiry into the frequency of bladder stones in Great Britain and Ireland' *Medico-Chir. Trans.* (1820) 11, p 20. The problem has now almost disappeared.

42. A. Nicholson 'The McBeths – hereditary physicians of the Highlands' *Trans. Gaelic Soc. Glasg.* (1958) 5, 94–111.

43. Duncan (ref 24) p 54.

44. *Diary of George Ridpath 1755–1761* Scottish History Society 1922, p 33. The Mss contains additional material since the editor removed 'a mass of sickroom details which is quite unprintable'.

45. P. Lowe *Chirurgerie* London 1596.

46. Descriptions of the surgical apprenticeship are found in Duncan (ref 24) p 49, C.H. Creswell *The Royal College of Surgeons of Edinburgh 1505–1905* Edinburgh 1926, pp 17, 28 and 137; other apprenticeships are described in R.E. Wright-St. Clair *Doctors Monro* London 1964. A 17th century apprenticeship document is given in full in the Erskine Diary – *Miscellany of the Scottish History Society* vol. 2, p 371, Edinburgh 1904.

47. Smollett's use of his medical training has been closely studied: D.M. Musher 'The medical views of Dr. Tobias Smollett' *Bull. Hist. Med.* (1967) 41, 455–462, C.E. Jones 'Tobias Smollett (1721–71) – the doctor as man of letters' *J. Hist. Med.* (1957) 12, 337–348. For a general account see M.A. Goldberg *Smollett and the Scottish School* Albuquerque 1959.

48. For the struggle of the Paris surgeons for recognition see V.L. Bullough *The Development of Medicine as a Profession* New York 1966, p 85.

49. Drummond (ref 35) p 2.

50. R.S. Moncrieff 'Note on the Incorporation of Surgeons and Barbers' *Ed. Med. J.* (1912) 9, 524–530.

51. Ducnan (ref 24) p 237.

52. Moncrieff (ref 50) p 530.

53. Only the Royal College of Physicians of Edinburgh have retained their original title throughout their existence. The Edinburgh surgeons did not use a fixed title in the 16th and 17th century, using the term 'Incorporation' or 'Calling' with or without the Barbers added to the title. In the early 18th century they were known as the Incorporation of Surgeons and became the Royal College of Surgeons of Edinburgh in 1778. In Glasgow the Faculty of Physicians and Surgeons became the Royal Faculty in 1909 and the Royal College of Physicians and Surgeons of Glasgow in 1962. The terminology is even more confused since the universities in Glasgow and Edinburgh were called 'College' until the early 18th century, and the original professoriate there were collectively known as the 'Faculty' until the mid-19th century reforms.

54. For a general history, see C.H. Creswell (ref 46).

55. Duncan (ref 24) gives a thoughtful history of the Glasgow College.

56. J. Finlayson *Life and Works of Maister Peter Lowe* Glasgow 1889: A.L. Goodall 'The Royal Faculty of Physicians and Surgeons Glasgow' *J. Hist. Med.* (1955) 10, 207– 225: L.D.W. Scott *Royal College of Physicians and Surgeons of Glasgow Bulletin* (1979) 8, 11–17 and 9, 12–19.

57. A comprehensive history of the College is given in W.S. Craig *History of the Royal College of Physicians of Edinburgh* Oxford 1976.

58. An earlier history of the College is R. Peel Ritchie *The Early Days of the Royall Colledge of Physitians of Edinburgh* Edinburgh 1899.

59. This account of the early days of the College is taken from Craig (ref 57) p 18.

60. J.D. Marwick *Extracts from the Records of the Convention of Royal Burghs in Scotland* Edinburgh 1878 vol 3, 441–469.

61. Craig (ref 57) p 58.

62. Early itinerants visiting Scotland are mentioned in Comrie (ref 15) pp 228 and 261. See also R. Thin 'Medical quacks in Edinburgh in the seventeenth and eighteenth centuries' *Book of the Old Edinburgh Club* 22 132–159 and L.G. Matthews 'Licensed mountebanks in Britain *J. Hist. Med.* (1964) 19, 30–45.

63. W. Barclay *Callirhoe, Commonly called the Well of Spa* Aberdeen 1615 p 21.

64. Thin (ref 62) op 135.

65. W.R. McDonald 'Scottish 17th century almanacs' *The Bibliotheck* (1963) 4, 257–278.

66. J. Ferguson 'Seventeenth Century Receipts' *Scot. Hist. Rev.* (1915) 13, 219–228.

67. E.A. Underwood 'English-speaking students at Leyden' *Nature* (1969) 221, 810–814. The ministers and parishes are Alexander Anderson (Duffus), David Cooper (Auchinleck) and James Wilson (Gamrie) – personal communication from Dr. Underwood.

68. F.F. MacKay *MacNeill of Carskey: His Estate Journal 1703–1743* Edinburgh 1955, p 103.

69. Mentioned in D. Guthrie 'The literature of Domestic Medicine' *Edinburgh Bibliographical Society Tans.* (1938) 2, 445–447.

70. *The Diary of Alexander Brodie of Brodie* Spalding Club Aberdeen 1873, p 327.

71. Martin Martin *A Description of the Western Isles of Scotland* London 1703 passim.

72. There is a substantial literature on Scottish traditional medicine and folk-healing: D. McKenzie *The Infancy of Medicine* London 1927; J.G. Dalyell *The Darker Superstitions of Scotland* Glasgow 1834, J.M. McPherson *Primitive Beliefs in the North-East of Scotland* London 1929 and W.D. Hand 'The folk-healer: calling and endowment' *J. Hist. Med.* (1971) 26, 263–275. The survival of traditional methods into the 20th century is mentioned in S. Parman 'Curing beliefs and practices in the Outer Hebrides' *Folklore* (1977) 88, 107–109. A compendium of gaelic charms is found in A. Carmichael *Carmina Gadelica* Edinburgh 1900, and a commentary on it in F.G. Thompson 'The folklore elements in Carmina Gadelica' *Trans. Gaelic Soc. Inverness* (1964) 44, 226–255.

73. Details of these healers is given in Hand (ref 72).

74. Dalyell (ref 72) p 62 describes touching by the King in Scotland, and for a description of touching in Britain see F.H. Garrison *History of Medicine* 4th Edition 1929 p 288.

75. Martin (ref 71) describes this empiric and his status. David Gregory (1627–1720), the Aberdeen inventor, father of David Gregory, Savilian professor at Oxford and skilled medical practitioner, was investigated by the Kirk Session. Whether this was the result of his remarkable cures or his ability to fortell the weather using his barometer is not clear.

76. J.K. Hewison *The Isle of Bute in the Olden Time* Edinburgh 1895, vol 2, p 264. Duncan (ref 24) p 75 also gives details of a warning to a female healer in 1657.

77. This account of witchcraft in Scotland is taken from C. Larner *Enemies of God* London 1980, and C. Larner, C.H. Lee and H.V. McLachlan *A Source-book of Scottish Witchcraft* Glasgow 1977. Brief accounts of the healing carried out by witches are found in Smout (ref 1) p 198, MacPherson (ref 72) p 235, Dalyell (ref 4) p 50. For Sir Walter Scott's use of witchcraft see C.C. Parsons *Witchcraft and Demonology in Scott's Fiction* Edinburgh 1964.

78. W.R. Rhind *Sketches of Moray* Edinburgh 1889, p 419.

79. G.R. Reid *Annals of Auchterarder* Crieff 1899, p 195.

80. I. Adam *Witch Hunt: the Great Scottish Witchcraft Trials of 1697* London 1978, p 175.

81. G. Tourney 'The physician and witchcraft in Restoration England' *Med. Hist.* (1972) 16, 143–155.

82. J.M. Mackinlay *Folklore of Scottish Lochs and Springs* Glasgow 1893. Other references are given in Chapt. 1.

83. MacKinlay (ref 82) p 269 and local convictions are given in W. Crammond *Extracts from the Records of the Kirk Session of Elgin* n.d., under the year 1596.

84. Brodie Diary (ref 70) p 333.
85. For a general account of this and the early mineral wells in Scotland and the literature on them see W.G. Aitchison Robertson 'Some ancient mineral wells in Scotland' *Ed. Med. J.* (1923) 30, pp 246, 276 and 368. The early literature on Kinghorn, Moffat, Aberdeen and the Edinburgh well is listed. For an early description of the Peterhead spa see A.M., Student in Medicine *The Discovery of St. Peters Well, at Peterhead in Scotland* Edinburgh 1636.
86. G.F. Black 'Scottish charms and amulets' (1892) *Proc. Soc. Ant. Scot.* 27, 433–526.
87. Black (ref 86) p 496.

Chapter 4: The rise of the professional: 18th century

1. For an analysis of the changes in 18th century Scottish population see M. Flinn (ed) *Scottish Population History* Cambridge 1977 part 4.
2. Descriptions of social life in Scotland in the 18th century can be found in M. Plant *The Domestic Life of Scotland in the Eighteenth Century* Edinburgh 1952.
3. R.L. Blanco 'The Diary of Jonathan Potts' *Transactions and Studies of the College of Physicians of Philadelphia* (1977) 44, 119–130.
4. W. Mercer 'The contribution of Edinburgh to early American medicine' *J. Roy. Coll. Surg. Ed.* (1961) 7, 180–194.
5. For a description of the temporary decline in Edinburgh see A.J. Youngson *The Making of Classical Edinburgh* Edinburgh 1966 p 20.
6. Descriptions of Glasgow are given in D. Defoe *A tour thro' the Whole Isle of Great Britain* London 1753 and E. Burt *Letters from a Gentleman in the North of Scotland* London 1815.
7. This account of the famine relief is taken from Flinn (ref 1) p 11, and T.C. Smout in L.M. Cullen and T.C. Smout *Comparative Aspects of Scottish and Irish Economics and Social History* Edinburgh 1977, p 21.
8. M.D.L. Finlay 'Was ague malaria?' *Royal College of Physicians of Edinburgh Chronicle* (1979) 9, 14–19. See also J.D. Comrie *History of Scottish Medicine* London 1932 p 430 and J.H.F. Brotherston *Observations on the Early Public Health Movement in Scotland* London 1952, p 26.
9. Brotherston (ref 8) p 25 and the remarkable collection of health statistics in Flinn (ref 1).
10. R. Watt *An Inquiry into the Relative Mortality of the Principal Diseases of Children . . .* Glasgow 1813. The problem of smallpox is discussed throughout the first *Statistical Account*.
11. A. Monro *An Account of the Inoculation of Smallpox in Scotland* Edinburgh 1765.
12. R.W. Chapman (ed) Johnson's *Journey to the Western Isles of Scotland* Oxford 1924 p 63.
13. C.H. Creswell *The Royal College of Surgeons of Edinburgh* Edinburgh 1926, p 254.
14. T. Ferguson *The Dawn of Scottish Social Welfare* London 1948 p 237.
15. R. Klibansky and E.C. Mossner *New Letters of David Hume* Oxford 1954, p 175.
16. *The Account Book of Sir John Foulis of Ravelston 1671–1707* Edinburgh 1894, p xxxv. Foulis still used the Scots pound in his accounts and in 1980 values the £12 Scots doctor fee would be about £60. For conversion of Scottish into English

money see Foulis p xxxiii and Comrie (ref 8) p 223. To convert early fees to 20th century prices see E.H.P. Brown and S.V. Hopkins *Economica* (1956) 23, 296–314, and P. Wilsher *The Pound in Your Pocket* London 1970.

17. G.B. Risse 'Doctor William Cullen, Physician, Edinburgh' *Bull. Hist. Med.* (1974) 48, 338–351.
18. Examples of surgeon-apothecaries bills are found in G.R. Gibson 'An Edinburgh Medical Family' *Ed. Med. J.* (1929) 36, 419–427 and E. D. Dunbar *Social Life in Former Days* Edinburgh 1865 p 20.
19. I.E. McCracken 'Eighteenth century medical care: a study of Roxburghshire' *Proc. Roy. Soc. Med.* (1949) 42, 410–416.
20. *Ridpath's Diary 1755–1761* Scottish History Society 1922.
21. For general accounts of the British Spas see F. Alderson *The Inland Resorts and Spas of Britain* Newton Abbot 1973.
22. The chemists interest in the mineral wells is analysed in J. Eklund 'Of a spirit in the water: some early ideas on the aerial dimension' *Isis* (1976) 67, 527–550.
23. For individual analyses of Scottish spas see Eklund (ref 22).
24. An expedition to study folk-healing methods and the plants of Scotland was funded by the Commissioners for Annexed Estates at the suggestion of John Hope: see SRO E 727/47 and 728/43.
25. Foulis (ref 16) p xxxv. He also used water from a well near Linlithgow.
26. Peterhead is omitted from all complications on British spas: but see J.T. Findlay *A History of Peterhead* 1933, p 200.
27. Burns letters from the spa are in J.G. Lockhart *The Life of Robert Burns* Liverpool 1914, vol 2, p 166.
28. Plant (ref 2) p 226 and M. Lochhead *The Scots Household in the Eighteenth Century* Edinburgh 1948 p 332.
29. For the survival of these supernatural beliefs see J.M. McKinlay *Folklore of Scottish Lochs and Streams* Glasgow 1893, p 117.
30. The quacks of the 18th century are dealt with in R. Chambers *Domestic Annals of Scotland* Edinburgh 1858, vol 2, 149, 347, 383, 458, 483; Comrie (ref 8) p 158; *Glasgow Past and Present* Glasgow 1890, vol 2, 87–92. For a general account of the medical quacks see L.G. Matthews 'Licensed Mountebanks in Britain' *J. Hist. Med.* (1964) 19, 30–45, and R. Thin 'Medical Quacks in Edinburgh in the seventeenth and eighteenth centuries' *Book of The Old Edinburgh Club* (1938) 12, 132–159.
31. W. Grossart *Historic Notices and Domestic History of the Parish of Shotts* Glasgow 1880 p 66.
32. Thin (ref 30) p 141.
33. Thin (ref 30) p 149.
34. The Scottish poorhouses are described in R.A. Cage *The Scottish Poor Law 1745–1845*: Ph.D. thesis University of Glasgow 1974, J.M. MacPherson *The Kirk's Care of the Poor* Aberdeen n.d. (?1945) p 130 and J. Lindsay *The Scottish Poor Law* Ilfracombe 1975, p 81.
35. The Edinburgh hospital is well served by A.L. Turner *Story of a Great Hospital: the Royal Infirmary of Edinburgh 1729–1929* Edinburgh 1937.
36. Unfortunately no account of the Aberdeen Royal Infirmary exists.

37. The apothecaries shop in the Edinburgh Royal has a place in history since Joseph Black spent much of his student time there watching the chemical methods: see J.B. Eklund and A.B. Davis 'Joseph Black matriculates: medicine and magnesia alba' *J. Hist. Med.* (1972) 27, 396–417.
38. Voluntary hospitals' annual report have detailed clinical statistics.
39. There is a confident description of a Dundee Dispensary set up in 1735 – see H.J.C. Gibson 'The old infirmary of Dundee, 1798–1855' *Ed. Med. J.* (1949) 56, 285–303.
40. The Edinburgh Dispensary is described by R. Scott in G. McLachlan (ed) *Medical Education and Medical Care: a Scottish-American Symposium* Oxford 1977 p 57.
41. Hume quoted in A.C. Chitnis *The Scottish Enlightenment* London 1976 p 12.
42. E.A. Underwood *Boerhaave's Men at Leyden and After* Edinburgh 1977 p 24.
43. Underwood (ref 42) p 25.
44. This analysis of the Enlightenment uses ideas from T.C. Smout (ref 1) c.19, J.B. Morrell 'Reflections on the history of Scottish science' *Hist. Sci.* (1974) 12, 81–94, J.R.R. Christie 'The origins and development of the Scottish scientific community' *Hist. Sci.* (1974) 12, 122–147 and S. Shapin 'The audience for science in eighteenth century Edinburgh' *Hist. Sci.* (1974) 12, 95–121.
45. P. Gay *The Enlightenment: an Interpretation* London 1967 vol 2, 12–23. Gay discusses the place of medicine in the Enlightenment: he identifies Cullen as Scotland's 'greatest surgeon'.
46. This suggestion that private practice declined in Edinburgh is given some support by noting the mysterious decline in the fortunes of the Incorporation of Surgeons in mid-century. This role of private practice may also help explain the failure of Glasgow to develop teaching, since Glasgow medical practice did not depend on the parliament and aristocracy, and hence the Union produced no crisis.
47. Christie (ref 44) makes this point.
48. The upper middle class origins of the literati is shown in V. Bullough and B. Bullough 'The causes of the Scottish medical renaissance of the eighteenth century' *Bull. Hist. Med.* (1971) 45, 13–28, and is also discussed by D.J. Witherington in N.T. Phillipson and R. Mitchison (eds) *Scotland in the Age of Improvment* Edinburgh 1970, p 172.
49. The early days of the Edinburgh medical school are discussed in many of the works given in the General Bibliography q.v. This account is mainly from Underwood (ref 42) p 88, A. Bower *The History of the University of Edinburgh* Edinburgh 1817, A.R. Cunningham *Aspects of medical education in Britain in the seventeenth and early eighteenth centuries*: unpublished Ph.D. Thesis University College London 1974 and A.L. Donovan *Philosophical Chemistry in the Scottish Enlightenment* Edinburgh 1975 p 7.
50. The Monro dynasty is described by R.E. Wright-St Clair *Doctors Monro: a medical saga* London 1964, p 64.
51. Christie (ref 44) p 127 makes this point.
52. Bower (ref 49) vol 2, p 185. No extended biography of Drummond exists.
53. It was about 1685 that the Town's College changed its name to 'university'.

54. J. Struthers Historical Sketch of *The Edinburgh Anatomical School* Edinburgh 1867, p 29.

55. D. Sloan *The Scottish Enlightenment and the American College Ideal* New York 1971.

56. The American links are dealt with fully in McLachlan (ref 40).

57. Bowers in McLachlan (ref 40) p 8.

58. J.R. McCulloch (ed) *Adam Smith: An Inquiry into the Wealth of Nations* 4th Edition, Edinburgh 1850, p 588.

59. Chitnis (ref 41) p 176.

60. This *Lernfreiheit* is analysed in J.B. Morrell (ref 44).

61. The Royal Medical Society has had close attention in J. Gray *History of the Royal Medical Society* Edinburgh 1952.

62. For the medical services of the armies of the '45 see M.M. Whittet 'Medical Resources of the Forty-five' *Trans. Gaelic Soc. Inverness* (1964) 44, 1–44.

63. This account is from Turner (ref 35) p 39.

64. Such a collection was not uncommon: parishes were often asked to support distant public works.

65. When Glasgow Royal Infirmary opened much later, parishes like Shotts near Glasgow were noted to have used the Royal Infirmary in Glasgow regularly.

66. The events in Glasgow are described in A. Duncan *Memorials of the Faculty of Physicians and Surgeons of Glasgow* Glasgow 1896 p 124, and in J. Coutts *A History of the University of Glasgow* Glasgow 1909, p 476.

67. W.B. Howie 'Samuel Benion – Glasgow University's first doctor of medicine' *Scot. Med. J.* (1979) 24, 76–79.

68. This account is from Donovan (ref 49) p 8.

69. W. Mercer 'The contribution of Edinburgh to early American medicine' *J. Roy. Col. Surg. Ed.* (1961) 7, 180–194, A.R. Riggs 'The colonial American medical student at Edinburgh' *Univ. Edin. J.* (1961) 20, 141–153, and J. Duffy *The Healers: a History of American Medicine* New York 1976.

70. The Glasgow and Aberdeen graduates are listed in W.J. Bell 'North American and West Indian graduates of Glasgow and Aberdeen to 1800' *J. Hist. Med.* (1965) 20, 411–415.

71. F.R. Packard 'How London and Edinburgh influenced medicine in Philadelphia in the eighteenth century' *Ann. Med. Hist.* (1932) 4, 219–244.

72. For the influence of Scotland on Canada see H.E. MacDermot 'The Scottish influence in Canadian practice' *Practitioner* (1959) 183, 84–91, and W. Mercer 'Edinburgh and Canadian medicine' *Canadian Med. Ass. J.* (1961) 84, 1241 and 1313.

73. A number of lists of distinguished Edinburgh medical men exist: see R.H. Girdwood in McLachlan (ref 40) p 35., and R.H. Girdwood 'The Royal Infirmary of Edinburgh 1729–1979' *Scot. Med. J.* (1979) 24, 154–158.

74. See Chapt. 3 ref 46 and J.H. Appleby 'British doctors in Russia 1657–1807' Unpublished Ph.D. East Anglia University 1979.

75. Marat is confidently claimed as an Edinburgh student in Gray (ref 61) but nowhere else.

76. R.D. Thornton *William Maxwell to Robert Burns* Edinburgh 1979.

77. P. Mathias in J.M. Winter (ed) *War and Economic Development* Cambridge 1975, 73–90, and R. Stott 'A Scottish dimension of Enlightenment medicine' *Society for the Social History of Medicine Bulletin* (in press).
78. Lind is described in L.H. Roddis *James Lind, Founder of Nautical Medicine* New York 1950.
79. S. Selwyn 'Sir John Pringle' *Med. Hist.* (1966) 10, 266–274.
80. All the stars of the Enlightenment produced texts and were well paid for them. This included the first Edinburgh sex manual, John Armstrong's *The Economy of Love* Edinburgh 1736, of which it was later said that 'it was quite properly omitted from all books of poetry thereafter'.
81. D.L. Cowen 'The Edinburgh Pharmacopoeia' *Med. Hist.* (1957) 1, 123–139. The *Edinburgh Dispensatory* – a pharmacopoeia plus explanatory comment – was possibly even better known in its field. See D.L. Cowen 'The Edinburgh Dispensatories' *Papers of the Bibliographical Society of America* (1951) 45, 85–96.
82. C. Alston *Lectures on Materia Medica* Edinburgh 1770, vol ii, p 498. Alston may have unfortunately picked the wrong substance to ridicule since toads' skin contains a digitalis-like substance.
83. See C.J. Lawrence 'William Buchan: medicine laid open' *Med. Hist.* (1975) 19, 20–35.
84. This point is made by Brotherston (ref 8) p 22.
85. There is little known of the early Edinburgh publishers, but the instrument makers are described in D.J. Bryden *Scottish Instrument Makers 1600–1900* Edinburgh 1972.
86. The Scottish medical societies are described in Christie (ref 44).
87. For the early British medical periodicals see 'British periodicals of medicine' *Bull. Hist. Med.* 5 (1937) 735–758.
88. E.C. Mossner *The Life of David Hume* Oxford 1970 p 589.
89. The accounts of Cullen are still unsatisfactory but see: J. Thomson *An Account of the Life, Letters and Writings of William Cullen, M.D.* Edinburgh 1852: Donovan (ref 49) and R.W. Johnstone 'William Cullen' *Med.Hist.* (1959) 3, 33–45.
90. Joseph Black has had slightly better attention than Cullen. See Donovan (ref 49), Eklund and Davis (ref 22) and W. Ramsay *The Life and Letters of Joseph Black* London 1918.
91. Black's movements and experiments prior to his great discovery have been closely documented by historians of science. See H. Guerlac 'Joseph Black and Fixed Air' *Isis* (1957) 48, 124–155, and 433–456: also J.B. Eklund and A.B. Davis 'Joseph Black matriculates: medicine and magnesia alba' *J. Hist. Med.* (1972) 27, 396–417. The earlier work in Edinburgh on lime water by Whytt and Alston is described in R.K. French *Robert Whytt, the Soul and Medicine* London 1969.
92. Gay (ref 45) p 22.
93. Brown is described in Thomson (ref 89) and G. Risse 'Scottish medicine on the continent: John Brown's system in Germany 1796–1806' *Proc. 23rd Cong. Hist. Med.* (1974) 682–687.
94. A.H.T. Robb-Smith in F.N.L. Poynter (1966) *The Evolution of Medical Education in Britain* London 1966, p 94.

95. This account is taken from W.N. Boog Watson 'Four Monopolies and the surgeons of London and Edinburgh' *J.Hist. Med.* (1970) 25, 311–322, and W.N. Boog Watson 'The Guinea trade and some of its surgeons' *J. Roy. Coll. Surg. Ed.* (1969) 14, 203–214.

96. This account is taken from I. Waddington 'The struggle to reform the Royal College of Physicians 1767–71' *Med. Hist.* (1973) 17, 107–126, and G. Clark *A History of the Royal College of Physicians*, Oxford, 1964, vol 2, pp 543, 566.

97. Clark (ref 96) vol 1, p 193.

98. Waddington (ref 96) p 113.

99. The satire is found in the collected *Dramatic Works of S. Foote* vol 2 London 1788.

100. Fothergill's discomfit is analysed in B.C. Corner 'Dr. Melchisedech Broadbrim and the playwright' *J. Hist. Med.* (1952) 7, 122–135.

101. V.S. Doe (ed) *The Diary of James Clegg of Chapel en le Frith 1708–55* Chesterfield 1978.

102. J. Thomson (ref 89)vol 1, pp 473 and 660 gives the letters between Cullen, Hunter and Smith, as does McCulloch (ref 59) p 587.

103. R.N. Smart in G.W.S. Barrow (ed) *The Scottish Tradition* Edinburgh 1974 p 91. It was alleged that the itinerant 'Dr.' Green had a St Andrews degree: it cannot be traced in the university archives.

Chapter 5: The industrial revolution: 19th century (1)

1. These numbers are only approximate, since the early records are poor and many students did not chose to graduate. The later figures are complicated by the success of the extramural schools, whose output is even less well documented. For the figures available see J. Struthers *Historical Sketch of the Edinburgh Anatomical School* Edinburgh 1867, A.L. Turner *Sir W. Turner, a Chapter in Medical History* Edinburgh 1919, and the Glasgow figures are found in J.D. Comrie *History of Scottish Medicine* London 1932 p 514 and in A. Duncan *Memorials of the Faculty of Physicians and Surgeons of Glasgow* Glasgow 1896 p 183.

2. C. Newman in F.N.L. Poynter (ed) *The Evolution of Medical Education in Britain* London 1957, p 49.

3. P. Manson-Bahr 'Scottish poineers in tropical medicine' *Ed. Med. J.* (1948) 55, 220–231.

4. For lists of distinguished Edinburgh trained medical men see Chapt. 4 ref 73. Unfortunately it is not possible to quantify the dominance of British medicine by the Scottish trained men, since the M.D. was optional at the end of the course in the early 19th century and for the armed forces or Indian Medical Service a diploma from the London Colleges was still desirable. These problems make analysis of the origins of British doctors impossible: thus little can be concluded from the carefully collected data in, for instance D.G. Crawford *Roll of the Indian Medical Service 1615–1930* London 1936.

5. R.E. Wright-St Clair *Proc. 23rd Cong. Hist. Med.* (1974) 748–753.

6. Conan Doyle used the observative Edinburgh surgeon Joseph Bell as his model for Sherlock Holmes: see J.A. Ross *The Edinburgh School of Surgery after Lister* Edinburgh 1978, p 70.

7. N. Cantlie and G. Seaver *Sir James Cantlie* London 1939 p 96.

8. R.L. Blanco 'Henry Marshall (1775–1851) and the health of the British Army' *Med. Hist.* (1970) 14, 260–276.
9. The Edinburgh extramural schools are described in D. Guthrie *Extramural Medical Education in Edinburgh* Edinburgh 1965 and R. Thin 'Edinburgh medical school a hundred years ago' *Ed. Med. J.* (1940) 47, 585–600.
10. Glasgow's extramural schools are described in Duncan (ref 1) p 178 and vigorously defended in D.C. McVail 'An Address on Scottish medical teaching' *Glas. Med. J.* (1882) 18, 419–439.
11. J. Muir *John Anderson* Glasgow 1950.
12. Duncan (ref 1) p 182.
13. Newman (ref 2) p 49.
14. For a full account of the Burke and Hare scandal see I. Rae *Knox, the Anatomist* London 1964, and Knox is portrayed in Bridie's *The Anatomist* and the events were used in Stevenson's *The Body-snatcher*. The Glasgow grave-robbing is described in P. MacKenzie *Reminiscences of Glasgow*, 1890, vol 2, p 462, and the precautions against grave-robbing are listed in G.A.G. Mitchell 'Anatomical and resurrectionist activities in northern Scotland' *J. Hist. Med.* (1949) 4, 417–430. See also H.P. Tait 'Some Edinburgh medical men at the time of the resurrectionists' *Ed. Med. J.* (1948) 55, 115–123. There were protests from Edinburgh over lack of consultation and remoteness of government during the passage of the Anatomy Act: see *Ed. Med. Surg. J.* (1829) 32, 211–219.
15. A brief analysis of the decline is given by J.B. Morrell 'The rise and fall of Scottish Science' *Times Higher Educational Suppl.* 8 April 1977, p 5. This period and its troubles are described in detail in *The Report made to His Majesty by a Royal Commission of Inquiry into the State of the Universties of Scotland* Parliamentary Papers Oct. 7 1831, vol 12. The evidence given in each university was later published separately in Parliamentary Papers 1837 vols 35, 36, 37 and 38.
16. *Lancet* (1827) vol 12, pp 343 and 463.
17. This account is from L.J. Saunders *Scottish Democracy 1815–1840* Edinburgh 1950, p 315.
18. J.B. Morrell 'Thomas Thomson: professor of chemistry and university reformer' *Brit. J. Hist. Sci.* (1969) 4, 245–269.
19. Practical chemistry was even more neglected in Edinburgh and attempts to introduce it failed: see J.B. Morrell 'Practical chemistry in the University of Edinburgh 1779–1843' *Ambix* (1969) 16, 66–80.
20. *Scottish Review* (1894) vol 23, p 380. For a recent defence of St Andrews see R.N. Smart in G.W.S. Barrow (ed) *The Scottish Tradition* Edinburgh 1974 p 91, who has counted 1,375 M.D. degrees granted on testimonials only between 1747–1897.
21. See Saunders (ref 17) p 323.
22. For two conflicting Scottish views on Germany see *Ed. Med. Surg. J.* (1808) 4, 69–73 and *Ed. Med. Surg. J.* (1843) 59, 271–291. The success of the French chemists is discussed in the *Ed. Med. Surg. J.* (1842) vol 57, 496–501.
23. G.N. Cantor 'The Edinburgh phrenology debate 1803–1828' *Ann. Sci.* (1975) 32, 195–218.

24. The hostility to vivisection is described in G.L. Geison 'Social and institutional factors in the stagnancy of English physiology 1840–1870' *Bull. Hist. Med.* (1972) 46, 30–58, and M.N. Ozer 'The British vivisection controversy' *Bull. Hist. Med.* (1966) 40, 158–167. The problems of a biographer of a Scottish atheist vivisector are seen in G. Wilson *Life of Dr. John Reid* Edinburgh 1852: Reid recanted on his death bed – the book was then possible.

25. B. Spector 'Sir Charles Bell and the Bridgewater Treatises' *Bull. Hist. Med.* (1942) 12, 314–322.

26. T.N. Bonner *American Doctors and German Universities* Lincoln, Nebraska 1963.

27. The litigation between the Faculty and University are described in J. Coutts *A History of the University of Glasgow* Glasgow 1909 p 546 and Duncan (ref 1) p 162.

28. The Apothecaries Act is discussed in S.W.F. Holloway 'The Apothecaries Act 1815: a reinterpretation' *Med. Hist.* (1966) 10, 107–129 and 221–236.

29. Holloway (ref 28) p 223.

30. The problems arising for the Scottish medical schools as a result of the Apothecaries Act were repeatedly discussed at length in the *Edinburgh Medical and Surgical Journal*: see the following major editorial reviews (1826) 25, 407–424: (1833) 40, 209–239: (1837) 47, 234–270.

31. Commission of Inquiry Report (ref 15) p 66.

32. *Ed. Med. Surg. J.* (1833) 40, 210.

33. This attempt is described fully in E. Harrison *An address delivered to the Lincolnshire Benevolent Medical Society . . . in 1809*, 1810.

34. The problem of the Scottish doctors with the Royal College of Physicians in London was dealt with at length in the *Ed. Med. Surg. J.* (1820) 16, 481–509; (1835) 44, 205–220; (1844) 62, 514–547.

35. *Ed. Med. Surg. J.* 44, 216.

36. *Ed. Med. Surg. J.* 13, 225–229.

37. Hamilton almost certainly was the author of the work: see J.H. Young 'James Hamilton (1767–1839) obstetrician and controversialist' *Med. Hist.* (1963) 7, 62–73.

38. Cockburn says of Gregory that 'the controversies were rather too numerous; but they never were for any selfish end, and he was never entirely wrong. Still, a disposition towards personal attack was his besetting sin.' *Memorials of his Time* Edinburgh 1910 reprint p 97.

39. J.A. Shepherd *Simpson and Syme of Edinburgh* Edinburgh 1969 p 1–17.

40. F.B. Smith *The People's Health 1830–1910* London 1979 has accounts of early 19th century therapy.

41. *Ed. Med. Surg. J.* (1842) vol 58, 155–186; (1846) vol 66, 481–493; (1852) vol 77, 451–464.

42. F.N.L. Poynter 'Thomas Anderson, pioneer of vaccination in Scotland' *Rep. Proc. Soc. Hist. Med.* (1959) 12–21.

43. The temporarily successful movement against vaccination was led by Dr. T. Brown in *An Inquiry into the Antivariolous power of Vaccination* Edinburgh 1809.

44. M.W. Flinn (ed) *Scottish Population History* Cambridge 1977 p 394.

45. J. Syme 'Superior maxillary bone excised' *Ed. Med. Surg. J.* (1829) 32, 218–220. This article supports the judgement that he 'never wasted a drop of ink or blood.'

46. For other tariffs see *Rules for the Regulation of Medical Charges in the County of Fife* Cupar 1828 and *Prices fixed by the Physicians and Surgeons of Glasgow for Medicines and Attendance* Glasgow 1799. Dundee fees are listed in *Brit. Med. J.* (1914) I, 1254. The 1980 equivalent of the early 19th century guinea is about £20 – see chapt. 4 ref 16.
47. *Rules Adopted by the Medical Society of the North the Regulation of their Fees* Inverness 1818.
48. *Statement regarding the Existing Deficiency of Medical Practitioners in the Highlands and Islands* Edinburgh 1852. The original returns are held in the Library of the Royal College of Physicians of Edinburgh.
49. T. Garnett *Observations on a Tour through the Highlands* . . . London 1811.
50. Statement etc (ref 49) p 5.
51. For the social services in the Highlands before the changes resulting from the Dewar Report see J.P. Day *Public Administration in the Highlands and Islands of Scotland* London 1918.
52. Highland folk medicine is described in D. Masson 'Popular domestic medicine in the Highlands fifty years ago' *Trans. Gaelic Soc. Inver.* (1887–88) 14, 298–313; K. Whyte Grant 'Old Highland therapy' *Cal. Med. J.* (1902–04) 5, 356–378. There is much use of folk medicine by Sir Walter Scott in his novels – see C.O. Parsons *Witchcraft and Demonology in Scott's Fiction* London 1964.
53. W. Gourlay 'History of the epidemic fever . . .' *Ed. Med. Surg. J.* 15, 329–344.
54. A good contemporary view of the voluntary hospitals is given by J.K. Walker 'Short view of the statistics and mortality of the hospitals of Scotland' *Ed. Med. Surg. J.* (1847) 67, 345–383. The Royal Infirmary of Edinburgh is well described by A.L. Turner *Story of a Great Hospital* Edinburgh 1937, and Glasgow Royal Infirmary is dealt with in the *Glasg. Med. J.* (1832) 5, 395–416., and J. Patrick *A Short History of the Glasgow Royal Infirmary* Glasgow 1940.
55. This point is made by M.J. Peterson *The Medical Profession in Mid-Victorian London* London 1978, p 143.
56. H.J.C. Gibson 'The old Infirmary of Dundee, 1798–1855' *Ed. Med. J.* (1949) 56, 285–303.
57. *Regulations for the Town's Hospital of Glasgow* Glasgow 1830.
58. J. Cleland 'An Account of the Former and Present State of Glasgow' *Transactions of the Glasgow and Clydesdale Statistical Society* 1837, part 1, p 1: R. Cowan *Vital Statistics of Glasgow* 1838.
59. A straightforward account of the Glasgow brothels is given in 'Shadow's' *Midnight Scenes and Social Photographs* Glasgow 1858, p 126.
60. Cholera and its problems are described in A.A. MacLaren in A.A. MacLaren (ed) *Social Class in Scotland* Edinburgh 1976 p 36 and R.J. Morris *Cholera 1832* London 1976 and A. Briggs 'Cholera and society in the nineteenth century' *Past and Present* (1961) 19, 76–96.
61. T. Ferguson *The Dawn of Scottish Social Welfare* London 1948 p 123.
62. This account is taken entirely from J. Hunter *The Making of the Crofting Community* Edinburgh 1976 and Flinn (ref 44).

63. Conditions on the emigrant ships are described in H. MacPhee 'The trail of the emigrants' *Trans. Gaelic Soc. Inver.* (1969) 46, 170–191. The early Passenger Acts have attracted attention as early examples of government intervention – see O. MacDonagh *A Pattern of Government Growth 1800–1860* London 1961.

64. A ships 'surgeon' was and is a general practitioner with surgical skills. The term arose in the 19th century as a physician would never be found in this type of work.

65. For a history of the use of the potato see R.N. Salaman *The History and Social Influence of the Potato* Cambridge 1949, and the influence in the Highlands is discussed by Flinn (ref 44) p 421.

66. The most isolated Scottish community was St Kilda, and they escaped most of the problems of the mainland including the epidemics, unless a ship delivered the disease to them. The health of the island is dealt with in T. Steel *The Life and Death of St Kilda* Edinburgh 1975.

67. For a comparison of the responses to the Irish and Scottish famines see L.M. Cullen and T.C. Smout *Comparative Aspects of Scottish and Irish Economic and Social History 1600–1900* Edinburgh 1977 p 21.

68. Hunter (ref 62) p 61.

69. Hunter (ref 62) p 66.

70. Most authorities agree that there was no large scale loss of life – Flinn (ref 44) p 36 and Hunter (ref 62) p 60.

71. These figures are from T. Stratton *Ed. Med. Surg. J.* (1849–9) 70, 101–113, and 71, 92–99.

72. The old Scottish Poor Law is described in R. Mitchison 'The making of the old Scottish Poor Law' *Past and Present* (1974) No. 63, 58–93. The conclusion that it was a mean organisation is challenged by R.A. Cage *Past and Present* (1975) 69, 113–118 and in his Ph.D. Thesis, University of Glasgow 1974 'The Scottish Poor Law 1745–1845'.

73. A full description is given in Saunders (ref 17) p 222.

Chapter 6: The entry of the state: 19th century (2)

1. Alison is briefly described in *Ed. Med. J.* (1859) 5, 469–486. and in W.T. Gairdner *The Physician as Naturalist* Glasgow 1889 p 388.

2. A. Buchanan 'Report of the diseases which prevailed among the poor of Glasgow . . .' *Glasg. Med. J.* (1830) 3, 435–450.

3. R. Perry 'Facts and observations on the sanatory state of Glasgow . . .' *Ed. Med. Surg. J.* (1844) 62, 81–95.

4. H. Hunter (ed) *T. Chalmers: Problems of Poverty* London 1912 p 370.

5. An account of these legal absurdities is found in the analysis of the Scottish public health movement by G.F.A. Best in H.J. Dyos and Wolff (eds) *The Victorian City* London 1973, 389–411.

6. For a comparison of Alison and Chadwick see M.J. Cullen *The Statistical Movement in Early Victorian Britain* Hassocks 1975 and the Introduction to M.W. Flinn (ed) *Edwin Chadwick's Report on the Sanitary Condition of the Labouring Population of Gt. Britain* Edinburgh 1965.

7. W.S. Craig *History of the Royal College of Physicians of Edinburgh* Edinburgh 1976, p 203.
8. H.P. Tait 'Sir Henry Duncan Littlejohn' *The Medical Officer* (1962) 108, 183–190.
9. G.A. Gibson *The Life of Sir William Tennant Gairdner* Glasgow 1912.
10. *Glasgow Medical Examiner* (1869) 2, p 5. This journal opposed all change and attacked everyone in Glasgow. It had two short runs from 1831–32 and 1869–71. For an account of the editor in the later period see J. Steven 'John Reid, surgeon' *Glasg. Med. J.* (1895) 43, 321–332.
11. J. Brownlee 'Biographical scetch of the late James B. Russell' *Proc. Roy. Phil. Soc. Glasg.* (1905) 36, 86–94.
12. R. Hunter *The Water Supply of Glasgow* Glasgow 1933.
13. A. Paterson *Poor Law Relief Administration in Edinburgh City Parish 1845–1891.* Unpublished Ph.D. Thesis University of Edinburgh 1973.
14. Best (ref 5) p 394.
15. F. McKichan 'A burgh's response to the problems of urban growth: Stirling 1780–1880' *Scot. Hist. Rev.* (1978) 57, 68–86.
16. *Sanitary Journal for Scotland* 1 March 1877 p 230.
17. A milkman acquitted on a technically after spreading scarlet fever in Glasgow in 1885 was given a testimonial dinner, a timepiece and a purse of sovereigns by his colleagues: *Glasg. Med. J.* (1885) 23, p 278.
18. A.L. Turner *Sir W. Turner, a Chapter in Medical History* Edinburgh 1867 p 285.
19. *Glasg. Med. J.* (1870) 3, 561.
20. J.B. Morrell 'The patronage of mid-Victorian science in the University of Edinburgh' *Sci. Stud.* (1973) 3, 353–388.
21. R.M. MacLeod 'The support of Victorian Science' *Minerva* (1971) 9, 197–230.
22. W.S. Craig (ref 7) p 105.
23. This quote is from *The State of the Medical Profession* Dublin 1875. The events in Edinburgh are described in E.H.C.M. Bell *Storming the Citadel* London 1953, Sophia Jex-Blake *Medical Women: Two Essays* Edinburgh 1872 and one of the lesser known activists is described in E. Lutzker 'Edith Pechey-Phipson, M.D.: an untold story' *Med. Hist.* (1967) 11, 41–45. The resistance by Edinburgh University is detailed in Turner (ref 18) p 262.
24. No less than five books deal with Dr. Inglis and her hospitals: H.P. Tait *Elsie Maud Inglis, a Great Lady Doctor* Edinburgh 1964, F. Balfour *Dr. Elsie Inglis* London 1918, E.S. McLaren *A History of the Scottish Women's Hospital* London 1919, Y. Fitzroy *With the Scottish Nurses in Roumania* London 1918 and M. Lawrence *Shadow of Swords* London 1971. See also A. de Navarro *The Scottish Women's Hospital* London 1918.
25. O. Checkland *Philanthropy in Victorian Scotland: Social Welfare and the Voluntary Principle* Edinburgh 1980 and C.I. Pennington *Mortality Public Health and Medical Improvements in Glasgow 1855–1911*, unpublished Ph.D. thesis, University of Stirling 1977, and *Med. Hist.* 23, 442–450.
26. *Glasgow Medical Examiner* (1876) vol 2 p 151 has the attack on Dr Wolfe.
27. See ref 25 for descriptions of the improvements in nursing in Scotland.
28. The dispensary is described in J. Miller *Medical Missions* Edinburgh 1849.

29. Pennington (ref 25) p 266 gives this account of the Glasgow Dispensaries.

30. I.A. Porter 'The Perth Dispensaries' *Practitioner* (1973) 210, 432–436.

31. For the mental health services see Checkland (ref 25); A MacNiven 'The first commissioners: reform in the mid-nineteenth century' *J. Ment. Sci.* (1960) 106, 451–471, and D.A. Primrose 'The development of mental deficiency hospitals in Scotland' *Health Bull.* (1977) 35, 63–67.

32. No serious studies of the Scottish Temperance Movement exist but short accounts are given in E. Morris *History of the Temperance Societies in Glasgow* Glasgow 1855 and M.B. MacGregor *Towards Scotland's Social Good* Edinburgh 1949.

33. This threat is contained in the *Report of the Departmental Committee . . . relating to Inebriates . . .* 1909, Cd 4766, and analysis of these attitudes is given in C. Greenland 'Habitual drunkards in Scotland 1879–1913' *Quart. J. Stud. Alcohol* (1960) 21, 135–139.

34. Report (ref 33) p 88.

35. A full account of the Scottish medical missionary work does not exist but there are short descriptions in K.J. McCracken 'Scottish medical missionaries in Central Africa' *Med. Hist.* (1973) 17, 188–191, A.L. Drummond and J. Bulloch *The Church in Victorian Scotland 1843–74* Edinburgh 1975 and M. Gelfand *Lakeside Pioneers: a Socio-medical Study of Nyasalnd* Oxford 1964. Individual missionaries like Livingstone, Laws and Macvicar are described in a number of biographies.

36. E.A. Underwood 'Dumfries and the early history of surgical anaesthesia' *Ann. Sci.* (1967) 23, 35–75, and T.W. Baillie *From Boston to Dumfries* Dumfries 1966.

37. J.A. Shepherd *Simpson and Syme of Edinburgh* Edinburgh 1969 pp 1–17 and A.J. Youngson *The Scientific Revolution in Victorian Medicine* London 1979.

38. H.J.C. Gibson, 'The old Infirmary of Dundee, 1798–1855' *Ed. Med. J.* (1949) 56, 298.

39. For discussion of the 'hospitalism' problem see J. Woodward *To Do the Sick No Harm* London 1974, chapt. 9.

40. The best of the Lister biographies are R.J. Godlee *Lord Lister* London 1917 and R.B. Fisher *Joseph Lister 1827–1912* London 1977.

41. The opponents and supporters of Lister in Edinburgh are described in J.A. Ross *The Edinburgh School of Surgery after Lister* Edinburgh 1978, and Youngson (ref 37).

42. J.C. McVail 'Dr. John Borland' *Glasg. Med. J.* (1923) 99, 1–18.

43. A.K. Bowman *The Life and Teaching of Sir William Macewen* London 1942.

44. Pennington (ref 25) p 110.

45. The fees of the Southern Medical Society showed little change from those of 1800: Pennington (ref 25) p 284 and Chapter 5 ref 47.

46. The friendly societies are described in T. Ferguson *Scottish Social Welfare 1864–1914* Edinburgh 1958, p 335.

47. These levels of health care are described in A. Cox *Among the Doctors* London 1950, p 56.

48. These analyses come from the British Medical Association's campaign against the patent medicine sellers in *Secret Remedies* London 1909 and *More Secret Remedies* London 1912.

49. For a description of the Scottish Poor Law services see A. Paterson in D. Fraser (ed) *The New Poor Law in the Nineteenth Century* London 1976, p 171–192, and M.W. Flinn at p 45 in the same volume. There are other details in T. Ferguson (ref 46) p 436. The Scottish Poor Law records are SRO HH 23–26, and 58/2. *The Poor Law Medical Services Report* is Cd 2008.
50. The Scottish poorhouses are described in Ferguson (ref 46) p 294 and in C. Harvey *Ha'penny Help* Glasgow 1976.
51. For nursing in the poorhouses see Pennington (ref 25) p 196.

Chapter 7: The rise of the state: 20th century.

1. For health statistics see *Registrar General for Scotland Annual Reports* and *Scottish Health Services Statistics*. International data comes from World Health Organisation *World Health Statistics Annuals*. Changes in patterns of disease in the early 20th century are found in M.W. Flinn *Scottish Population History* Cambridge 1977.
2. For these reforms see H.P. Tait *The Doctor and Two Policemen* Edinburgh 1974.
3. J.E. Hoskings (ed) *Nursing Homes – A Directory* London 1932.
4. Nursing homes can also be traced in contemporary Post Office directories.
5. For an account of his own canvassing to be appointed to Stobhill Hospital see James Bridie *One Way of Living* London 1939.
6. L. MacQueen and A.B. Kerr *The Western Infirmary 1874–1974* Glasgow 1974, p 15.
7. For an account of the debate see B.B. Gilbert *The Evolution of National Insurance in Great Britain, the Origins of the Welfare State* London 1966.
8. *Report of the Royal Commission on Physical Training (Scotland)* 1903, Cd 1507.
9. Scotch Education Department *The physical condition of Children Attending the Public Elementary Schools of the School Board for Glasgow* (1907) Cd 3637.
10. *Report of the Interdepartmental Committee on Physical Deterioration* London 1904, Cd 2175.
11. That children grew quickly when fed properly in hospital was shown by A.S.M. MacGregor 'Physique of Glasgow children' *Proc. Roy. Phil. Soc. Glasg.* (1908) 40, 156–172.
12. J.B. Orr *Food Health and Income* London 1936. Orr's own account of the events at this time are given in his autobiography *As I Recall* London 1966. An account of the politics of nutrition in this period is given in H.D. Kay 'John Boyd Orr' *Biographical Memoirs of Fellows of the Royal Society* (1972) 18, 43–81.
13. The Scheme is described in B.B. Gilbert (ref 7) and E.S. Turner *Call the Doctor* London 1958. A factual account of the Scheme in Scotland is found in the *Sixth Annual Report of the Scottish Board of Health 1924*, Cmnd 2416.
14. *Glasgow Herald* 11 Dec. 1912. The *Glasgow Herald* has a useful index which covers the events.
15. *Brit. Med. J.* 1912, ii, Suppl. p 682.
16. R. Titmus in H.N Bunbury *Lloyd George's Ambulance Wagon* London 1957, p 31.
17. *Glasgow Herald*, March 28th 1913.

18. *Brit. Med. J.* 8 Feb 1913 Suppl. p 137.

19. The Dewar Report is the *Report of the Committee on the Highlands and Islands Medical Services* 1912 Cd 6559. The papers are SRO HH 65 but have been heavily culled.

20. *Brit. Med. J.* 1913, i, p 247.

21. In 1967 the Birsay Report on *General Medical Services in the Highlands and Islands* Cmnd 3257 could find no major defects.

22. The Dawson Report is the *Interim Report of the Consultative Council on the Future Provision of Medical and Allied Services* 1920, Cmnd 693.

23. *Interim Report of the Consultative Committee on Medical and Allied Services on a Scheme of Medical Service for Scotland* 1920, Cmnd 1039.

24. The Cathcart Report is *Report of a Committee on Scottish Health Services* 1935–36, Cmnd 5204.

25. For a commentary on it see E.R.C. Walker 'The forgotten report' *Ed. Med. J.* (1949) 56, 493–501.

26. T. Johnston *Memories* London 1952, p 148.

27. For Johnston methods in the Cabinet see H. Morrison *An autobiography* London 1960 p 199.

28. A detailed account of the EMS is given in C.L. Dunn *History of the Second World War: the Emergency Medical Services, vol 2: Scotland* London 1952. There is brief comment on it in R.M. Titmuss *Problems of Social Policy* London 1950. The papers are SRO HH 64 and 65, but have been heavily culled.

29. The Clyde Basin experiment is described in *Health and Industrial Efficiency*, Department of Health for Scotland 1943.

30. See the Hetherington Report: *Report of the Committee on Post-War Hospital Problems in Scotland* Cmnd 6472.

31. For general accounts of the NHS see H. Eckstein *The English Health Service* Boston 1959, and J.S. Ross *The NHS in Great Britain; an Historical and Descriptive Study* London 1952.

32. These quotes are from M. Foot. *Aneurin Bevan: a Biography* London 1973 vol 2, p 102.

33. The papers for the Scottish Bill are SRO HH 102/501–3 and others are in the Public Records Office MH 77/158.

34. *Brit. Med. J.* 1948, i, 893.

35. Walker (ref 25) p 500

36. *The Health Service in Scotland: The Way Ahead* Edinburgh 1976,and B. Abel-Smith *National Health Service: the First Thirty Years* HMSO 1978.

37. For a defence of the Scottish reorganisation see D. Hunter in M.G. Clarke and H.M. Drucker *Our Changing Scotland: A Yearbook of Scottish Government 1976–1977* Edinburgh 1976.

38. See H.J. Hanham 'The creation of the Scottish Office' *Juridicial Review* (1965) 10, 205–244.

39. For an account of the Boards see F.M.G. Willson 'Ministries and Boards' *Public Administration* (1955) 33, 43–57.

40. See Hanham (ref 38) p 219.

41. For a factual account of the devolved administration see D. Milne *The Scottish Office* London 1957, and for an analysis see J.G. Kellas *The Scottish Political System* Cambridge 1973.

42. For statistical sources see ref 1.
43. P.N. Lee *Statistics of Smoking in the United Kingdom* Tobacco Research Council, 1977.
44. The problems of the health of west-central Scotland are dealt with in D.N.H. Hamilton in H.M. Drucker and M.G. Clarke (eds) *The Scottish Government Yearbook 1978*, Edinburgh 1978, p 77.
45. P. Wedge and H. Prosser *Born to Fail?* London 1973.
46. *Glasgow Herald* 23 May 1955.
47. T.S. Wilson in JMA Lenihan *Health and the Environment* Glasgow 1976.
48. For a hint of concern see 'The Medical Schools of Scotland' *Scottish Review* (1894) 23, 1–31, and *Scot. Med. J.* (1962) 7, 245–249.
49. T.N. Bonner *American Doctors and the German Universities* Lincoln Nebraska 1963.
50. The extramural schools were abolished as a result of the Goodenough Committee, *Report of the Interdepartmental Committee on Medical Schools* HMSO London 1944.
51. Figures from the Royal Commission on Medical Education 1968, Cmnd 3569.
52. No less than four books describe the Polish Medical School: J. Brodzki *Polish Medical School of Medicine at the University of Edinburgh* Edinburgh 1942; J. Rostowski *History of the Polish School of Medicine* Edinburgh 1955; C. Pole *Medicine, Murder and Merriment* Pinner 1976. For a complete survey of the links see T. Tomaszewski (ed) *The University of Edinburgh and Poland: a Historical Review* Edinburgh 1969.
53. J.R. Peddie *The Carnegie Trust for the universities of Scotland* Edinburgh 1951.

Index